Acute Coronary Syndromes

Acute Coronary Syndromes

Edited by
K Sarat Chandra
AJ Swamy

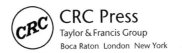

CRC Press is an imprint of the
Taylor & Francis Group, an **informa** business

First edition published 2020
by CRC Press
6000 Broken Sound Parkway NW, Suite 300, Boca Raton, FL 33487-2742

and by CRC Press
2 Park Square, Milton Park, Abingdon, Oxon, OX14 4RN

© 2021 Taylor & Francis Group, LLC

CRC Press is an imprint of Taylor & Francis Group, LLC

Library of Congress Cataloging-in-Publication Data
Names: Chandra, K. Sarat, editor. | Swamy, A. J., editor.
Title: Acute coronary syndromes / edited by K. Sarat Chandra, AJ Swamy.
Other titles: Acute coronary syndromes (Chandra)
Description: First edition. | Boca Raton : CRC Press, 2020. | Includes
    bibliographical references and index. | Summary: "Acute Coronary
    Syndromes (ACS) are a growing global menace with patients increasing in
    developing countries where tobacco and food play a major role. Its
    treatment guidelines and research results have proliferated in the
    academia but practical world application lags"-- Provided by publisher.
Identifiers: LCCN 2020006256 (print) | LCCN 2020006257 (ebook) | ISBN
    9780367135096 (hbk) | ISBN 9780367112226 (pbk) | ISBN 9780429025396 (ebk)
Subjects: MESH: Acute Coronary Syndrome--therapy | Percutaneous Coronary
    Intervention | Treatment Outcome
Classification: LCC RC685.C6 (print) | LCC RC685.C6 (ebook) | NLM WG 300 | DDC 616.1/2--dc23
LC record available at https://lccn.loc.gov/2020006256
LC ebook record available at https://lccn.loc.gov/2020006257

ISBN: 9780367135096 (hbk)
ISBN: 9780367112226 (pbk)
ISBN: 9780429025396 (ebk)

Typeset in Minion Pro
by Nova Techset Private Limited, Bengaluru & Chennai, India

Visit the Taylor & Francis Web site at
http://www.taylorandfrancis.com

and the CRC Press Web site at
http://www.crcpress.com

This book is dedicated to the memory of my late mother, Smt. K Visalakshi,
who encouraged me to take up medicine.

Dr K Sarat Chandra

Contents

Foreword

Acute coronary syndrome (ACS) is an important manifestation of cardiovascular disease with critical consequences and outcomes. This syndrome reflects a life-or-death situation that patients will survive with a timely and accurate diagnosis and immediate treatment; if the diagnosis is missed or delayed, patients are at risk of death.

Patients with ACS typically present to the emergency room and thus should be assessed thoroughly and immediately. The process of assessing patients with ACS in the emergency room has improved but is not without controversy. Many key questions remain unanswered, such as the role of biomarker stratification and clinical utility of diagnostic testing, particularly in the young and in those with no risk factors who present with normal ECGs and biomarkers.

To address the complexity of ACS, Dr K Sarat Chandra has assembled this timely and much needed handbook on acute coronary syndromes; he should be congratulated not only for conceiving the idea of bringing out this book, but also for organizing the chapters dealing with every aspect of ACS. I would venture to say that it is, in fact, not a "handbook" but rather a "treatise" filled with scientific information detailing the entire gamut of ACS. The reader will find that the book explores, synthesizes and examines the panoramic landscape of ACS – pathophysiology, symptomatology, haemodynamics, diagnostic methods, biomarkers and imaging techniques. To provide the clinicians a complete picture of therapeutic blueprints, Dr Chandra has put together schemes for therapeutic and interventional strategies, such as thrombolytic therapy, anti-platelet therapy, angioplasty, CABG and rehabilitation. The book contains a wealth of enlightened knowledge on the value of statin therapy, special populations and qualitative outcome measures. With the compilation of this book, Dr Chandra has filled an unmet need in the cardiology literature. Interpretive discussions, such as case-based scenarios are another treasure of this valuable dissertation.

I am sure that this book will become essential reading for teachers, educators, trainees and practitioners of modern cardiology. It is my optimistic estimation that this book will be an effective tool for providing improved care to patients with ACS and, thus, will reduce the burden of cardiovascular disease in the community.

In composing this book on ACS, Dr Chandra has intelligently embraced the lessons of the past to welcome the future into the present!

C Venkata S Ram, MD, MACP, FACC, FASH
Apollo Institute for Blood Pressure Management
Apollo Hospitals and Apollo Medical College
World Hypertension League/South Asia Office
Hyderabad, India

and

Texas Blood Pressure Institute
University of Texas Southwestern Medical School
Dallas, Texas, USA

and

India Campus
Macquarie University Medical School
Sydney, Australia

Preface

Acute coronary syndrome (ACS) forms a large part of the cardiology practice today. It represents a life-threatening manifestation of atherosclerosis and is characterised by sudden and critical reduction in myocardial blood supply. Prompt restoration of myocardial blood flow is crucial for minimizing myocardial damage and improving clinical outcomes in patients who present with ACS. The complex interplay of pathophysiological processes involved in the development of ACS renders it a challenging condition to tackle, but at the same time, it also provides several therapeutic targets that can be intervened on. Not surprisingly, therefore, ACS has been an area of intense research in cardiology. Numerous preclinical to large clinical, randomized trials have been undertaken in the recent past to unravel every aspect of ACS. As a result, our understanding of this commonly encountered clinical problem has vastly improved over the last several years. There have been many advances in the management of ACS, especially in drug therapy. Interventional therapy has also improved considerably, with advances in both the procedural understanding and the available hardware and adjunctive pharmacotherapy to support these procedures. Consequently, percutaneous coronary interventions are now being performed in the vast majority of patients, with improved outcomes. This book is an attempt to bring together in one place all of these recent advances in a simple way and to act as a ready reckoner for students and practitioners of cardiology.

K Sarat Chandra
AJ Swamy

Acknowledgements

The editors are deeply indebted to all the authors of different chapters in this book who contributed articles despite their busy schedules. Dr Dayasagar Rao, senior cardiologist, Hyderabad has been a friend, philosopher and guide in all academic matters over the last 25 years, and I hereby express my sincere gratitude to him. Ms. Shivangi Pramanik and Ms. Himani Dwivedi of the publishers CRC Press/Taylor & Francis have been of great help in bringing out this book. My sincere thanks to Ms. Bharathi for her secretarial assistance. Finally, my wife, Dr Rekha, helped me at various stages, including proofreading.

Dr K Sarat Chandra

Editors

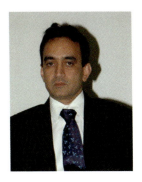

Dr K Sarat Chandra is one of the most experienced interventional cardiologists of India. Since completing his DM from the Postgraduate Institute of Medical Education & Research, Chandigarh in 1989, he has been working in Hyderabad, India. He is one of the early interventional cardiologists of India and did the first device closure of congenital heart disease in Hyderabad along with the first case of rotational atherectomy in 1994. He has a special interest in left main artery interventions. He has many publications in the area of interventional cardiology. He was Chairman of the National Interventional Council of India during the years 2008 and 2009. He was Editor of the *Indian Heart Journal* from 2012 to 2014. He was elected President of the Cardiological Society of India in 2018.

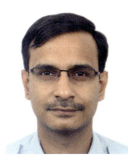

Dr AJ Swamy is an accomplished interventional cardiologist with a strong research background and wide-ranging experience with a variety of complex cases. He completed his graduate and postgraduate degrees from the Armed Forces Medical College, joined the Indian Air Force and completed his DM Cardiology from PGIMER, Chandigarh in 2006. He was awarded gold medals for his research work both for his MD and DM and has won the best case award at APICON, NIC and IJCTO, among others. He was awarded a Senior Scientist Fellowship by the Indian Council of Medical Research in 2016. He has always been an enthusiastic and eager student of cardiology, keen to learn and share knowledge at any forum. He has numerous publications in national and international journals and has been guiding students for more than a decade.

He is presently serving in the Indian Air Force with more than 25 years of service and is currently working as Professor of Cardiology at the Armed Forces Medical College and the Maharashtra University of Health Sciences in India.

Contributors

Rajiv Agarwal
Department of Cardiology
Max Smart Super Speciality Hospital
New Delhi, India

Rajeev Agarwala
Department of Cardiology
Jaswant Rai Speciality Hospital
Meerut, India

Shaheer Ahmed
Department of Cardiology
All India Institute of Medical Sciences
New Delhi, India

Thomas Alexander
Department of Cardiology
Kovai Medical Center and Hospital
Coimbatore, India

Ankit Bansal
Department of Cardiology
Govind Ballabh Pant Institute of Postgraduate Medical
    Education and Research (GIPMER)
New Delhi, India

Manish Bansal
Department of Cardiology
Medanta – The Medicity
Gurgaon, India

Dinkar Bhasin
Department of Cardiology
All India Institute of Medical Sciences
New Delhi, India

Keshavamurthy Ganapathy Bhat
Department of Cardiology
Command Hospital Air Force
Bangalore, India

Davinder Singh Chadha
Department of Cardiology
Command Hospital Air Force
Bangalore, India

K Sarat Chandra
Department of Cardiology
Virinchi Hospital and Indo-US Super Speciality Hospital
Hyderabad, India

Vivek Chaturvedi
Department of Cardiology
Narayana Superspeciality Hospital
Gurugram, India

Nishad Chitnis
Department of Cardiology
Aster Aadhar Hospital
Kolhapur, India

Ramesh Daggubati
Division of Cardiology
NYU Winthrop Hospital
Mineola, New York

Niteen Vijay Deshpande
Department of Cardiology
Spandan Heart Institute and Research Center
Nagpur, India

Kiran Gaur
Department of Cardiology
Govt SKN Agriculture University
Jaipur, India

Rajeev Gupta
Department of Cardiology
Eternal Heart Care Centre and Research
    Institute
Jaipur, India

SS Iyengar
Department of Cardiology
Manipal Hospital
Bangalore, India

RK Jain
Department of Cardiology
KIMS Hospitals
Secunderabad, India

PB Jayagopal
Department of Cardiology
Lakshmi Hospital
Palakkad, Kerala, India

Saubhik Kanjilal
Department of Cardiology
Vivekananda Institute of Medical Sciences
Kolkata, India

Upendra Kaul
Department of Cardiology
Batra Hospital and Medical Research
    Centre
New Delhi, India

Varsha Koul
Department of Cardiology
Batra Hospital and Medical Research
    Centre
New Delhi, India

Leela Krishna
Department of Cardiology
Krishna Institute of Medical Sciences
Hyderabad, India

Soumitra Kumar
Department of Cardiology
Vivekananda Institute of Medical
    Sciences
Kolkata, India

Suraj Kumar
Department of Cardiology
Government Medical College & Hospital
Chandigarh, India

Kunal Mahajan
Department of Cardiology
Indira Gandhi Medical College & Hospital
Shimla, India

Geetesh Manik
Department of Cardiology
Teerthanker Mahaveer University
Moradabad, India

PP Mohanan
Department of Cardiology
Westfort Hi-Tech Hospital
Thrissur, India

Ajit S Mullasari
Institute of Cardiovascular Diseases
The Madras Medical Mission
Chennai, India

Nitish Naik
Department of Cardiology
All India Institute of Medical Sciences
New Delhi, India

Srinivasan Narayanan
Institute of Cardiovascular Diseases
The Madras Medical Mission
Chennai, India

Nitin Parashar
Department of Cardiology
All India Institute of Medical Sciences
New Delhi, India

Sakalesh Patil
Department of Cardiology
Lakshmi Hospital
Palakkad, India

Yashasvi Rajeev
Department of Cardiology
Sagar Hospital
Bangalore, India

Sivasubramanian Ramakrishnan
Department of Cardiology
All India Institute of Medical Sciences
New Delhi, India

Shraddha Ranjan
Department of Cardiology
Medanta – The Medicity
Gurgaon, India

B Hygriv Rao
Department of Cardiology
KIMS Hospitals
Hyderabad, India

Dayasagar Rao
Department of Cardiology
Krishna Institute of Medical Sciences
Hyderabad, India

Avanti Gurram Reddy
Division of Cardiology
NYU Winthrop Hospital
Mineola, New York

Gianluca Rigatelli
Cardiovascular Diagnosis and Endoluminal
    Interventions Service
Rovigo General Hospital
Rovigo, Italy

JPS Sawhney
Department of Cardiology
Dharma Vira Heart Centre
Sir Ganga Ram Hospital
New Delhi, India

Simran Sawhney
Department of Medicine
St. Stephen's Hospital
New Delhi, India

Smit Shrivastava
Department of Cardiology
Advanced Cardiac Institute
Pt JNM Medical College & Dr BRAM Hospital
Raipur, India

Deepti Siddharthan
Department of Cardiology
All India Institute of Medical Sciences
New Delhi, India

Abhikrishna Singh
Cardiology Clinic
Raipur, India

Vijayakumar Subban
Institute of Cardiovascular Diseases
The Madras Medical Mission
Chennai, India

AJ Swamy
Department of Cardiology
MH CTC (AFMC)
Pune, India

Suma M Victor
Institute of Cardiovascular Diseases
The Madras Medical Mission
Chennai, India

Gagandeep Singh Wander
Department of Cardiology
Medanta – The Medicity
Gurgaon, India

Gurpreet S Wander
Department of Cardiology
Hero DMC Heart Institute
Dayanand Medical College & Hospital
Ludhiana, India

Prashant Wankhade
Department of Cardiology
Dharma Vira Heart Centre
Sir Ganga Ram Hospital
New Delhi, India

Sushant Wattal
Department of Cardiology
Max Smart Super Speciality Hospital
New Delhi, India

OP Yadava
Department of Cardiology
National Heart Institute
New Delhi, India

Epidemiology of acute coronary syndromes in India

RAJEEV GUPTA AND KIRAN GAUR

INDIA: CORONARY CAPITAL OF THE WORLD

Cardiovascular diseases, especially coronary or ischaemic heart disease (IHD), are epidemics in India [1]. A decade ago, it was predicted that by the year 2020 India would gain the dubious distinction of being the coronary capital of the world [2]. Perusal of the current data from the Global Burden of Disease (GBD) Study and others shows that this prediction has already come true. The Registrar General of India has reported that mortality from cardiovascular diseases is rapidly increasing in the country [3]. The World Health Organization (WHO) and the Global Burden of Disease (GBD) Study have highlighted secular increase in mortality, years of life lost (YLLs) and disability-adjusted life years (DALYs) from IHD in India [4,5]. In India, studies have reported increasing coronary heart disease (CHD) prevalence over the last 60 years, from 1% to 9%–10% in urban populations and from <1% to 4%–6% in rural populations [6–8]. Using more stringent criteria (clinical diagnosis and/or Q waves), the current prevalence varies from 1% to 2% in rural populations and 2%–4% in urban populations [1]. All these calculations were based on limited data using a small number of regional studies. The Million Death Study in India has been using the Indian Sample Registration System data and verbal autopsy to assess causes of death in different states of the country since the year 2003 [9,10]. For the last two decades the GBD group and others have been systematically collating IHD morbidity and mortality data, globally and in India, from various sources to produce estimates of nationwide and state-specific IHD burden in the country [11,12].

The GBD Study has reported an annual absolute burden of IHD mortality and DALYs as well as rates per 100,000 persons in more than 190 countries. To compare the total mortality and death rates from IHD as well as disease burden estimated as DALYs we used the 2017 GBD database (Table 1.1) [13]. We collated mortality and disease burden data from the 10 most populous nations of the world – China, India, the United States, Indonesia, Brazil, Pakistan, Nigeria, Bangladesh, Russian Federation and Japan – at different levels of epidemiological and sociodemographic transition. The number of deaths in the years 1990, 2005 and 2017 is shown in Figure 1.1. China and India lead the tally in terms of absolute numbers. Trends show that while IHD mortality is increasing in the lower- to middle-income countries such as China, India and South Asian and African countries, it is declining in high income countries such as the United States and lately Russia (Table 1.1). Data also shows that there are variations in the rate of change of the absolute number of people dying of IHD in these countries (Figure 1.2). All the countries in South Asia show a rapid increase, with Bangladesh showing the most rapid increase of 128% from 1990 to 2005, while from years 2005 to 2017 India and Bangladesh have the most rapid increase in absolute number of IHD deaths.

Detailed data on IHD deaths, death rate/100,000, DALYs and DALY rate/100,000 are shown in Table 1.1. High IHD death rates/100,000 population is observed in India especially during the more recent period of estimation from 2005 to 2017. DALYs are a more useful estimate of disease burden [14]. The number of DALYs lost in India is 36.99 million in the year 2017 and is more than China (30.11 million), the United States (8.03 million) and Russia (9.60 million). The DALY rate/100,000 population in India is 2679/100,000. This is more than other large countries excluding Russia (6569/100,000).

Clearly, these data support our contention that India has already become the coronary capital of the world with the second highest number of total and incident IHD patients and the largest DALY burden. In this chapter we focus on epidemiology of acute coronary syndromes (ACS) in India, which are the most important cause of death in IHD and can be prevented by a multitude of public health and clinical approaches [15].

Table 1.1 Number of IHD deaths, rate/100,000, DALYs and DALY/100,000 in 10 large countries

Country (2018 population in millions)	Year	Deaths '000	Death rate/100,000	DALYs '000,000	DALY rate/100,000
China (1394.5)	1990	580.58	48.50	13.36	1116.45
	2005	1069.37	80.18	20.18	1513.32
	2017	1750.03	123.90	30.11	2131.45
	% change (1990–2005)	84.19	65.30	51.04	35.55
	% change (2005–2017)	63.65	54.53	49.16	40.85
India (1343.3)	1990	682.04	78.27	18.75	2152.10
	2005	914.98	79.47	23.51	2042.15
	2017	1540.32	111.57	36.99	2679.17
	% change (1990–2005)	34.15	1.54	25.37	−5.11
	% change (2005–2017)	68.35	40.39	57.32	31.19
USA (328.7)	1990	605.60	238.98	9.77	3853.49
	2005	539.60	183.24	8.15	2768.67
	2017	533.16	164.13	8.03	2470.71
	% change (1990–2005)	−10.90	−23.32	−16.51	−28.15
	% change (2005–2017)	−1.19	−10.43	−1.56	−10.76
Indonesia (268.1)	1990	99.65	53.64	2.67	1438.92
	2005	172.50	75.84	4.37	1921.52
	2017	235.00	90.94	5.72	2214.98
	% change (1990–2005)	73.10	41.40	63.48	33.54
	% change (2005–2017)	36.23	19.91	30.83	15.27
Brazil (210.2)	1990	129.01	86.34	2.96	1980.66
	2005	140.08	75.19	3.10	1663.23
	2017	176.00	82.99	3.68	1736.59
	% change (1990–2005)	8.58	−12.91	4.70	−16.03
	% change (2005–2017)	25.64	10.37	18.71	4.41
Pakistan (203.6)	1990	95.27	87.80	2.20	2029.02
	2005	162.50	101.43	4.08	2550.82
	2017	217.00	101.23	5.39	2513.52
	% change (1990–2005)	70.57	15.52	85.32	25.72
	% change (2005–2017)	33.54	−0.20	32.01	−1.46

(Continued)

Table 1.1 (Continued) Number of IHD deaths, rate/100,000, DALYs and DALY/100,000 in 10 large countries

Country (2018 population in millions)	Year	Deaths '000	Death rate/100,000	DALYs '000,000	DALY rate/100,000
Nigeria (193.4)	1990	35.14	39.14	0.69	762.90
	2005	41.72	29.29	0.84	590.26
	2017	51.00	24.80	1.04	502.57
	% change (1990–2005)	18.72	−25.17	22.63	−22.63
	% change (2005–2017)	22.24	−15.33	23.30	−14.86
Bangladesh (166.0)	1990	31.83	29.23	0.76	700.53
	2005	72.75	53.12	1.87	1367.40
	2017	131.00	83.44	3.11	1982.94
	% change (1990–2005)	128.52	81.73	145.12	95.20
	% change (2005–2017)	80.07	57.08	66.46	45.02
Russia (146.8)	1990	491.96	325.20	9.26	6120.10
	2005	733.71	500.32	14.90	10,163.93
	2017	563.00	385.06	9.60	6568.82
	% change (1990–2005)	49.14	53.85	60.93	66.07
	% change (2005–2017)	−23.27	−23.04	−35.55	−35.37
Japan (126.3)	1990	123.48	98.11	2.02	1602.95
	2005	127.80	98.45	1.86	1438.89
	2017	151.00	117.68	1.83	1427.39
	% change (1990–2005)	3.50	0.35	−7.80	−10.23
	% change (2005–2017)	18.15	19.53	−1.49	−0.80

Abbreviations: DALYs, disability-adjusted life years.

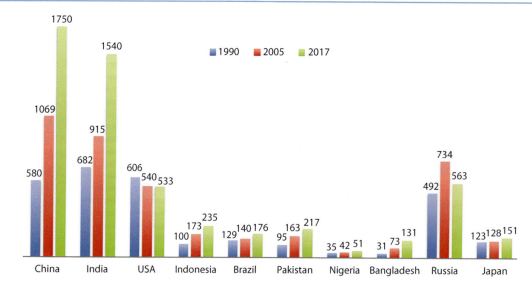

Figure 1.1 Absolute number of persons (men and women, in thousands) with IHD deaths in 10 most populous countries in the GBD Study [13].

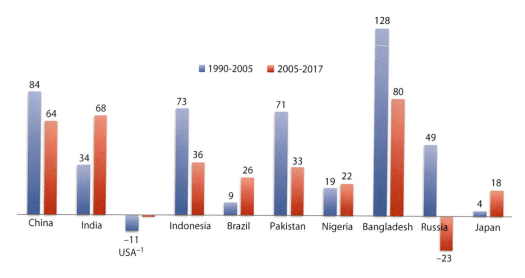

Figure 1.2 Percent change in absolute mortality from IHD in various countries from 1990–2005 and 2005–2017 in the GBD Study [13].

ACUTE CORONARY SYNDROMES IN INDIA

There are no reliable data on incidence and prevalence of ACS in India. Some years ago, using data from population-based epidemiological studies and crude statistical methods we predicted an annual incidence of 9–10 million cases a year [7]. Recently, the GBD Study and India State-Level Disease Burden Initiative Collaborators have reported annual incidence of IHD in India from the years 1990 to 2017 [12].

ACS is the primary form of presentation of IHD and could be ST-elevation myocardial infarction (STEMI), non ST-elevation myocardial infarction (NSTEMI) or unstable angina (UA) [16]. The pathophysiology of these syndromes is different [17,18]. The biology and clinical spectrum of these disorders are not described in this chapter and are available elsewhere in this monograph.

The annual incidence of IHD, i.e. ACS, has been reported for India as well as different states within the country in the GBD

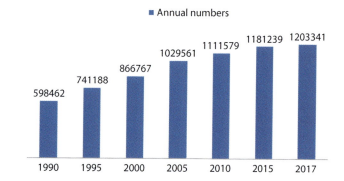

Figure 1.3 Quinquennial trends in annual incidence (absolute numbers) of IHD in India according to the GBD estimates [13].

Study [13,19]. There has been a steady increase in the number of ACS in India from 1990 to 2017 (Figure 1.3). The estimated numbers were 598.5 thousand in 1990 and have increased to 1203.3 thousand in 2017, an increase of 101.1%. This increase is much

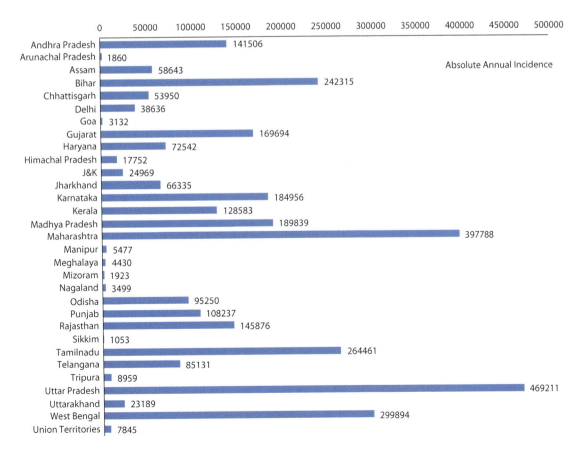

Figure 1.4 Secular trends in annual incidence of IHD (numbers/100,000) in India in men, women, and overall according to the GBD Study [13].

GEOGRAPHIC EPIDEMIOLOGY

A unique feature of IHD epidemiology in India is that there are large regional variations [1]. Epidemiological studies in the past have reported a major urban-rural difference, with rural IHD prevalence being less than half of the urban [8]. This urban-rural difference is a well-known feature of low and lower- to middle-income countries in the developing world [4]. On the other hand, in most high income countries IHD occurs more in rural populations as compared to urban. At a macrolevel, IHD mortality, incidence and prevalence is much higher in low income regions than in large high- and middle-income regions such as the USA, UK, China and Russia [21–24]. In the United States, the prevalence and incidence of IHD is much higher in the southern and south-eastern states [21] while in the UK it is much higher in deprived counties of Scotland and Northern England [22].

India State-Level Disease Burden Initiative Collaborators and GBD Compare have reported state-level incidence of IHD events for the year 2016 [19]. There are large differences in the absolute annual incidence of IHD events (Figure 1.5). Large numbers of annual IHD events are observed in large states such as Uttar Pradesh (469,211), Maharashtra (397,788), West Bengal (299,894), Tamilnadu (264,461), Bihar (242,315), Madhya Pradesh (184,956), Karnataka (184,956), Gujarat (169,694), Rajasthan (145,896) and Andhra Pradesh (141,506).

Rates of IHD events per 100,000 persons as estimated by the GBD Study shows a different picture (Figure 1.6). Overall, in India

more than in most countries of the world. The increasing trends in incidence of IHD events in India contrast with most of the developed countries where the absolute numbers of ACS events are declining [20].

Quinquennial trends in annual incidence of IHD events (ACS/100,000 population) in men, women and overall are shown in Figure 1.4. There has been a steady increase in incident IHD from 1990 to 2005, however, the incidence rates have levelled off in recent years. An important finding is that while the rates have plateaued in men, they continue to increase in women. The greater increase in IHD events in women and male-female convergence is similar to many developed countries.

Figure 1.5 Estimated absolute number of IHD events in different states of India in 2016 (GBD).

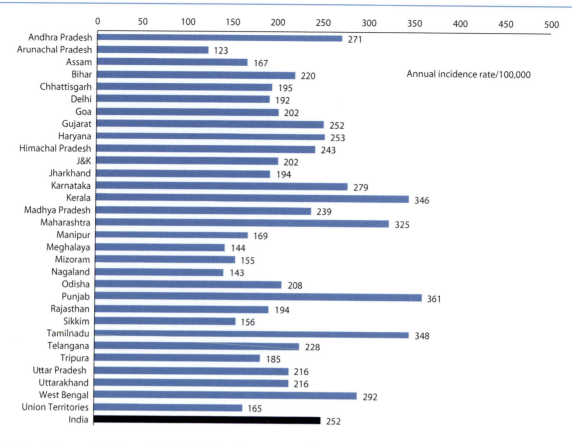

Figure 1.6 Estimated annual incidence of IHD/100,000 in different states of the country (GBD Study).

the rate of IHD events was 252/100,000 in the year 2016 with a two-fold difference in various states of the country. High rates (>250/100,000) are observed in states of Punjab (361), Tamilnadu (348) Kerala (346), Maharashtra (325), West Bengal (292) and Andhra Pradesh (271) while low rates (<150/100,000) are observed in many north-eastern Indian states. Data also show that the states with greater prevalence of IHD have higher IHD incidence rates with a strong correlation coefficient ($R^2 = 0.86$) (Figure 1.7).

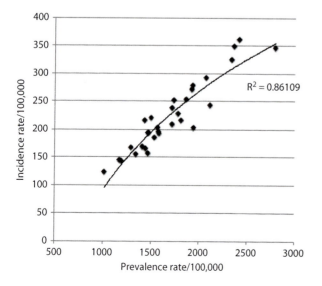

Figure 1.7 Correlation of IHD prevalence in different Indian states with its incidence.

Macrolevel analysis of ACS incidence with sociodemographic features indicates that the event rate is greater in states with a better human development index. We correlated the state level human development index with IHD mortality, ACS incidence and IHD prevalence in India (Figure 1.8) using logarithmic correlation. Significant positive correlation (R^2 value) is observed with various IHD parameters. A linear relationship of IHD prevalence and ACS incidence with human development suggests that prosperity is associated with greater ACS incidence and higher prevalence of IHD. This relationship is similar to the data on association of the human development index in India with obesity and hypertension prevalence as reported earlier [25]. This contrasts with most of the developed countries where there is an inverse correlation of development with IHD parameters. However, association of IHD mortality is hyperbolic, suggesting that highly developed states have lower IHD mortality. This indicates better quality of care in these states (Kerala, Tamilnadu and Maharashtra) which is associated with development attenuates IHD mortality. Maybe there are lessons to be learnt from the 'Kerala model' or 'Tamilnadu model' of cardiovascular care [26]. More studies are required to explain these findings.

Epidemiological studies have also reported that while IHD and ACS were more common among the higher socioeconomic status (SES) individuals in the last century in India, there has been a shift in its epidemiology in the present century associated with epidemiological transition [27]. Greater prevalence of risk factors (unhealthy diet, smoking/tobacco, hypertension, etc.) was reported in the mid-1990s among rural and urban participants in Jaipur Heart Watch studies [28,29]. Similar trends in risk factors were observed in a

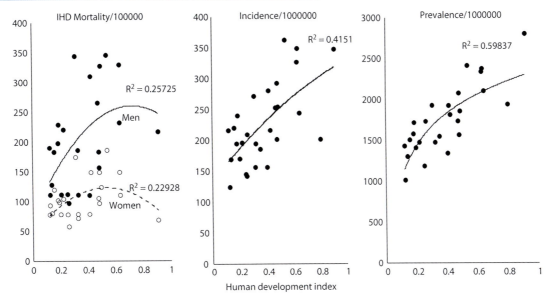

Figure 1.8 Logarithmic correlation of state-level human development index with IHD mortality, IHD prevalence, and ACS incidence.

country-wide study among industrial workers [30]. The Mumbai Cohort Study reported greater cardiovascular disease mortality among men with no or sub-primary educational status [31]. Low SES status individuals in the CREATE registry had a greater than 30-day mortality following an ACS [2]. This was primarily due to lower use of evidence-based therapies among these patients, as the differences in mortality attenuated following adjustment for risk factors and use of evidence-based therapies (thrombolysis, beta blockers, ACE inhibitors, statins and coronary interventions) [2]. The Prospective Urban Rural Epidemiology (PURE) study also reported greater cardiovascular mortality in low income countries of South Asia (mainly India) [32]. Cardiovascular mortality was the highest in low SES rural participants [32]. Socioeconomic disparities in epidemiology, presentation and management of ACS in India need more studies.

CLINICAL AND PHARMACOEPIDEMIOLOGY

Although acute coronary syndrome is a major health problem in India and IHD leads to the largest number of deaths, there are almost no data on its clinical epidemiology from population-based registries. For example, there are no data on incidence of ACS in the general population apart from the estimates provided by the GBD Study *vide supra*. There are no representative data on primary care-based ACS registries from different locations of the country. There are a few hospital-based registries but they are confined to secondary and tertiary care centres. Models of the population-based ACS registries are available in the United States and Europe [33,34].

There has been substantial change in the type of ACS in developed countries. More than 50 years ago, the predominant ACS was STEMI and was the presenting feature in more than 60%–70% of ACS patients [18,34]. This has changed, and presently NSTEMI/unstable angina is the predominant ACS presentation [17,35]. In contrast to these findings, the nationwide CREATE registry reported that more than 60% of patients with ACS were STEMI [2]. However, more recent registries from developed states (Kerala [36], DEMAT [37], Kerala-ACS [38] and Tamilnadu [39]) have reported that NSTEMI is the predominant form of ACS similar to developed countries (Table 1.2). Data from lesser-developed states (Himachal [40] and Assam [41]) and among young ACS patients

Table 1.2 Pharmacological agents used in ACS patients in hospital/at discharge in different registries in India

Pharmacological agents	Sites	Patient number	STEMI (%)	Thrombolysis (% in STEMI)	PCI (%)	Anti-platelets (%)	Beta-blockers (%)	ACE Inhibitors/ ARB (%)	Statins (%)
CREATE [2]	86	20,967	61	56	7	98	58	57	52
Kerala [36]	1	1,865	56	69	—	94	80	67	72
DEMAT [37]	8	1,565	55	45	49	96	79	67	93
Kerala ACS [38]	125	25,748	37	41	12	79	63	26	70
Himachal [40]	33	4,953	46	36	<1	99	82	84	88
Assam [41]	1	704	72	39	13	99	90	91	99
Chennai [39]	1	1,468	34	23	53	98	83	51	96
CADY [42]	22	680	51	NA	36	81	55	36	81

Abbreviations: STEMI, ST-elevation myocardial infarction; PCI, percutaneous coronary intervention; ACE, angiotensin converting enzyme; ARB, angiotensin receptor blocker.

(CADY) [42] have reported persistence of STEMI as the predominant form of ACS. More such studies involving a larger sample are required. The Indian Council of Medical Research supported MACE registry [43] has a much greater regional spectrum and may provide more nuanced data.

The pharmacoepidemiology of ACS in India has not been well studied. Registries have reported on revascularization therapies and pharmacological agents during hospitalisation and at-discharge with short term outcomes (Table 1.2). No long-term studies (>12 months) that have reported outcomes associated with different pharmacotherapies exist. The pattern of use of various evidence-based medicines in ACS patients at index hospitalisation in various registries is shown in Table 1.2. Pharmacological thrombolysis rates in STEMI are low, and coronary intervention rates vary from <1% in government hospitals [36] to >50% in non-government corporate [39] hospitals. Larger studies similar to European and US-based registries that have enrolled hundreds of thousands of patients are needed [44]. Also needed are long-term follow-up data to identify changing trends in the use of various evidence-based therapies among ACS patients.

GENETIC EPIDEMIOLOGY

Genetic factors have been hypothesised to explain the greater risk of IHD in Indians. Studies among emigrant South Asians have reported that cardiovascular risk factors and coronary artery disease are heritable [45]. Initial studies among emigrant Indians in Southeast Asia, Oceania and the UK suggested that standard risk factors do not explain greater incidence, and it was speculated that some genetic factors were involved [45]. Subsequent studies reported that higher insulin resistance and diabetes in these populations explained this greater risk [46,47].

Multiple genetic studies, almost all in patients with ACS, have been performed in India and have reported associations with many single nucleotide polymorphisms (SNPs) [48]. All these studies are underpowered. Genetic analyses using Genome-Wide Association Studies (GWAS) have failed to replicate the results of most of these studies [49]. GWAS have identified a number of SNPs as important coronary atherosclerosis at different pathways

(Table 1.3) [50]. This list keeps on growing as more information is available including studies that identified genes important in South Asians [50,51]. These individual variants have a modest effect size with odds ratios of 1.05 to 1.30 per risk allele and in aggregate account for only a small proportion of the total predicted genetic variance. However, these findings do not exclude a role for genetic factors since the GWAS approach is not well designed to identify either low frequency or rare variants. Moreover, the South Asian genome, although similar to Caucasian populations to certain extents, is unique [52,53], and more research is required in this direction.

IHD and vascular atherosclerosis are multifactorial diseases. Risk predictive capability of individual genetic risk factors with IHD incidence has been found to be inferior to classical cardiovascular risk factors. Therefore, recent focus has shifted from SNP-based models to gene risk score models [50,54]. The initial reports combined only a few SNPs for risk prediction [54,55]. As knowledge has evolved, more and more SNPs have been added to create various polygenic risk scores. These SNPs are involved in not only inflammatory and thrombogenic pathways (important in ACS) but also in pathways involved in various major cardiovascular risk factors, namely hypertension, dyslipidemias and diabetes. Complex trait diseases such as IHD may have omnigenic rather than polygenic pathways. Recent reports suggest that an omnigenic gene risk prediction model, especially in ACS patients, with incorporation of 50K–100 K SNPs is a better predictor than classical cardiovascular risk scores [56]. Indeed, there has been a progressive increase in the number of SNPs in each risk score and current genome-wide polygenic risk scores are based on millions of SNPs [57,58].

Presently, there are no studies that have specifically identified genomic risk factors in South Asians or Indians using GWAS, Whole Genome Studies (WGS), Whole Exome Sequencing (WES) or Next-Generation Sequencing (NGS). The GWAS study among the PROMIS cohort in Pakistan did not report any unique SNP associations with IHD and risk factors [59]. The genetic structure of human populations does not change in a few decades and it would be more important to study gene functions as well as gene-gene and gene-environment interaction [50]. Very limited information exists in these areas of research, especially in Indians and South

Table 1.3 Genes identified for atherosclerosis and its pathways

LDL cholesterol and lipoprotein(a)	Triglyceride-rich lipoproteins	Inflammation	Cellular proliferation and vascular remodelling	Vascular tone and nitric oxide signalling
SORT1	LPL	IL6R	COL4A1-COL4A2	CUCY1A3
PCSK9	TRIB1	CXCL12	MIA3	EDNRA
APOB	APOA5		REST-NOA1	NOS3
ABCG5-ABCG8	APOA4		ZC3HC1	
LPA	APOC4		9p21	
LIPA	APOA1		PDGFD	
LDLR	ANGPTL4		AWAP70	
APOE			KSR2	
			ADAMTS7	
			BCAS3	
			FLT1	
			SMAD3	

Asians. The study of gut microbiome and its influence on atherosclerosis is also important in this regard [60]. Also required is the study of epigenetic factors that are known to alter the gene function but are not the result of changes in the DNA sequence. Gene-environment interactions can lead to adverse epigenetic influences that can promote atherosclerosis. For example, physical inactivity and harmful nutrients are known to promote atherosclerosis via epigenetic changes, and both these risk factors are rapidly increasing in India [1,4]. Ambient air pollution and use of industrial and agricultural toxins is also increasing in India. Both may affect the epigenetic factors responsible for IHD [11]. More studies are required in our country to elucidate mechanistic pathways for ACS involving genes, gene-gene and gene-environment interaction.

CONCLUSION

Acute coronary syndromes are major public health and clinical problems in India. The Million Death Study [10] and the Global Burden of Diseases Study [12] have established IHD as the most important cause of mortality and morbidity in the country. Comparative epidemiology data suggest that India has one of the highest IHD burdens in the world (Table 1.1). The GBD Study has estimated that there were more than 1.2 million incident IHD patients in 2017. There is a large regional variation with more than two-fold differences in ACS incidence/100,000 persons in more developed versus less developed states. No large nationwide registry has identified ACS types and patterns of therapies. Multisite and regional registries have reported that the major form of ACS in India is still STEMI. The in-hospital mortality from ACS varies from 5% to 15% with a high event rate at 3–6 months follow-up [2,38,40,41]. These are much more than the data from developed countries in North America and Europe. Registries have shown that ACS occurs about 10 years earlier in Indian patients as compared to other countries [61]. More studies on pharmacoepidemiology of ACS in India are required to identify gaps in cardiovascular care. Also required are interventional studies to improve cardiovascular care, similar to the ACS-QUIK study in Kerala [62]. Decreasing the high mortality from ACS in India will need universal primary care for prevention and early identification of the disease [63,64]. We require a vibrant and affordable secondary and tertiary health care system with focus on high quality care, training and research [65,66]. Only then will the dream of attenuating the massive burden of IHD and ACS in the country be realised.

REFERENCES

1. Gupta R, Mohan I, Narula J. Trends in coronary heart disease epidemiology in India. *Ann Global Health*. 2016;82:307–315.
2. Xavier D, Pais P, Devereaux PJ et al. Treatment and outcomes of acute coronary syndromes in India (CREATE): A prospective analysis of registry data. *Lancet*. 2008;371:1435–1442.
3. Gupta R, Khedar RS, Gaur K, Xavier D. Low quality cardiovascular care is important coronary risk factor in India. *Indian Heart J*. 2018;70(Suppl 3):s419–s430.
4. World Health Organization. *Global Status Report on Non-Communicable Diseases 2014*. Geneva: World Health Organization. 2014.
5. GBD 2017 Causes of Death Collaborators. Global, regional, and national age-sex specific mortality for 282 causes of death, 1980–2017: A systematic analysis for the Global Burden of Disease Study 2017. *Lancet*. 2018;392:1736–1788.
6. Gupta R, Gupta VP. Meta-analysis of coronary heart disease prevalence in India. *Indian Heart J*. 1996;48:241–245.
7. Gupta R. Recent trends in coronary heart disease epidemiology in India. *Indian Heart J*. 2008;60(Suppl B): B4–B18.
8. Gupta R, Joshi PP, Mohan V, Reddy KS, Yusuf S. Epidemiology and causation of coronary heart disease and stroke in India. *Heart*. 2008;94:16–26.
9. Ram U, Jha P, Gerland P et al. Age-specific and sex-specific adult mortality risk in India in 2014: Analysis of 0·27 million nationally surveyed deaths and demographic estimates from 597 districts. *Lancet Glob Health*. 2015;3:e767–e775.
10. Ke C, Gupta R, Xavier D et al. Divergent trends in ischemic heart disease and stroke mortality in India from 2000 to 2015: A nationally representative mortality survey. *Lancet Glob Health*. 2018;6:e914–e923.
11. India State-Level Disease Burden Initiative Collaborators. Nations within a nation: Variations in epidemiological transition across the states in India 1990–2016, in the Global Burden of Disease Study. *Lancet*. 2017;390:2437–2460.
12. India State-Level Disease Burden Initiative Collaborators. The evolution of cardiovascular diseases and their risk factors in the states of India: The Global Burden of Disease Study 1990–2016. *Lancet Glob Health*. 2018;6:e1339–e1351.
13. Global Health Data Exchange. Available at: http://ghdx.healthdata.org/gbd-results-tool. Accessed 7 March 2019.
14. Vos T, Murray CJL. Measuring the health of populations: The Global Burden of Disease Study methods. In: Detels R, Gulliford M, Abdool Karim Q, Tan CC. *Oxford Textbook of Global Public Health*. Oxford: Oxford University Press. 2015; 634–644.
15. Geilen S, De Backer G, Peipoli MF, Wood D. *The ESC Textbook of Preventive Cardiology*. Oxford: Oxford University Press & European Society of Cardiology. 2015; 273–342.
16. Loscalzo J. Approach to the patients with possible cardiovascular disease. In: Jameson JL, Kasper DL, Longo DL, Fauci AS, Hauser SL, Loscalzo J, Editors. *Harrison's Textbook of Internal Medicine*, 20th ed. New York: McGraw Hill. 2018; 1649–1651.
17. Giugliano RP, Cannon CP, Braunwald E. Non-ST-segment elevation acute coronary syndrome. In: Jameson JL, Kasper DL, Longo DL, Fauci AS, Hauser SL, Loscalzo J, Editors. *Harrison's Textbook of Internal Medicine*, 20th ed. New York: McGraw Hill. 2018; 1866–1872.
18. Antman EM, Loscalzo J. ST-segment elevation myocardial infarction. In: Jameson JL, Kasper DL, Longo DL, Fauci AS, Hauser SL, Loscalzo J, Editors. *Harrison's Textbook of Internal Medicine*, 20th ed. New York: McGraw Hill. 2018; 1872–1885.
19. GBD India Compare. Available at: https://gbd2016.healthdata.org/gbd-compare/india. Accessed 8 March 2019.

20. Gaziano TA, Gaziano JM. Epidemiology of cardiovascular disease. In: Jameson JL, Kasper DL, Longo DL, Fauci AS, Hauser SL, Loscalzo J, Editors. *Harrison's Textbook of Internal Medicine*, 20th ed. New York: McGraw Hill. 2018; 1662–1666.

21. Global Burden of Cardiovascular Diseases Collaboration, Roth GA, Johnson CO et al. The burden of cardiovascular diseases among the US states 1990–2016. USA regional differences. *JAMA Cardiol.* 2018;3:375–389.

22. Steel N, Ford JA, Newton JN et al. Changes in health in the counties of the UK and 150 English Local Authority areas 1990–2016: A systematic analysis for the Global Burden of Disease Study 2016. *Lancet.* 2018;392:1647–1661.

23. Zhang G, Yu C, Zhou M, Wang L, Zhang Y, Lou L. Burden of ischemic heart disease and attributable risk factors in China from 1990 to 2015: Findings from the Global Burden of Disease 2015 Study. *BMC Cardiovasc Disord.* 2018;18:18.

24. GBD 2016 Russia Collaborators. The burden of disease in Russia from 1980–2016: A systematic analysis for the Global Burden of Disease Study. *Lancet.* 2018;392:1138–1146.

25. Gupta R, Gaur K, Ram CVS. Emerging trends in hypertension epidemiology in India. *J Hum Hypertension.* 2019;33:575–587.

26. Zachariah G, Mohanan PP, Narayanan KM. A Kerala model for cardiovascular research. *Indian Heart J.* 2016;68:862–865.

27. Gupta R, Gupta KD. Coronary heart disease in low socioeconomic status subjects in India: An evolving epidemic. *Indian Heart J.* 2009;61:358–367.

28. Gupta R, Gupta VP, Ahluwalia NS. Educational status, coronary heart disease and coronary risk factor prevalence in a rural population of India. *BMJ.* 1994;309:1332–1336.

29. Gupta R, Kaul V, Agrawal A, Guptha S, Gupta VP. Cardiovascular risk according to educational status in India. *Prev Med.* 2010;51:408–411.

30. Reddy KS, Prabhakaran D, Jeemon P et al. Educational status and cardiovascular risk profile in Indians. *PNAS.* 2007;104:16263–16268.

31. Pednekar M, Gupta R, Gupta PC. Illiteracy, low educational status and cardiovascular mortality in India. *BMC Public Health.* 2011;11:e568.

32. Yusuf S, Rangarajan S, Teo K et al. Cardiovascular risk and events in 17 low-, middle- and high-income countries. *N Engl J Med.* 2014;371:818–827.

33. Roger VL, Jacobsen SJ, Weston SA, Bailey KR, Kottke TE, Frye RL. Trends in heart disease deaths in Olmsted County, Minnesota, 1979–1994. *Mayo Clin Proc.* 1999;74:651–657.

34. Degano IR, Salomaa V, Veronesi G et al. Twenty five year trends in myocardial infarction attack and mortality rates, and case-fatality in six European population. *Heart.* 2015;101:1413–1421.

35. Benjamin EJ, Muntner P, Alonso A et al. Heart disease and stroke statistics—2019 update: A report from the American Heart Association. *Circulation.* 2019;139:e56–66.

36. Misriya KJ, Sudhayakumar N, Khader SA, George R, Jayaprakash VL, Pappachan JM. The clinical spectrum of acute coronary syndromes: Experience from a major centre in Kerala. *J Assoc Physicians India.* 2009; 57:377–383.

37. Pagidapatti N, Huffman M, Jeemon P et al. Association between gender, process of care measures, and outcomes in ACS in India: Results from the Detection and Management of Coronary Heart Disease (DEMAT) Registry. *PLoS One.* 2013;8:e062061.

38. Mohanan PP, Mathew R, Harikrishnan S et al. Presentation, management and outcomes of 25748 acute coronary syndrome admissions in Kerala, India: Results from the Kerala ACS Registry. *Eur Heart J.* 2013;34:121–129.

39. Isezuo S, Subban V, Krishnamoorthy J et al. Characteristics, treatment and one-year outcomes of patients with acute coronary syndrome in a tertiary hospital in India. *Indian Heart J.* 2014;66:156–163.

40. Negi PC, Merwaha R, Panday D, Chauhan V, Guleri R. Multicenter Himachal Pradesh ACS Registry. *Indian Heart J.* 2016;68:118–127.

41. Iqbal F, Barkataki JC. Spectrum of acute coronary syndrome in North Eastern India: A study from a major center. *Indian Heart J.* 2016;68:128–131.

42. Iyengar SS, Gupta R, Ravi S et al. Premature coronary artery disease in India: Coronary artery disease in the young (CADY) registry. *Indian Heart J.* 2017;69:211–216.

43. Sharma M, Bharani A, Chadha DS et al. Rationale, design and feasibility of a nationwide prospective registry of management of acute coronary events (MACE) in India. Abstract. *Am J Med.* 2016;11(Suppl.):e103.

44. Masoudi FA, Ponirakis A, De Lemos JA et al. Trends in US cardiovascular care: 2016 report from 4 ACC national cardiovascular data registries. *J Am Coll Cardiol.* 2017;69:1427–1450.

45. McKeigue PM, Miller GJ, Marmot MG. Coronary heart disease in south Asians overseas. *J Clin Epidemiol.* 1989;42:597–609.

46. Zabaneh D, Chambers JC, Elliott P, Scott J, Balding DJ, Kooner JS. Heritability and genetic correlations of insulin resistance and component phenotypes in Asian Indian families using a multivariate analysis. *Diabetologia.* 2009;52:2585–2589.

47. Tillin T, Hughes AD, Mayet J et al. The relationship between metabolic risk factors and incident cardiovascular disease in Europeans, South Asians and African Caribbean: SABRE (Southall and Brent Revisited): A prospective population based study. *J Am Coll Cardiol.* 2013;61:1777–1786.

48. Tan ST, Scott W, Panoulas V et al. Coronary heart disease in Indian Asians. *Global Cardiol Sci Pract.* 2014;2014:4.

49. Jeemon P, Pettigrew K, Sainsbury C, Prabhakaran D, Padmanabhan S. Implications of discoveries from genome-wide association studies in current cardiovascular practice. *World J Cardiol.* 2011;3:230–247.

50. Khera AV, Kathiresan S. Genetics of coronary artery disease: Discovery, biology and clinical translation. *Nat Rev Genet.* 2017;18:331–344.

51. Coronary Artery Disease (C4D) Genetics Consortium. A genome wide association study in Europeans and South Asians identifies five new loci for coronary artery disease. *Nat Genet.* 2011;43:339–344.

52. Chambers JC, Abbott J, Zhang W et al. The South Asian genome. *PLoS One.* 2014;9:e102645.

53. Nakatsuka N, Moorjani P, Rai N et al. The promise of discovering population specific disease associated genes in South Asia. *Nat Genetics.* 2017;49:1403–e101407.

54. Tada H, Melander O, Louie JZ et al. Risk prediction by genetic risk scores for coronary heart disease is independent of family history. *Eur Heart J.* 2016;37:561–567.

55. Khera AV, Emdin CA, Drake I et al. Genetic risk, adherence to a healthy lifestyle, and coronary disease. *N Engl J Med.* 2016;375:2349–2358.

56. Abraham G, Havulinna AS, Bhalala OG et al. Genomic prediction of coronary heart disease. *Eur Heart J.* 2016;37:3267–3278.

57. Boyle EA, Li YI, Pritchard JK. An expanded view of complex traits: From polygenic to omnigenic. *Cell.* 2017;169:1177–1186.

58. Khera AV, Chaffin M, Aragam KG et al. Genome wide polygenic score for common diseases identify individuals with risk equivalent for monogenic mutations. *Nature Genet.* 2018;50:1219–1224.

59. Salaheen D, Haycock PC, Zhao W A et al. Apolipoproein(a) isoform size, lipoprotein(a) concentration and coronary artery disease: A mendelian randomization analysis. *Lancet Diabetes Endocrinol.* 2017;5:524–533.

60. Jonsson AL, Backhed F. Role of gut microbiota in atherosclerosis. *Nature Rev Cardiol.* 2017;14:79–87.

61. Prabhakaran D, Jeemon P, Roy A. Cardiovascular diseases in India: Current epidemiology and future directions. *Circulation.* 2016;133:1605–1620.

62. Huffman MD, Mohanan PP, Devarajan R et al. Effect of a quality improvement intervention on clinical outcomes in patients in India with acute myocardial infarction: The ACS-QIUK randomized clinical trial. *JAMA.* 2018;319:567–578.

63. Rao M, Mant D. Strengthening primary healthcare in India: White paper on opportunities for partnership. *BMJ.* 2012;344:e3151.

64. Gupta R. Universal healthcare ahoy! *RUHS J Health Sciences.* 2018;3:179–e3181.

65. Swaminathan S, Qureshi H, Jahan MU, Baskota DK, De Alwis S, Dandona L. Health research priorities and gaps in South Asia. *BMJ.* 2017;357:j1510.

66. Gupta R, Yusuf S. Challenges in ischemic heart disease management and prevention in low socioeconomic status people in LMICs. *BMC Med.* 2019;17:e209. https://doi.org/10.1186/s12916-019-1454-y

2

Pathophysiology of acute coronary syndrome

JPS SAWHNEY, PRASHANT WANKHADE AND SIMRAN SAWHNEY

INTRODUCTION

The acute coronary syndromes constitute unstable angina, ST-elevation myocardial infarction [STEMI] and non-ST-elevation myocardial infarction. The first description of the clinical presentation of acute myocardial infarction (MI) was published by Obstrastzow and Straschesko [1]. Herrick [2] associated the clinical presentation of acute MI with thrombotic occlusion of the coronary arteries. MI alone is the main cause of death in most Western countries and cardiovascular disease will become a major global cause of death by 2020 [3]. Atherosclerotic plaque formation within the coronaries with subsequent lesion disruption, platelet aggregation and thrombus formation is the leading cause of acute coronary syndromes. MI in patients with normal coronary arteries (MINOCA) is becoming an increasingly recognised entity. This chapter reviews the pathogenesis of atherosclerosis and mechanisms responsible for the sudden conversion of stable atherosclerotic plaques into unstable life-threatening atherothrombotic lesions.

ATHEROGENESIS

Atherogenesis is the result of a complex process involving blood elements, abnormalities in the vessel wall and alterations in blood flow. Various pathologic mechanisms play an important role in the development of atherosclerotic plaque, which includes inflammation with activation of endothelial cells, monocyte recruitment, smooth muscle cell proliferation and matrix synthesis, lipid particles necrosis, calcification and thrombosis [4] (Figure 2.1). These diverse processes result in the formation of atheromatous plaques that form the nidus for future acute coronary syndromes.

It has been postulated that some form of injury to the arterial endothelium gives rise to atherosclerotic lesions. This injury results in an alteration in endothelial cell-cell attachment or endothelial cell-connective tissue attachment, which along with blood flow derived shear forces results in focal desquamation of the endothelium. This is followed by adherence, aggregation and release of platelets at the sites of focal injury. These platelets release a mitogenic factor which along with other plasma constituents causes focal intimal proliferation of smooth muscle cells. This intimal proliferation is accompanied by the synthesis of a new connective tissue matrix and the deposition of intracellular and extracellular lipids (Figure 2.2).

As the thrombosis serves as a trigger for acute myocardial ischaemia, it is important to know about the structure of plaques before thrombotic events occur and the reason behind conversion from a stable state to an unstable state.

THE CULPRIT PLAQUE

There are various stages of plaque maturation as described by the American Heart Association (AHA) [6]. The early stages, i.e. AHA types I–III, are not associated with evidence of structural damage to the endothelium. The fully developed fibro-lipid plaque, designated as type IV or type Va, has a core of lipid surrounded by a capsule of connective tissue. The core consists of an extracellular mass of lipid containing cholesterol and its esters. This core is surrounded by numerous macrophages, many of which are foam cells, i.e. macrophages containing abundant intracytoplasmic droplets of cholesterol. Monocytes which crossed the

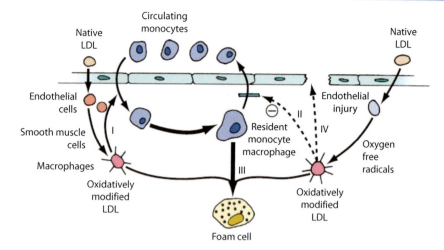

Figure 2.1 Mechanisms of atherogenesis [5].

endothelium from the arterial lumen serve as precursors for these macrophages. These macrophages are highly activated cells and produce a procoagulant tissue factor and various inflammatory cell mediators such as interleukins, tumour necrosis factor-α (TNF α) and metalloproteinases. Smooth muscle cells synthesise collagen which forms the connective tissue capsule surrounding this inflammatory mass. This portion of the capsule separating the core from the arterial lumen forms the plaque cap.

The endothelium over and between plaques shows enhanced replication compared to normal arteries, implying abnormal physiological function. The focal areas of endothelial denudation occur over the plaque which exposes the underlying connective tissue matrix and allows a platelet monolayer to adhere at the site. These ultramicroscopic thrombi are not visible on angiography, nor do they impede flow, but they can release a platelet derived growth factor which causes smooth muscle cell growth.

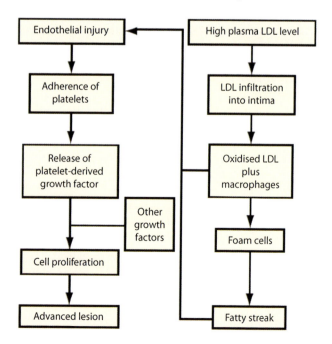

Figure 2.2 Linkage between the lipid infiltration hypothesis and the endothelial injury hypothesis [5].

MECHANISMS OF THROMBOSIS

Thrombosis over plaques occurs because of two processes described as follows [7] (Figure 2.3):

1. *Endothelial erosion*: The highly activated macrophages cause endothelial cell death by apoptosis and by the production of proteases which cut loose the endothelial cells from their adhesion to the vessel wall. This leads to endothelial denudation causing large areas of the surface of the subendothelial connective tissue of the plaque to expose to blood products. These exposed areas become nidus for thrombus formation which is adherent to the plaque surface.

2. *Plaque disruption*: The plaque cap tears to expose the lipid core to blood in the arterial lumen. This core area is highly thrombogenic, containing tissue factor, fragments of collagen, and crystalline surfaces, which accelerates coagulation. Initially the thrombus forms within the plaque which may then extend into the arterial lumen causing partial or complete occlusion of the arterial lumen. Like endothelial erosion, plaque disruption is a reflection of enhanced inflammatory activity within the plaque [8].

The cap of plaque: The tensile strength of connective tissue matrix depends upon the cap of plaque. It is a dynamic structure and is constantly being replaced and maintained by the smooth muscle cells. The inflammatory process reduces collagen synthesis by inhibiting the smooth muscle cells and causes its death by apoptosis [7].

Macrophages produce various metalloproteinases capable of degrading all the components of the connective tissue matrix, including collagen. These metalloproteinases are secreted within tissue in inactive form and subsequently activated by plasmin. Their production by macrophages is upregulated by inflammatory cytokines such as TNF α. Plaque disruption is therefore an auto-destruct phenomenon associated with an enhanced inflammatory activation.

The relative importance of disruption and erosion as triggers for thrombus formation may vary between different patient

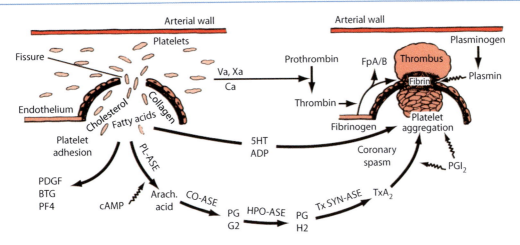

Figure 2.3 Schematic of ruptured unstable plaque with subsequent thrombus formation [5]. 5HT, Serotonin; ADP, adenosine diphosphate; BTG, β-thromboglobulin; cAMP, cyclic adenosine monophosphate; CO-ASE, cyclooxygenase; FpA/B, fibrinopeptide A and B; HPO-ASE, hydroperoxidase; PDGF, platelet-derived growth factor; PF4, platelet factor 4; PG, prostaglandin; PL-ASE, phospholipase A2; TxA2, thromboxane A2; Tx SYN-ASE, thromboxane synthetase.

groups. Disruption is the predominant cause (>85%) of major coronary thrombi in white males with high plasma concentrations of low-density lipoprotein (LDL) and low concentrations of high-density lipoprotein (HDL); whereas in women erosion of the endothelium is responsible for around 50% of major thrombi [9].

The distinction between erosion and disruption is not necessarily of major clinical importance. Both the processes are results of enhanced inflammatory activity within the plaque and appear equally responsive to lipid-lowering therapy. The intra-plaque component of disrupted plaque is more resistant to fibrinolytic treatment in contrast to erosion where the thrombus is more accessible. This potential advantage is, however, offset by the tendency of erosion to occur at sites where the pre-existing stenosis was more severe. There is another smoking related form of thrombosis caused by endothelial erosion over plaques which do not contain lipid or have a major inflammatory component [10]. This type of disease is rare and arguably is distinct from conventional atherosclerosis.

THE VULNERABLE PLAQUE CONCEPT

Pathological studies have described various features of vulnerable plaque [11]:

1. Large lipid core occupying at least 50% of the overall plaque volume
2. High density of macrophages
3. Low density of smooth muscle cells in the cap
4. High tissue factor content
5. Thin plaque cap in which the collagen structure is disorganised

The risk of a future acute event will depend on the number of vulnerable plaques rather than on the total number of plaques. This variation in number of vulnerable plaques explains why one individual has a series of infarcts at regular intervals while another individual has an infarct without further events for 10 or even 20 years [7].

THE SEQUENCE OF THROMBOTIC EVENTS

The thrombi which occur in the acute coronary syndrome setting are dynamic and evolve in stages. The initial stage occurs within the lipid core itself and is predominantly composed of platelets. As thrombus begins to protrude into the lumen, the fibrin component tends to increase, but any surface exposed to the blood will be covered by activated platelets. Clumps of activated platelets are swept down with the blood flow into the distal intramyocardial arteries as microemboli. This thrombus may continue to grow to occlude the artery leading to a final stage in which there is a loose network of fibrin entrapping large numbers of red cells. This final stage thrombus may propagate distally after the onset of myocardial infarction. The structure of the final stage of occlusive thrombus makes it very susceptible to either natural or therapeutic lysis, but the deeper and earlier thrombus is more resistant to lysis.

SYMPTOMOLOGY IN RELATION TO CORONARY THROMBI

Episodes of plaque disruption are associated with the onset or exacerbation of stable angina caused by a sudden increase in plaque volume.

Non-occluding thrombi projecting into the lumen (mural thrombi) are the basis of unstable angina. The intermittent attacks of myocardial ischaemia at rest are caused by various potential mechanisms:

1. The thrombus may intermittently wax and wane in size and become occlusive for relatively short periods of time.
2. Intense local vasoconstriction can further cause reduction in distal blood flow.
3. Platelet deposition is a known potent stimulus for local smooth muscle constriction.
4. Platelet aggregates can get distally embolised into the intramyocardial vascular leading to blockage of smaller arteries of sizes between 50 and 100 μm external diameter and cause

vasoconstriction within the myocardium. Necropsy studies show a strong correlation between such platelet thrombi and microscopic foci of myocyte necrosis [12].

PLAQUE DISRUPTION: THE HEALING PROCESS

The majority of episodes of plaque disruption do not cause a major event such as infarction or death. Minor episodes of erosion or disruption are usually clinically silent but do contribute to the progression of coronary artery disease (CAD) seen on sequential angiography.

The natural lysis process removes thrombus up to some extent. 'Passification' implies that the exposed collagen becomes less active in causing platelet adhesion, probably due to being coated by natural heparinoids. A residual thrombus persisting after 36 hours can provoke smooth muscle cell migration with subsequent production of new connective tissue which smoothes out the surface and restores plaque integrity. The final result will be a stable lesion ranging from chronic total occlusion to only a minor increase from the pre-existing degree of stenosis. This process takes weeks, and residual thrombi at the base of the exposed lipid core act as a nidus for a further thrombotic event up to 6 months.

If the culprit lesion has an irregular outline on the initial angiogram taken soon after the acute event of unstable angina or post-thrombolysis for acute myocardial infarction, then there is higher risk of progressing to complete occlusion [13].

IN VIVO CULPRIT LESION ASSESSMENT IN ACS BY OPTICAL COHERENCE TOMOGRAPHY

In humans, culprit coronary lesion morphology in acute coronary syndrome (ACS) was first reported using a 3.2 Fr prototype optical coherence tomography (OCT) catheter in 2005 [14].

OCT is a novel invasive imaging technology that allows *in vivo* assessment of the coronary wall with high resolution (approximately 15 micron). OCT studies in patients with ACS were able to confirm post-mortem histopathology findings and provide information about dynamic nature of atherosclerotic plaque formation, modification and rupture. *In vivo* OCT showed that the incidence of target lesion and remote thin cap fibroatheroma (TCFA) varies with the clinical syndrome and is more pronounced in patients with acute myocardial infarction as compared to patients with stable angina.

It has been observed that fibrous cap thickness and the site of rupture are different in the type of ACS [15], and it is thinner (50 m vs. 90 m, respectively) in rest-onset ACS compared with exertion-triggered ACS, and the rupture at plaque shoulder is more frequent in the latter (57% vs. 93%). Not only TCFA but also thick cap (up to 150 m) fibroatheroma (ThCFA) might have a chance to rupture, and a high-sensitive C-reactive protein level negatively correlates well in proportion to the thickness of the ruptured fibrous cap. Exercise-induced high shear stress at the site of the plaque shoulder might be a possible cause of fibrous cap disruption, although the demonstration of inflammation by commercially available OCT systems has not been established yet. However, the possibility of macrophage accumulation by OCT has been already described in the culprit lesion in ACS [16].

It has been reported that various classes of unstable angina, i.e. Braunwald's class I, II and III, respectively, has different frequency of plaque rupture (43% vs. 13% vs. 71%, p < 0.001) and plaque ulceration (32% vs. 7% vs. 8%, p = 0.003), fibrous cap thickness (140 m vs. 150 m vs. 60 m, p < 0.001), minimal lumen area (0.70 mm² vs. 1.80 mm² vs. 2.31 mm², p < 0.001) and frequency of thrombus (72% vs. 30% vs. 73%, p < 0.001) [17].

Stent thrombosis is a life-threatening cause of ACS, and TCFA within stent has been reported as a cause of very late stent thrombosis after bare-metal stent (BMS) implantation (Figure 2.4). OCT can define stent edge dissection, tissue protrusion, and stent malapposition better than IVUS. Presence of uncovered strut, incomplete strut apposition and positive remodelling of the vessel

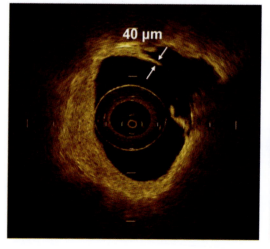
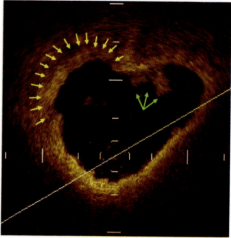

Figure 2.4 Optical coherence tomographic images of plaque rupture in acute coronary syndrome [17]. *Left*: The thickness of ruptured fibrous cap is 40 m and crater formation within plaque disruption. *Right*: Ulceration (yellow arrows) of thick fibrous cap with white thrombus (green arrows) in plaque erosion.

have been proposed as potential causes of late thrombosis after DES implantation [18].

Studies have demonstrated superiority of OCT compared to IVUS and angioscopy in the detection of plaque rupture (73% vs. 40% vs. 43%, p = 0.021) (Figure 2.2, left), erosion (23% vs. 0% vs. 3%, p = 0.003) (Figure 2.2, right) and thrombus (100% vs. 33% vs. 100%, p < 0.001) [19].

Lipid-lowering therapy by statins may have a potential to increase fibrous cap thickness and stabilise plaque vulnerability by reducing inflammation.

MYOCARDIAL INFARCTION WITH NON-OBSTRUCTIVE CORONARY ARTERIES

Approximately 1%–14% of myocardial infarction occur in the absence of obstructive (>50% stenosis) CAD. The demonstration of non-obstructive (<50%) CAD in the presence of features suggestive of acute myocardial infarction does not preclude an atherothrombosis aetiology, as thrombosis is a very dynamic phenomenon and the underlying atherosclerotic plaque can be non-obstructive.

The diagnosis of MINOCA is made in a patient who is fulfilling universal criteria for acute myocardial infarction with non-obstructive coronary arteries on coronary angiography without overt cause for the acute presentation [20].

There are multiple aetiologies causing MINOCA which can be grouped into: (1) secondary to epicardial coronary artery disorders (e.g. atherosclerotic plaque rupture, ulceration, fissuring, erosion, or coronary dissection with non-obstructive or no CAD) (MI type 1); (2) imbalance between oxygen supply and demand (e.g. coronary artery spasm and coronary embolism) (MI type 2); (3) coronary endothelial dysfunction (e.g. microvascular spasm) (MI type 2); and (4) secondary to myocardial disorders without involvement of the coronary arteries (e.g. myocarditis or Takotsubo syndrome). The outcome of MINOCA depends on the underlying cause; though, its overall prognosis is serious, with a 1-year mortality of about 3.5% [21].

Cardiac magnetic resonance (CMR) imaging is one very helpful imaging technique due to its unique non-invasive tissue characterisation, ability to identify wall motion abnormalities, presence of oedema, and myocardial scar/fibrosis presence and pattern. CMR within two weeks after onset of symptoms should be considered for identifying the aetiological cause of MINOCA [20].

CONCLUSION

Coronary atherosclerosis is the most common cause of ischaemic heart disease. Atherosclerosis is generally a benign disease unless complicated by erosion or disruption. Vulnerable plaques are more prone to rupture and are the ones that have a rich lipid core and a thin fibrous cap. Numerous factors, intrinsic and extrinsic to the plaque itself, interact to cause the formation of a vulnerable lesion and, ultimately, plaque disruption. Erosion, fissuring or

rupturing of plaques play a fundamental role in the onset of acute coronary syndromes whereas repetitive damage to the plaque with thrombosis and fibrotic organisation causes insidious progression of coronary artery disease. MINOCA is not uncommon, and the patient should undergo further evaluation to establish the cause, as failure to identify the underlying cause may result in inadequate and inappropriate therapy. Imaging techniques have added to our knowledge of pathophysiology of acute coronary syndrome and should be considered whenever feasible.

REFERENCES

1. Obstrastzow WP, Straschesko ND. Zur Kenntnis der Thrombose der Koronararterien des Herzens. *Z Klin Med.* 1910;71:116–132.
2. Herrick JB. Clinical features of sudden obstruction of the coronary arteries. *JAMA.* 1912;59:2015–2020.
3. Murray CJ, Lopez AD. Global mortality, disability, and the contribution of risk factors. Global Burden of Disease Study. *Lancet.* 1997;349:1436–1442.
4. Farugi RM, DiCorleto PE. Mechanisms of monocyte recruitment and accumulation. *Br Heart J.* 1993;69(suppl):S19–S29.
5. Sodhi N, Brown DL. Pathophysiology of acute coronary syndromes: Plaque rupture and atherothrombosis. In: Brown DL, editor. *Cardiac Intensive Care,* 3rd ed. Philadelphia, PA: Elsevier. 2019.
6. Stary H, Chandler A, Dinsmore R et al. A definition of advanced types of atherosclerotic lesions and a histological classification of atherosclerosis. A report from the committee on vascular lesions of the council on atherosclerosis, American Heart Association. *Circulation.* 1995;92:1355–1374.
7. Davies MJ. The pathophysiology of acute coronary syndrome. *Heart.* 2000;83:361–366.
8. Ross R. Atherosclerosis – An inflammatory disease. *N Engl J Med.* 1999;340:115–126.
9. Davies M. The composition of coronary artery plaques. *N Engl J Med.* 1997;336:1312–1313.
10. Arbustini E, Dal Bello P, Morbini P et al. Plaque erosion is a major substrate for coronary thrombosis in acute myocardial infarction. *Heart.* 1999;82:269–272.
11. Davies M. Stability and instability: Two faces of coronary atherosclerosis. The Paul Dudley White Lecture 1995. *Circulation.* 1996;94:2013–2020.
12. Davies M, Thomas A, Knapman P et al. Intramyocardial platelet aggregation in patients with unstable angina suffering sudden ischaemic cardiac death. *Circulation.* 1986;73:418–427.
13. Chen L, Chester M, Redwood S et al. Angiographic stenosis progression and coronary events in patients with 'stabilised' unstable angina. *Circulation.* 1995;91:2319–2324.
14. Jang IK, Tearney GJ, MacNeill B et al. In vivo characterization of coronary atherosclerotic plaque by use of optical coherence tomography. *Circulation.* 2005;111:1551–1555.
15. Tanaka A, Imanishi T, Kitabata H et al. Morphology of exertion-triggered plaque rupture in patients with acute coronary syndrome: An optical coherence tomography study. *Circulation.* 2008;118:2368–2373.

16. Tearney GJ, Yabushita H, Houser SL, Aretz HT, Jang IK, Schlendorf KH, Kauffman CR, Shishkov M, Halpern EF, Bouma BE. Quantification of macrophage content in atherosclerotic plaques by optical coherence tomography. *Circulation.* 2003;107:113–119.

17. Mizukoshi M, Imanishi T, Tanaka A et al. Clinical classification and plaque morphology determined by optical coherence tomography in unstable angina pectoris. *Am J Cardiol.* 2010;105.

18. Akasaka T, Kubo T, Mizukoshi M, Tanaka A, Kitabata H, Tanimoto T, Imanishi T. Pathophysiology of acute coronary syndrome assessed by optical coherence tomography. *J Cardiol.* 2010;56:8–14

19. Kubo T, Imanishi T, Takarada S et al. Assessment of culprit lesion morphology in acute myocardial infarction: Ability of optical coherence tomography compared with intravascular ultrasound and coronary angioscopy. *J Am Coll Cardiol.* 2007;50:933–939.

20. Ibanez B, James S, Agewall S, Antunes MJ, Bucciarelli-Ducci C, Bueno H, Caforio ALP. 2017 ESC Guidelines for the management of acute myocardial infarction in patients presenting with ST-segment elevation. *Eur Heart J.* 2018;39:119–177.

21. Pasupathy S, Air T, Dreyer RP, Tavella R, Beltrame JF. Systematic review of patients presenting with suspected myocardial infarction and nonobstructive coronary arteries. *Circulation.* 2015;131(10):861–870.

3

Current outcomes and outcome measures in acute coronary syndrome

DINKAR BHASIN, SHAHEER AHMED AND NITISH NAIK

INTRODUCTION

Acute coronary syndromes (ACS) have witnessed a significant improvement in outcomes over the past two decades due to significant improvements in therapeutic options and therapeutic strategies. Numerous trials have lowered mortality in ACS due to use of effective anti-platelet drugs as well as aggressive early interventional approaches. This chapter outlines current outcomes in ACS.

ST-ELEVATION MYOCARDIAL INFARCTION (STEMI)

Aggressive management of STEMI has been associated with improvements in both short-term and long-term outcomes. Immediate reperfusion with an invasive strategy is superior to fibrinolytic therapy. Many clinical trials have demonstrated superiority of routine early percutaneous intervention of the culprit artery in patients who receive fibrinolysis. Outcomes are superior if patients receive early reperfusion therapy as myocardial salvage is best within the first few hours. Relevant clinical outcomes in STEMI are outlined in Table 3.1.

MORTALITY

Mortality rate of STEMI differs among studies depending upon the population studied and nature of the study (controlled trials versus registries). There has been a progressive decline in the mortality rate after STEMI over the years in various registries [1,2]. In the national registry for myocardial infarction, which looked at trends of mortality rates related to STEMI in the United States, a decline in the mortality rate from 8.6% to 3.1% in those who underwent primary percutaneous coronary intervention (PCI) and declined from 7% to 6% in those who were thrombolysed [3,4] was noted. In a French registry of 6700 patients, there was a significant reduction in the crude mortality rates from 11.3% to 4.4% [5]. In the Indian context, the in-hospital mortality rate of STEMI was 8.2% in the Kerala ACS Registry and 8.6% in the CREATE registry [6,7]. Outcomes are better with early percutaneous intervention than with fibrinolytic therapy. Generally, only PCI of the infarct related artery is performed in STEMI. Intervention of non-infarct related arteries may be desirable in patients in cardiogenic shock. Routine revascularization of non-infarct related arteries may be considered before discharge in other patients. Routine percutaneous intervention has not been found useful in patients with occluded arteries beyond 48 hours (OAT trial). However, an ischaemia-guided strategy is useful in these patients.

EARLY REHOSPITALISATION

Early rehospitalisation (readmission within 30 days of STEMI) ranges between 15% and 25% in various studies [8–10]. However, there has been a trend towards reduction in the rates in the national readmissions database to 12.3% [11]. The predictors of

Table 3.1 Short-term and long-term outcomes after STEMI

Short-term outcomes	Long-term outcomes
Mortality	Mortality
Reinfarction	Sudden cardiac death
Rehospitalisation	Angina
Stroke	Recurrent MI
Bleeding	Stroke
Heart failure	

early rehospitalisation are diabetes mellitus, hypertension, atrial fibrillation, congestive heart failure, anaemia, and chronic kidney disease [12]. Prolonged hospital stay during the index hospitalisation and female sex are also strongly predictive of readmissions.

STROKE

The incidence of stroke in the immediate post-STEMI period is around 2% [13–15]. According to the Myocardial Infarction Study Group, the elderly and those with a past history of cerebrovascular accidents and atrial fibrillation were predictive of stroke [15].

HEART FAILURE

Incidence of heart failure ranges between 15% and 35% in various studies [16]. According to the National Registry of Myocardial Infarction, 20.4% of patients had presented with heart failure and a further 8.6% developed heart failure during hospitalisation [17]. In the National Cardiovascular Action Data Registry, 12% presented with heart failure, whereas 4% developed it during the course of a hospital stay [18]. Diabetes mellitus, left ventricular ejection fraction <30%, previous history of heart failure and female sex were independent predictors of heart failure. Patients in heart failure are more likely to receive thrombolysis and less likely to get PCI.

REINFARCTION

Reinfarction within 30 days of STEMI after successful primary PCI is seen in 1.8% of cases according to HORIZON AMI trial data and 2.1% in the PAMI trial [19,20]. After successful thrombolysis, 4.3% of patients experience re-occlusion [21,22]. Killip Class 2 or more, thrombocytosis, current smoking, stent length, final stenosis more than 30% and coronary dissection and left ventricular dysfunction are found to be independent predictors of reinfarction [19,20]. Reinfarction is an independent predictor of mortality after STEMI.

MAJOR BLEEDING

The rate of major bleeding postSTEMI varies between 0.9 and 8.9% in various studies, depending of the definition of major bleeding [23–25].

LONG-TERM OUTCOMES

MORTALITY

Long-term mortality in STEMI is better than NSTEMI in contrast to the short-term mortality [26–28]. The largest data comparing

mortality rates between STEMI and NSTEMI comes from the GUSTO IIb trial [29], which showed significantly higher 30-day mortality rates for STEMI (6.1% vs. 3.8%), which had reduced at 6 months and almost equalised at 1 year follow-up (9.6% vs. 8.8%).

SUDDEN CARDIAC DEATH

Out of the sudden cardiac deaths occurring in patients followed up after STEMI, around 50% occur in the first year and 25% in the first 3 months [30,31]. Risk factors for sudden death following STEMI are outlined in Table 3.2 [32–43].

OTHER OUTCOMES

In a study which followed patients of STEMI in 19 US centres, about 20% of patients reported to have angina at 1 year follow-up [44]. The risks of recurrent myocardial infarction and stroke at 3-year follow-up were 6%–7% and 1%–2%, respectively, according to the data from the HORIZON AMI trial [23].

RISK STRATIFICATION OF OUTCOMES

Various risk stratification tools have been devised based on data obtained from major clinical trials (Table 3.3). In addition, there are two risk stratification models proposed for patients undergoing primary PCI (Table 3.4) [49,50]. Based on these two scores, patients can be classified into low, intermediate and high risk.

Table 3.2 Risk factors for SCD after STEMI

LV dysfunction
Inducible ventricular tachycardia
NSVT on Holter
Late potentials on signal averaged ECG
Reduced heart rate variability
T wave alternans

Table 3.3 Risk models for STEMI

Risk stratification model [45–48]	Components
TIMI Risk Score	Age >65, diabetes, hypertension, angina, SBP<100 mmHg, HR > 100/min, Killip II and above, weight <67 Kg, anterior MI or LBBB, time to reperfusion > 4 hrs
PAMI Risk Score	Age >75, Killip >1, HR>100/min, diabetes, anterior MI or LBBB
TIMI Risk Index	(Heart rate) X [age/10]^2 / systolic blood pressure
GRACE Risk Model	Age, Killip Class, SBP, ST segment deviation, cardiac arrest, serum creatinine, elevated cardiac biomarkers and heart rate
Action Registry Score	Heart rate, low SBP, life-threatening presentations (cardiac arrest, cardiogenic shock or heart failure), low creatinine clearance, troponin levels

Table 3.4 Primary PCI risk scores

Zwolle Primary PCI Index	CADILLAC Risk Score
Killip Class	LVEF <40%
Post-PCI TIMI flow grade	Killip Class
Age	Creatinine clearance < 60 mL/min
Number of diseased vessels	TIMI flow grade after PCI 0–2
Location of infarction	Age >65 years
Time to reperfusion	Anaemia
	Triple vessel disease

Table 3.5 TIMI Risk Score for risk stratification of patients with NSTE-ACS[a]

Age ≥ 65 years
Presence of ≥ risk factors for CAD
Previous coronary artery lesion ≥ 50%
ST segment changes on initial ECG
At least two anginal episodes in previous 24 hrs
Elevated cardiac biomarker levels
Aspirin use in previous 7 days

[a] Each variable is given a score of 0 if absent and 1 if present. The total TIMI score is calculated by adding the points. A score of 0/1 is considered a low-risk score.

The mortality rate at 30 days ranges between 0.1% and 0.2% for low-risk cases to 6.6%–8% for high-risk cases. The risk stratification tools were compared in a study [51], which looked into the predictive accuracies of these scores for 1 year mortality. CADILLAC, TIMI and PAMI risk scores performed better, with the CADILLAC score being marginally better compared to other scores. The GRACE score had lower predictive accuracy for mortality.

NON-ST-ELEVATION MYOCARDIAL INFARCTION

Non-ST-elevation acute coronary syndrome (NSTE-ACS) represents a spectrum which includes unstable angina (UA) and non-ST-elevation myocardial infarction (NSTEMI). Unstable angina is defined as rest angina, which is more than 20 minutes in duration, new-onset angina, which limits physical activity, or crescendo angina (increased frequency, longer in duration or occurring with less exertion than before). Unstable angina with positive biomarkers qualifies as NSTEMI.

INCIDENCE AND OUTCOMES IN CONTEMPORARY CARE

Patients with UA have better outcomes compared to STEMI or NSTEMI with early mortality (<30 days) being less than 2%. Patients with NSTEMI have better short-term outcomes compared to STEMI but have worse long-term outcomes, which is likely related to higher age at presentation, comorbid conditions and possibly greater extent of disease.

RISK ASSESSMENT IN NSTEMI

Several risk assessment scores that allow triage of patients presenting with NSTE-ACS have been developed. The most widely used and validated scores are the TIMI risk score and GRACE (Global Registry of Acute Coronary Events) risk score. The TIMI risk score is a simple additive score consisting of seven points that can be easily calculated by hand (Table 3.5) [52]. The GRACE score consists of weighted risk factors and requires detailed calculation [53]. Long-term risk assessment after NSTE-ACS can be done using the TIMI stable ischaemic CAD risk score. It is based on nine risk factors and predicts the risk of cardiovascular events allowing intensification of medical therapy [54].

BASIC MANAGEMENT

Basic measures are similar to the management of STEMI and include adequate analgesia, oxygen administration if hypoxaemia is present, and use of nitrates and beta-blockers to decrease ischaemia. Beta-blockers should be used judiciously as their routine early use has not shown any major benefit.

ANTI-PLATELET THERAPY

All patients should receive a loading dose of 162–325 mg of chewable, non-enteric coated aspirin at diagnosis of NSTE-ACS. Dual anti-platelet therapy decreases major adverse cardiovascular events (MACE) and evidence comes from the CURE trial where addition of 300 mg clopidogrel immediately after diagnosis of ACS resulted in a 20% reduction in the hazard ratio for MACE [55]. There was an absolute risk reduction in MACE of 2.1% with an absolute risk increase of 1% of major bleeding with no significant difference in intracranial bleeding or fatal bleeding. This amounts to a net clinical benefit of 1% and hence is the recommended strategy for all patients with ACS (STEMI or NSTEMI). In patients undergoing PCI a total loading dose of 600 mg may further decrease MACE and is the recommended strategy whenever clopidogrel is used. Evidence for this comes from the CURENT OASIS 7 trial where a loading dose of 600 mg followed by 150 mg OD for one week after PCI resulted in lower rates of stent thrombosis [56]. A small but significant percentage of patients with NSTEMI requires CABG. In such patients, a delay of 5 days is suggested after the last dose of clopidogrel.

Newer anti-platelets such as prasugrel and ticagrelor have also been studied in NSTE-ACS.

The TRITON-TIMI 38 trial showed that in patients with ACS undergoing PCI, prasugrel (60 mg loading dose followed by 10 mg OD) results in 19% reduction in MACE over a 15 months period with significant reduction in risk of stent thrombosis [57]. However, the TRILOGY-ACS trial showed that there was no benefit of prasugrel over clopidogrel in patients who were medically managed [58]. Prasugrel is associated with increased risk of bleeding in patients older than 75 years or patients with previous TIA or stroke and is contraindicated in these subgroups. In patients with body weight <60 kg, 5 mg OD dose should be used. Prasugrel should be discontinued 7 days before planned cardiac surgery to decrease risk of bleeding.

The PLATO trial showed significant benefit with ticagrelor compared to aspirin in patients with NSTE-ACS (54% of the entire cohort of patients with ACS) [59]. There was significant reduction in overall MACE, stent thrombosis and total mortality. PEGASUS-TIMI 54 trial showed that long-term treatment with ticagrelor 60 mg BD may provide a net clinical benefit in patients with a history of ACS [60]. Cangrelor is a direct-acting antagonist of P2Y12 receptors administered intravenously (IV) and has a half-life of only 3 to 6 minutes. It is useful in patients who have not been preloaded with oral P2Y12 inhibitors or patients requiring bridging anti-platelet therapy before CABG. Routine use of GpIIb-IIIa inhibitors in patients with NSTEMI is not beneficial.

ANTI-COAGULATION

All patients with NSTE-ACS should receive anti-coagulation unless immediate invasive strategy is planned when anti-coagulation is given during the procedure. Use of unfractionated heparin (UFH) in addition to anti-platelets has shown in a meta-analysis to improve outcomes with reduction in composite of death or MI by 33% [61]. Therapy with UFH requires continuous IV infusion and frequent monitoring of activated partial thromboplastin time (aPTT) to maintain the value between 1.5 and 2.5 times control. Low molecular weight heparin allows easier dosing therapy with BD subcutaneous doses. Evidence from a meta-analysis showed that treatment with enoxaparin compared to UFH decreases new or recurrent MI without increase in major bleeding [62]. Fondaparinux is a useful alternative in patients with NSTE-ACS who are being managed conservatively, however, it provides suboptimal anti-coagulation for patients undergoing PCI and is not recommended in this setting. Anti-coagulation is recommended until PCI is performed in patients undergoing invasive management or until hospital discharge (at least 48 hours).

INVASIVE VERSUS CONSERVATIVE MANAGEMENT

Management options for NSTE-ACS include a routine early invasive management versus a conservative strategy that involves initial medical management followed by ischaemia-driven revascularisation (spontaneous ischaemia or stress-induced ischaemia). A 2006 meta-analysis showed that early invasive strategy resulted in significant reduction in all-cause mortality (4.9% vs. 6.5%; RR = 0.75, 95% CI 0.63–0.90) and recurrent MI (7.6 versus 9.1%, RR = 0.83, 95% CI 0.72–0.96) at 2 years [63]. Hence, most patients with NSTE-ACS should undergo coronary angiography although the timing may differ depending upon the estimated risk and presentation as discussed in the following section. However, a conservative approach may be optimal in patients who are at low risk with no ECG changes, negative biomarkers and no recurrence of angina. Such patients should be subjected to stress testing (preferably stress imaging) to guide treatment.

TIMING OF INVASIVE MANAGEMENT

Immediate invasive management is recommended in patients who have hemodynamic instability, heart failure, refractory angina or electrical instability (ventricular fibrillation or ventricular tachycardia).

The strategy of early invasive strategy versus delayed invasive strategy has been extensively debated. The largest trial to study this was the TIMACS trial which showed that routine early invasive strategy (≤24 hours) failed to improve the primary outcome compared to delayed invasive strategy (≥36 hours) but improved the secondary outcome, mainly driven by the decrease in refractory ischaemia [64]. However, the early invasive strategy improved outcomes in high-risk patients such as those with age >65 years, ST-changes, elevated biomarkers and a GRACE score >140. The evidence was most robust for patients with a GRACE score >140. A 2017 meta-analysis of eight RCTs showed no difference in mortality with a routine early invasive strategy (<24 hours) compared to delayed invasive strategy (12–108 hours) [65]. However, significant survival benefit was noted with early invasive strategy in high-risk patients such as patients with elevated biomarkers (HR 0.76, 95% CI 0.58–1.00), diabetes (HR 0.67, 95% CI 0.45–0.99), GRACE score >140 (HR 0.70, 95% CI 0.52–0.95) and age ≥75 years (HR 0.65, 95% CI 0.46–0.93).

The latest RCT to study timing of invasive strategy was the VERDICT trial. Early invasive (<12 hours) versus standard invasive (48–72 hours) treatment was compared in patients in whom angiography was clinically indicated and follow-up was done for over 4 years [66]. There was no difference in outcomes in the entire cohort, however, there was significant improvement in outcomes in patients with a GRACE score >140 (HR 0.81, 95% CI 0.67–1.00). There was no difference in bleeding or procedural complication rates. Hence, early invasive strategy is as safe as delayed invasive strategy but may be beneficial only in selected patients. The recommendations regarding timing of intervention are summarised in Table 3.6.

CULPRIT VESSEL VERSUS MULTI-VESSEL PCI

Patients with NSTEMI often have co-existent disease in other vessels. The optimal management of these patients has been questioned. Unlike STEMI, where the culprit vessel is obvious, identification of the culprit vessel in NSTEMI may be difficult in patients with multi-vessel disease. No randomised trial has strictly tested this question. A recent observation study of more than 20,000 patients showed that patients undergoing complete revascularisation had lower mortality compared to patients undergoing culprit only revascularisation (22.9% versus 25.9%; HR 0.90, 95% CI 0.85–0.97) at a median follow-up of 4.1 years [67]. Other observational studies have shown similar results [68,69].

Table 3.6 Timing of invasive strategy in management of NSTE-ACS

Immediate invasive	Early invasive (<24 hrs)	Routine invasive (<72 hrs)	Conservative or early stress test
Refractory angina	Positive biomarkers (rise or fall)	Diabetes mellitus	No recurrence of angina
Hemodynamic compromise	Dynamic ST-T changes	Renal failure (eGFR <60 mL/min/1.73 m²)	No ECG change
Serious arrhythmias	GRACE score >140	LV dysfunction (EF <40%)	Biomarker negative
Heart failure		Post-MI angina	GRACE ≤109
Recurrent ST-T changes		Post CABG	
		PCI in prior 6 months	
		GRACE risk score >109 and <140	

PCI VERSUS CORONARY ARTERY BYPASS GRAFTING

Randomised trials comparing CABG with PCI using current generation DES are lacking. However, based on data from stable CAD, CABG is recommended over PCI in patients with diabetes mellitus, multi-vessel disease (involving all three arteries or left anterior descending plus one other major artery) or left ventricular (LV) dysfunction (ejection fraction <40%). A heart team approach should be taken. Factors favouring PCI would include prior surgery, high peri-operative mortality risk and chronic kidney disease (CKD). Characteristics favouring CABG are complex coronary artery disease, diabetes, LV dysfunction and increased risk of bleeding with dual anti-platelet therapy.

REFERENCES

1. Krumholz HM, Wang Y, Chen J et al. Reduction in acute myocardial infarction mortality in the United States: Risk-standardized mortality rates from 1995–2006. *JAMA*. 19 Aug 2009;302(7):767–773.
2. Myerson M, Coady S, Taylor H, Rosamond WD, Goff DC, ARIC Investigators. Declining severity of myocardial infarction from 1987 to 2002: The Atherosclerosis Risk in Communities (ARIC) Study. *Circulation*. 3 Feb 2009;119(4):503–514.
3. Rogers WJ, Canto JG, Lambrew CT et al. Temporal trends in the treatment of over 1.5 million patients with myocardial infarction in the US from 1990 through 1999: The National Registry of Myocardial Infarction 1, 2 and 3. *J Am Coll Cardiol*. Dec 2000;36(7):2056–2063.
4. Gibson CM, Pride YB, Frederick PD et al. Trends in reperfusion strategies, door-to-needle and door-to-balloon times, and in-hospital mortality among patients with ST-segment elevation myocardial infarction enrolled in the National Registry of Myocardial Infarction from 1990 to 2006. *Am Heart J*. Dec 2008;156(6):1035–1044.
5. Puymirat E, Simon T, Steg PG et al. Association of changes in clinical characteristics and management with improvement in survival among patients with ST-elevation myocardial infarction. *JAMA*. 12 Sep 2012;308(10):998–1006.
6. Mohanan PP, Mathew R, Harikrishnan S et al. Presentation, management, and outcomes of 25 748 acute coronary syndrome admissions in Kerala, India: Results from the Kerala ACS Registry. *Eur Heart J*. Jan 2013;34(2):121–129.
7. Xavier D, Pais P, Devereaux PJ et al. Treatment and outcomes of acute coronary syndromes in India (CREATE): A prospective analysis of registry data. *Lancet Lond Engl*. 26 Apr 2008;371(9622):1435–1442.
8. Curtis JP, Schreiner G, Wang Y et al. All-cause readmission and repeat revascularization after percutaneous coronary intervention in a cohort of Medicare patients. *J Am Coll Cardiol*. 1 Sep 2009;54(10):903–907.
9. Dunlay SM, Weston SA, Killian JM, Bell MR, Jaffe AS, Roger VL. Thirty-day rehospitalizations after acute myocardial infarction: A cohort study. *Ann Intern Med*. 3 Jul 2012;157(1):11–18.
10. Joynt KE, Orav EJ, Jha AK. Thirty-day readmission rates for Medicare beneficiaries by race and site of care. *JAMA*. 16 Feb 2011;305(7):675–681.
11. Krumholz HM, Merrill AR, Schone EM et al. Patterns of hospital performance in acute myocardial infarction and heart failure 30-day mortality and readmission. *Circ Cardiovasc Qual Outcomes*. Sep 2000;2(5):407–413.
12. Kim Luke K, Yeo I, Cheung JW et al. Thirty-day readmission rates, timing, causes, and costs after ST-segment–elevation myocardial infarction in the United States: A national readmission database analysis 2010–2014. *J Am Heart Assoc*. 18 Sep 2018;7(18):e009863.
13. Becker RC, Burns M, Gore JM et al. Early assessment and in-hospital management of patients with acute myocardial infarction at increased risk for adverse outcomes: A nationwide perspective of current clinical practice. The National Registry of Myocardial Infarction (NRMI-2) Participants. *Am Heart J*. May 1998;135(5 Pt 1):786–796.
14. Fibrinolytic Therapy Trialists' (FTT) Collaborative Group. Indications for fibrinolytic therapy in suspected acute myocardial infarction: Collaborative overview of early mortality and major morbidity results from all randomised trials of more than 1000 patients. *Lancet Lond Engl*. 5 Feb 1994;343(8893):311–322.
15. Wienbergen H, Schiele R, Gitt AK et al. Incidence, risk factors, and clinical outcome of stroke after acute myocardial infarction in clinical practice. MIR and MITRA Study Groups. Myocardial Infarction Registry. Maximal Individual Therapy in Acute Myocardial Infarction. *Am J Cardiol*. 15 Mar 2001;87(6):782–785, A8.
16. Hellermann JP, Jacobsen SJ, Gersh BJ, Rodeheffer RJ, Reeder GS, Roger VL. Heart failure after myocardial infarction: A review. *Am J Med*. Sep 2002;113(4):324–330.

17. Spencer FA, Meyer TE, Gore JM, Goldberg RJ. Heterogeneity in the management and outcomes of patients with acute myocardial infarction complicated by heart failure. *Circulation*. 4 Jun 2002;105(22):2605–2610.

18. Shah RV, Holmes D, Anderson M et al. Risk of Heart Failure Complication During Hospitalization for Acute Myocardial Infarction in a Contemporary Population. *Circ Heart Fail*. 1 Nov 2012;5(6):693–702.

19. Stone SG, Serrao GW, Mehran R et al. Incidence, predictors, and implications of reinfarction after primary percutaneous coronary intervention in ST-Segment–Elevation myocardial infarction. *Circ Cardiovasc Interv*. 1 Aug 2014;7(4):543–551.

20. Kernis SJ, Harjai KJ, Stone GW et al. The incidence, predictors, and outcomes of early reinfarction after primary angioplasty for acute myocardial infarction. *J Am Coll Cardiol*. 1 Oct 2003;42(7):1173–1177.

21. Hudson MP, Granger CB, Topol EJ et al. Early reinfarction after fibrinolysis: Experience from the global utilization of streptokinase and tissue plasminogen activator (alteplase) for occluded coronary arteries (GUSTO I) and global use of strategies to open occluded coronary arteries (GUSTO III) trials. *Circulation*. 11 Sep 2001;104(11):1229–1235.

22. Gibson CM, Karha J, Murphy SA et al. Early and long-term clinical outcomes associated with reinfarction following fibrinolytic administration in the Thrombolysis in Myocardial Infarction trials. *J Am Coll Cardiol*. 2 Jul 2003;42(1):7–16.

23. Stone GW, Witzenbichler B, Guagliumi G et al. Bivalirudin during primary PCI in acute myocardial infarction. *N Engl J Med*. 22 May 2008;358(21):2218–2230.

24. Kwok CS, Rao SV, Myint PK et al. Major bleeding after percutaneous coronary intervention and risk of subsequent mortality: A systematic review and meta-analysis. *Open Heart*. 1 Feb 2014;1(1):e000021.

25. Giugliano RP, Giraldez RR, Morrow DA et al. Relations between bleeding and outcomes in patients with ST-elevation myocardial infarction in the ExTRACT-TIMI 25 trial. *Eur Heart J*. 1 Sep 2010;31(17):2103–2110.

26. Behar S, Haim M, Hod H et al. Long-term prognosis of patients after a Q wave compared with a non-Q wave first acute myocardial infarction. Data from the SPRINT Registry. *Eur Heart J*. Oct 1996;17(10):1532–1537.

27. Yan AT, Tan M, Fitchett D et al. One-year outcome of patients after acute coronary syndromes (from the Canadian Acute Coronary Syndromes Registry). *Am J Cardiol*. 1 Jul 2004;94(1):25–29.

28. Haim M, Behar S, Boyko V, Hod H, Gottlieb S. The prognosis of a first Q-wave versus non-Q-wave myocardial infarction in the reperfusion era. *Am J Med*. 1 Apr 2000;108(5):381–386.

29. Armstrong PW, Fu Y, Chang WC et al. Acute coronary syndromes in the GUSTO-IIb trial: Prognostic insights and impact of recurrent ischemia. The GUSTO-IIb Investigators. *Circulation*. 3 Nov 1998;98(18):1860–1868.

30. Marchioli R, Barzi F, Bomba E et al. Early protection against sudden death by n-3 polyunsaturated fatty acids after myocardial infarction: Time-course analysis of the results of the Gruppo Italiano per lo Studio della Sopravvivenza nell'Infarto Miocardico (GISSI)-Prevenzione. *Circulation*. 23 Apr 2002;105(16):1897–1903.

31. Kannel WB, Cupples LA, D'Agostino RB. Sudden death risk in overt coronary heart disease: The Framingham Study. *Am Heart J*. Mar 1987;113(3):799–804.

32. Mukharji J, Rude RE, Poole WK et al. Risk factors for sudden death after acute myocardial infarction: Two-year follow-up. *Am J Cardiol*. 1 Jul 1984;54(1):31–36.

33. Zaret BL, Wackers FJ, Terrin ML et al. Value of radionuclide rest and exercise left ventricular ejection fraction in assessing survival of patients after thrombolytic therapy for acute myocardial infarction: Results of Thrombolysis in Myocardial Infarction (TIMI) phase II study. The TIMI Study Group. *J Am Coll Cardiol*. Jul 1995;26(1):73–79.

34. Burns RJ, Gibbons RJ, Yi Q et al. The relationships of left ventricular ejection fraction, end-systolic volume index and infarct size to six-month mortality after hospital discharge following myocardial infarction treated by thrombolysis. *J Am Coll Cardiol*. 2 Jan 2002;39(1):30–36.

35. Buxton AE, Lee KL, DiCarlo L et al. Electrophysiologic testing to identify patients with coronary artery disease who are at risk for sudden death. Multicenter Unsustained Tachycardia Trial Investigators. *N Engl J Med*. 29 Jun 2000;342(26):1937–1945.

36. Schmitt H, Hurst T, Coch M, Killat H, Wunn B, Waldecker B. Nonsustained, asymptomatic ventricular tachycardia in patients with coronary artery disease: Prognosis and incidence of sudden death of patients who are noninducible by electrophysiological testing. *Pacing Clin Electrophysiol PACE*. Aug 2000;23(8):1220–1225.

37. Bigger JT, Fleiss JL, Rolnitzky LM. Prevalence, characteristics and significance of ventricular tachycardia detected by 24-hour continuous electrocardiographic recordings in the late hospital phase of acute myocardial infarction. *Am J Cardiol*. 1 Dec 1986;58(13):1151–1160.

38. Anderson KP, DeCamilla J, Moss AJ. Clinical significance of ventricular tachycardia (3 beats or longer) detected during ambulatory monitoring after myocardial infarction. *Circulation*. May 1978;57(5):890–897.

39. Gang ES, Lew AS, Hong M, Wang FZ, Siebert CA, Peter T. Decreased incidence of ventricular late potentials after successful thrombolytic therapy for acute myocardial infarction. *N Engl J Med*. 14 Sep 1989;321(11):712–716.

40. Pedretti R, Laporta A, Etro MD et al. Influence of thrombolysis on signal-averaged electrocardiogram and late arrhythmic events after acute myocardial infarction. *Am J Cardiol*. 1 Apr 1992;69(9):866–872.

41. Farrell TG, Bashir Y, Cripps T et al. Risk stratification for arrhythmic events in postinfarction patients based on heart rate variability, ambulatory electrocardiographic variables and the signal-averaged electrocardiogram. *J Am Coll Cardiol*. Sep 1991;18(3):687–697.

42. Kleiger RE, Miller JP, Bigger JT, Moss AJ. Decreased heart rate variability and its association with increased mortality after acute myocardial infarction. *Am J Cardiol*. 1 Feb 1987;59(4):256–262.

43. Armoundas AA, Tomaselli GF, Esperer HD. Pathophysiological basis and clinical application of T-wave alternans. *J Am Coll Cardiol*. 17 Jul 2002;40(2):207–217.

44. Maddox TM, Reid KJ, Spertus JA et al. Angina at 1 year after myocardial infarction: Prevalence and associated findings. *Arch Intern Med*. 23 Jun 2008;168(12):1310–1316.

45. McNamara RL, Kennedy KF, Cohen DJ et al. Predicting in-hospital mortality in patients with acute myocardial infarction. *J Am Coll Cardiol*. 09 2016;68(6):626–635.

46. Addala S, Grines CL, Dixon SR et al. Predicting mortality in patients with ST-elevation myocardial infarction treated with primary percutaneous coronary intervention (PAMI risk score). *Am J Cardiol*. 1 Mar 2004; 93(5):629–632.

47. Morrow DA, Antman EM, Charlesworth A et al. TIMI risk score for ST-elevation myocardial infarction: A convenient, bedside, clinical score for risk assessment at presentation: An intravenous nPA for treatment of infarcting myocardium early II trial substudy. *Circulation*. 24 Oct 2000;102(17):2031–2037.

48. Morrow DA, Antman EM, Giugliano RP et al. A simple risk index for rapid initial triage of patients with ST-elevation myocardial infarction: An InTIME II substudy. *Lancet Lond Engl*. 10 Nov 2001;358(9293):1571–1575.

49. Halkin A, Singh M, Nikolsky E et al. Prediction of mortality after primary percutaneous coronary intervention for acute myocardial infarction: The CADILLAC risk score. *J Am Coll Cardiol*. 3 May 2005;45(9):1397–1405.

50. De Luca G, Suryapranata H, van 't Hof AWJ et al. Prognostic assessment of patients with acute myocardial infarction treated with primary angioplasty: Implications for early discharge. *Circulation*. 8 Jun 2004;109(22):2737–2743.

51. Lev EI, Kornowski R, Vaknin-Assa H et al. Comparison of the predictive value of four different risk scores for outcomes of patients with ST-elevation acute myocardial infarction undergoing primary percutaneous coronary intervention. *Am J Cardiol*. 1 Jul 2008;102(1):6–11.

52. Antman EM, Cohen M, Bernink PJ et al. The TIMI risk score for unstable angina/non-ST elevation MI: A method for prognostication and therapeutic decision making. *JAMA*. 16 Aug 2000;284(7):835–842.

53. Fox KAA, Dabbous OH, Goldberg RJ et al. Prediction of risk of death and myocardial infarction in the six months after presentation with acute coronary syndrome: Prospective multinational observational study (GRACE). *BMJ*. 25 Nov 2006;333(7578):1091.

54. Bohula EA, Bonaca MP, Braunwald E et al. Atherothrombotic risk stratification and the efficacy and safety of Vorapaxar in patients with stable Ischemic heart disease and previous myocardial infarction. *Circulation*. 26 Jul 2016;134(4): 304–313.

55. Yusuf S, Zhao F, Mehta SR et al. Effects of clopidogrel in addition to aspirin in patients with acute coronary syndromes without ST-segment elevation. *N Engl J Med*. 16 Aug 2001;345(7):494–502.

56. Mehta SR, Tanguay J-F, Eikelboom JW et al. Double-dose versus standard-dose clopidogrel and high-dose versus low-dose aspirin in individuals undergoing percutaneous coronary intervention for acute coronary syndromes (CURRENT-OASIS 7): A randomised factorial trial. *Lancet Lond Engl*. 9 Oct 2010;376(9748):1233–1243.

57. Wiviott SD, Braunwald E, McCabe CH et al. Prasugrel versus clopidogrel in patients with acute coronary syndromes. *N Engl J Med*. 15 Nov 2007;357(20):2001–2015.

58. Roe MT, Armstrong PW, Fox KAA et al. Prasugrel versus clopidogrel for acute coronary syndromes without revascularization. *N Engl J Med*. 4 Oct 2012;367(14):1297–1309.

59. Wallentin L, Becker RC, Budaj A et al. Ticagrelor versus clopidogrel in patients with acute coronary syndromes. *N Engl J Med*. 10 Sep 2009;361(11):1045–1057.

60. Bonaca MP, Bhatt DL, Cohen M et al. Long-term use of ticagrelor in patients with prior myocardial infarction. *N Engl J Med*. 7 May 2015;372(19):1791–1800.

61. Eikelboom JW, Anand SS, Malmberg K, Weitz JI, Ginsberg JS, Yusuf S. Unfractionated heparin and low-molecular-weight heparin in acute coronary syndrome without ST elevation: A meta-analysis. *Lancet Lond Engl*. 3 Jun 2000;355(9219):1936–1942.

62. Antman EM, McCabe CH, Gurfinkel EP et al. Enoxaparin prevents death and cardiac ischemic events in unstable angina/non-Q-wave myocardial infarction. Results of the Thrombolysis In Myocardial Infarction (TIMI) 11B trial. *Circulation*. 12 Oct 1999;100(15):1593–1601.

63. Bavry AA, Kumbhani DJ, Rassi AN, Bhatt DL, Askari AT. Benefit of early invasive therapy in acute coronary syndromes: A meta-analysis of contemporary randomized clinical trials. *J Am Coll Cardiol*. 3 Oct 2006;48(7):1319–1325.

64. Mehta SR, Granger CB, Boden WE et al. Early versus delayed invasive intervention in acute coronary syndromes. *N Engl J Med*. 21 May 2009;360(21):2165–2175.

65. Jobs A, Mehta SR, Montalescot G et al. Optimal timing of an invasive strategy in patients with non-ST-elevation acute coronary syndrome: A meta-analysis of randomised trials. *Lancet*. 19 Aug 2017;390(10096):737–746.

66. Kofoed KF, Kelbæk H, Hansen PR et al. Early versus standard care invasive examination and treatment of patients with Non-ST-Segment elevation acute coronary syndrome. *Circulation*. 11 Dec 2018;138(24):2741–2750.

67. Rathod KS, Koganti S, Jain AK et al. Complete versus culprit-only lesion intervention in patients with acute coronary syndromes. *J Am Coll Cardiol*. 15 Oct 2018;72(17):1989–1999.

68. Shishehbor MH, Lauer MS, Singh IM et al. In unstable angina or non-ST-segment acute coronary syndrome, should patients with multivessel coronary artery disease undergo multivessel or culprit-only stenting? *J Am Coll Cardiol*. 27 Feb 2007;49(8):849–854.

69. Gaffar R, Habib B, Filion KB, Reynier P, Eisenberg MJ. Optimal timing of complete revascularization in acute coronary syndrome: A systematic review and meta-analysis. *J Am Heart Assoc*. 10 Apr 2017;6(4).

4

Clinical syndromes in acute coronary syndrome
Angina and its equivalents

LEELA KRISHNA AND DAYASAGAR RAO

INTRODUCTION

Acute coronary syndromes (ACS) refer to a spectrum of clinical presentations compatible with myocardial ischaemia and are usually due to an abrupt decrease in coronary blood flow. Acute ischaemic manifestations include unstable angina and myocardial infarction (NSTEMI and STEMI) and sudden cardiac death (SCD). The variable clinical presentations represent the range of myocardial ischaemia from transient, reversible to complete cessation of coronary blood flow.

A historical perspective of coronary artery disease (CAD) reveals the prevailing concept of those times. James Herrick recognised angina on effort and MI as manifestation of the same underlying disease process. The clinical differentiation of angina from MI was done by the Russian physicians Obrastzov and Straschesko who stated that 'differential diagnosis of coronary thrombosis and angina is made by presence of status angiosus in coronary thrombosis and its absence with isolated attacks of angina indicating distinct etiopathological entities' [1]. This distinction between angina and MI began to blur as several clinical observers noted the presence of prolonged angina that often preceded the development of MI in some patients. This pattern of symptoms was variably referred to as pre-infarction angina or crescendo angina, which has led to the concept that coronary circulation is insufficient to meet all demands at rest and this pre-infarct angina is sufficient to prevent MI [2].

William Heberden first described angina pectoris in 1768 and suggested this could be the origin of coronary artery disease [3]. In 1858, Rudolph Virchow proposed that injury to the inner wall of a blood vessel and inflammation can lead to plaque formation [4]. Smapson, Eliason and Feil, in 1937, hypothesised that a gradually

forming thrombus was the reason for pre-infarction angina [5,6]. They advised, 'effort should be made to improve coronary blood flow'. In 1966, Constantinides [7] described plaque fissuring in total coronary obstruction and hypothesized that breaks in the plaque were a precipitating cause of acute coronary thrombosis. In 1985, Davies and Thomas initiated the concept of vulnerable plaques [8]. These plaques had thin fibrous caps over a lipid pool containing inflammatory cells. When these plaques rupture, acute myocardial infarction, sudden cardiac death and crescendo angina can ensue.

The term *intermediate coronary syndrome* was suggested in 1951 by Vakil [9] in India and Graybiel [10] in the United States. Vakil [9,11] observed that patients with prolonged chest pain and recognisable clinical and electrocardiographic characteristics were strongly predisposed to development of MI in three months. Because of this high predisposition to MI, the term *pre-infarction syndrome* was considered a more appropriate subtitle to intermediate coronary syndrome. Vakil went further by investigating the role of anticoagulant therapy as a prophylaxis against onset of MI. The term unstable angina was coined by Fowler in 1971, and first guidelines on its diagnosis and management were published in 1994 [12].

The knowledge regarding CAD, and in particular ACS, continues to grow. The advent of new technology led to intravascular imaging to evaluate the proximate cause of ACS (it found luminal thrombus over atheroma plaque in the majority of ACS). The advent of sensitive and specific markers of myocardial cell injury – troponins – has redefined the criterion of myocardial infarction and introduced the term myocardial injury elevated biomarkers without evidence of ischaemia. Thus, for diagnosis of ACS there must be objective evidence of ischaemia with compatible symptoms.

PATHOPHYSIOLOGY

Virtually all acute coronary syndromes are caused by thrombosis developing on a culprit coronary atherosclerotic plaque, resulting in acute reduction of coronary blood flow. If it results in total obstruction it may cause infarction with corresponding regional myocardial necrosis. The occurrence of infarct with subtotal obstruction as in NSTEMI, is due to distal embolisation of thrombi (usually platelet thrombi). Rarely, total obstruction may not result in infarct, because of the presence of rich collaterals. The vast majority of myocardial infarctions occurs in patients with coronary atherosclerosis with more than 90% associated with superimposed luminal thrombi. Arbustini et al. [13] found coronary thrombi in 298 of patients dying with clinically documented acute myocardial infarction. Of these thrombi, 74 were caused by plaque erosion. The proximate cause of this luminal thrombus – ruptured plaque or plaque erosion – is variable and is influenced by age and gender.

Acute coronary syndrome (ACS) includes the clinical manifestations of the whole range of myocardial ischaemia from the transient imbalance of supply versus demand of oxygen to the myocardium to the prolonged duration of ischaemia resulting from combination of vascular spasm and fixed obstruction. Understanding determinants of coronary blood flow and factors that influence oxygen demands of the myocardium helps to appreciate the pathophysiology of angina.

The heart of normal adults weighs approximately 250–300 grams and receives approximately 5% cardiac output (expressed as 0.96–1.2 mL/gm/mt). The myocardium extracts most of the oxygen in the arterial blood, leaving no oxygen useful in the venous system. Increase in oxygen demand has to be met by increased coronary blood flow.

The heart is an obligatory aerobic organ, and an estimation of myocardial oxygen consumption serves as a measure of total energy utilisation. Myocardial oxygen consumption determinants will help to understand the physiologic basis of ischaemia and the therapeutic potential by modulating these parameters (in the relief of ischaemic manifestation).

The major determinants of myocardial oxygen needs are as follows:

- Heart rate
- Aortic pressure
- Inotropy
- Wall stress
- Cavity and wall thickness

The basal oxygen consumption is approximately 20% of the contracting heart, and the cost of depolarisation is approximately 0.5% of total oxygen consumed by the working heart. The oxygen cost of pressure work is much higher than flow work (volume movement) and there is a close relationship between tension – time index – and myocardial oxygen consumption.

Buckberg et al. [14] in 1972 showed that the index based on LV and aortic pressure could predict subendocardial ischaemia. The area between the diastolic aortic and LV pressure (DPTI) represented diastolic coronary flow (oxygen supply) and the systolic LV pressure curve (SPTI) represented oxygen demand by the myocardium. When the ratio DPTI/SPTI was <0.45, evidence of ischemia was present (Figure 4.1).

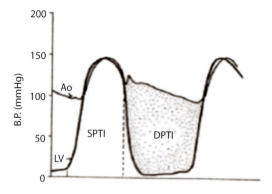

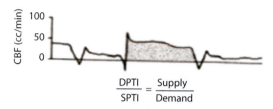

$$\frac{DPTI}{SPTI} = \frac{Supply}{Demand}$$

Figure 4.1 Myocardial oxygen supply: Demand index. (Reproduced from Buckberg GD et al. *Circ Res.* 1972;30:67–81 [14].)

ISCHAEMIC CASCADE

The impact of ischaemia on the myocardium is gradual and progressive if unrelieved. The earliest change is biochemical and histological, followed by mechanical dysfunction (initially diastolic followed by systolic) and preceded by electrical changes – ST/T deviations and finally to symptoms. All these changes regress, including rapid reversal of mechanical dysfunction once coronary blood flow is restored and ischaemia is relieved. Not infrequently, the recovery of cardiac muscle function may be delayed despite immediate restoration of blood flow. This delayed recovery of function is called myocardial stunning. The recovery of a dysfunctional myocardium may take a few hours to days. Rarely, episodes of ischaemia may result in metabolic changes in myocardial cells which result in resistance to ischaemic insult, which is labelled as ischaemic pre-conditioning. In patients with persistent and severe decrease in CBF, myocardial cells might adapt in a way that results in decreased function without necrosis called hibernation. The recovery in function follows improvement of CBF. Thus, ischaemic LV dysfunction may have reversible (stunning and hibernation) and irreversible (necrosis and MI) components. The proportion of each component defines the extent of recovery of function following the improvement of CBF.

The relationship between ischaemia and anginal pain may be seen as a bell shaped distribution, in which totally painless ischaemia is at one end and microvascular angina is at the other end.

Thus, myocardial ischaemia can manifest as:

1. *Angina:* Painful precordial distress with one of many variations of distribution of anginal discomfort.
2. *Anginal equivalents:* Painless but symptomatic – either due to ischaemic LV dysfunction, or due to dysrhythmias manifesting as dyspnea/palpitation/fatigue or syncope.

3. *Silent:* Totally silent, with no clinical manifestation, usually identified by either ECG or cardiac imaging.
4. From the pathophysiology point of view, it is important to know the pattern of recurrence of angina and the circumstances under which it occurs.

FIXED THRESHOLD ANGINA

Exertional angina develops whenever a given level of effort is exceeded and relieved promptly by rest. This usually is due to fixed flow limiting coronary artery stenosis.

VARIABLE THRESHOLD ANGINA

Variable thresholds are those with predictable angina at a given level of effort and also for efforts that are usually well tolerated and occasionally at rest. This variability in anginal threshold usually indicates a combination of fixed flow limiting coronary obstruction over which dynamic vasoconstriction occurs, resulting in marked decrease in coronary flow and thus worsening of angina.

UNSTABLE ANGINA

Acute worsening of ischaemic symptoms is usually consequent to complications of atheroma plaque rupture/erosion with superadded thrombosis and portends to be the onset of myocardial infarction. It often indicates critical reduction of coronary blood flow consequent to thrombus.

PRINZMETAL (VARIANT) ANGINA

Rest angina usually in early mornings and of short duration, occurring in clusters of two to three episodes within hours, associated with ST elevation on ECG. It is usually due to segmental coronary spasm and is often associated with dysrhythmias and conduction disturbances.

POST-PRANDIAL ANGINA

Angina is precipitated by ingestion of a meal and is thought to be due to diversion of blood from the coronaries to the gut. Alternative explanations included inappropriate rise in heart rate and systolic blood pressure in post-prandial state, at rest and on effort at reduced anginal threshold. Studies using radiolabelled water (H2o15) revealed an appropriate increase in CBF (for greater cardiac work) but with abnormal regional blood flow to the myocardium – more blood to normal coronary segments, with less blood to diseased segment resulting in angina. Thus it is due to maldistribution of CBF (steal phenomenon) rather than decrease in flow.

WALK-THROUGH ANGINA: SECOND WIND PHENOMENON

Walk-through angina is usually defined as occurrence of angina during initial stages of effort with disappearance of discomfort with continued effort. This is found in two subsets of patients: those with variant angina where the initial coronary spasm causing angina is relieved on continued exercise, and patients with severe CAD where the relief of angina is due to delayed vasodilatation of collaterals.

NOCTURNAL ANGINA

Nocturnal angina is caused by increased demands during the night. It can be a subtle manifestation of LV dysfunction with worsening of increased LV EDV in a recumbent posture consequent to increased venous return. Changes in heart rate during REM sleep and dreams causing adrenergic surges are implicated. Rarely, coronary spasms at night are implicated as a cause of nocturnal angina.

MICROVASCULAR ANGINA

Microvascular angina is a clinical syndrome of angina but with normal epicardial coronary arteries. It is due to dysfunctional microcirculation – decreased microvascular dilation (abnormal vasodilator reserve) which results in decreased oxygen supply to the myocardium. The diagnosis is confirmed by reversible myocardial ischaemic segments on MPI (myocardial perfusion imaging), with normal epicardial coronary vessels on angiogram. This syndrome is more frequent in women.

POST-INFARCT ANGINA

Early post-infarct angina (2–15 days) occurs in 10%–15% of patients following MI and more frequently in patients with NSTEMI and who usually have more extensive CAD. Angina occurs at rest or on minimal activity, after an asymptomatic period following the index event. These patients generally have unstable angina, preceding AMI. Post-infarct angina identifies patients at high risk of mortality, especially in patients with remote ischaemia (non-infarct area). These patients need more aggressive investigation and management.

SECONDARY ANGINA

In patients with secondary angina there is no significant obstructive CAD, but they still develop angina, because of increased demands – aortic valve disease, especially aortic stenosis and conditions characterised by severe LVH (like HCM). Rarely, angina can occur in patients with severe anaemia because of decreased oxygen carrying capacity. A description of angina is based on clinical variables like severity, clinical circumstances and intensity of treatment. Integrating these three variables, Braunwald has designed a classification to facilitate communication and aid in diagnostic and therapeutic decision, much like onco-classification of tumours (TNM) [15].

GRADING SEVERITY OF ANGINA (BY THE CANADIAN CARDIOVASCULAR SOCIETY)

Grading severity of angina (by the Canadian Cardiovascular Society) is a functional classification of angina and is a clinical tool to assess the severity of angina. This classification is useful in determining the urgency and impact of treatment (by change in functional class).

Class I: Ordinary physical activity doesn't cause angina (e.g., activities such as walking and climbing stairs). Angina occurs at strenuous or rapid or prolonged exertion at work or recreation.

Class II: Slight limitation of ordinary physical activity. Walking or climbing stairs rapidly, walking uphill, walking or stair climbing after meals or in cold or in wind or under emotional stress or only during the few hours after awakening. Walking more than two blocks on the level and climbing more than one flight of ordinary stairs at a normal pace and in normal conditions.

Class III: Marked limitation of ordinary physical activity. Walking one or two blocks on the level and climbing one flight of stairs in normal conditions and at normal pace.

Class IV: Inability to carry on any physical activity without discomfort; anginal symptom may be present at rest.

The history must be concise, yet expeditious so as not to delay implementation of therapy.

CHEST DISCOMFORT/PAIN

Of all the symptoms for which patients seek emergency medical care, chest pain or discomfort is one of the most common and complex, accounting for about 5.6 million emergency department visits annually [16]. Many people will not admit having chest pain but will acknowledge the presence of chest discomfort, because of their definition of pain. Published reports suggest that up to 5% of visits to the emergency department involve complaints relating to chest discomfort [17]. The complaint of chest discomfort encompasses many varying conditions, ranging from insignificant to high-risk in terms of threat to the patient's life, including but not limited to acute coronary syndromes, thrombotic disease, aortic dissection and pneumothorax. Chest discomfort/pain may be perceived as with descriptions such as crushing, vice-like constriction, a feeling equivalent to an elephant sitting on the chest, tightness, pressure, heart burn or indigestion or as discomfort most noticeable for its radiation to an adjacent area of the body, such as neck, jaw, intrascapular area, upper extremities or epigastrium. Elderly patients or those patients who have diabetes may have altered ability to specifically localise the discomfort [19]. Individuals of each gender and different cultural groups vary in their expression of pain and ability to communicate with health professionals, so that presentation may range from mainly bothersome to cataclysmic for conditions that seem nearly equivalent when objective criteria are matched. The level of discomfort does not necessarily correlate with the severity of illness, making identification of potentially life-threatening conditions difficult in certain patients.

It is sometimes difficult to distinguish cardiac from non-cardiac chest discomfort, even though chest pain is the hallmark of acute coronary syndrome. Taking time to elicit the character of the sensation (without prompting the patient, if possible) and any pattern of radiation (if present) is most helpful. Typically, the chest discomfort of acute ischaemia has a deep visceral character, preventing the patient from localising the discomfort to a specific region of the chest.

It is often described as a pressure or heavy weight on the chest, a tightness, a constriction about the throat or an aching sensation that comes on gradually, reaches its maximum intensity over a period of 2–3 minutes, does not last longer than 15 minutes, rather than seconds. It may wax and wane and may be remitting but generally not worsen by trunk movement or deep inspiration. The discomfort might worsen on lying flat and might be relieved by sitting with legs hanging at the edge of the bed.

Sometimes it may be described as indigestion and occasionally may be relieved by belching. Pope and colleagues found that 76% of patients who presented with the complaint of chest pain or chest discomfort (including arm, jaw or equivalent discomfort) had a 29% incidence of acute coronary syndrome at final diagnosis (10% AMI,19% UAP). In 69% of patients, chest pain or discomfort was the chief complaint, and this group had a 31% incidence of ACS (10% AMI, 21% UAP). In 21% of patients, it was the only complaint, and this group had a 32% incidence of ACS (9% AMI, 23% UAP). Sharp, stabbing or positional pain is less likely to represent ischaemia, but does not exclude it [24].

Lee and colleagues [20] found that among patients in the ED who had sharp or stabbing pain, 13% had acute ischaemia (6% AMI, 7% UAP) and among those who had pleuritic pain none was shown to have acute ischaemia. Of the patients whose pain was fully reproduced by palpation, 7% had ischaemia (5% AMI, 2% UAP). 24% of patients who had pain partially reproduced with palpation had ischaemia (6% AMI, 18% UAP). Patients who described their discomfort as similar to previous episodes of cardiac ischaemia were more likely to have ACS. Combinations of variables improved discrimination in these patients.

Exact location of chest pain is not significantly different in patients who have or do not have AMI [23], but pain radiating to arms and neck does increase the likelihood. In a study done by Sawe that looked at admitted patients who had AMI, 71% had pain radiation to arms and neck [22], where 39% of admitted patients, who expressed pain radiation, did not have AMI. Consistent with classical description, 33% of patients who proved to have infarction had radiation to both arms, 29% had pain radiating to the left arm only, 2% to the right arm only.

Some investigators believe that a significant number of patients who have cardiac ischaemia can present with abdominal pain as their chief complaint [21,24]. Pope and colleagues [24] have found that 14% of study patients had this complaint. This group had a 15% incidence of acute coronary syndrome at final diagnosis (6% AMI, 9% UAP). Abdominal pain as a chief complaint or presenting symptom was associated with higher incidence of a non-ACS final diagnosis.

Thus, location and duration of chest discomfort might lead one to coronary artery disease but none of the characteristics (duration and radiation) are diagnostic of ACS. The reproducibility of discomfort by palpation does not rule out ACS, just as the probability of CAD cannot be predicted by the response to sublingual NTG (Nitroglycerin). Perhaps the location, progression (gradual worsening in <5 minutes) and worsening by physical effort and relieved by rest are more reliable predictors of CAD.

Aesophageal reflux and motility disorders are common masqueraders of acute coronary syndrome. In a study done by Aneskog et al. [25] of all patients discharged from CCU with undetermined causes of chest pain, over half had esophageal dysfunction.

ANGINAL PAIN EQUIVALENTS

Angina equivalents are symptoms other than chest discomfort and are consequences of acute ischaemic ventricular dysfunction, such as shortness of breath (dyspnaea), diaphoresis (sweating), extreme fatigue, or pain at a site other than the chest, occurring in a patient at high cardiac risk. Angina equivalents are considered to have the same importance as angina pectoris in patients presenting with elevation of cardiac biomarkers or certain ECG changes.

Dyspnaea presents in about 1/3rd of patients who have infarction [21] and is the most important angina equivalent. In a study done by Pope and colleagues, 16% of patients who had suspected ACS [24] presented with the chief complaint of shortness of breath (SOB) and had an 11% incidence of ACS at a final diagnosis (6% AMI, 5% UAP); in 8% this was the only complaint. ACS should be considered as a cause of unexplained SOB. Diaphoresis and vomiting when associated with chest pain increase the likelihood of infarction [26,27].

Diaphoresis occurs in 20%–50% of patients who have AMI. Pope and colleagues [24] found nausea in 28% of patients who had suspected ACS. Patients who had nausea as presenting symptoms had a 26% incidence of ACS as the final diagnosis (10% AMI, 16% UAP). So-called soft clinical features, such as fatigue, weakness, malaise, dizziness and clouding of mind are surprisingly frequent, occurring in 11% to 40% of patients who have AMI [27,28]. Prodromal symptoms occurring in preceding days or weeks are also frequent. 40% report unusual fatigue or weakness, 20%–39% dyspnaea, 14% to 20% emotional changes, 20% a change in appearance (looked pale) and 8–10% dizziness [21]. Pope and colleagues [24] found that 28% of patients who had suspected ACS presented to the emergency department with dizziness and had a 16% incidence of ACS (5% AMI, 11% UAP). Dizziness or fainting as a chief complaint were more commonly associated with the final diagnosis of non-ACS. ECG evaluation is helpful in low prevalence patients who have these vague complaints.

ATYPICAL PRESENTATIONS

These are fatigue, dyspnaea, abdominal discomfort, nausea, syncope. Among hospitalised patients who have AMI, 13%–26% have no chest pain or have chief complaints other than chest pain. A study done by Coronade and colleagues [18] found pain to be absent in 6.2% of patients who had acute ischaemia and 9.8% of patients who had AMI. Independent predictors of atypical presentation for patients who had UAP were older age, had a history of dementia and absence of prior myocardial infarction, hypercholesterolaemia or family history of heart disease. Patients who had atypical presentation received aspirin, heparin and beta-blocker therapy less aggressively, but there was no difference in mortality.

In women with MI, the typical presentation differs from that of men in many ways. Women are less likely to present with chest pain and may instead show atypical symptoms. Women also receive different final diagnoses. Female study subjects were less likely than men to have received a diagnosis of NSTEMI or unstable angina. We need to fully understand these gender-based differences in presentation to ensure that they do not worsen women's outcomes.

Diagnosis of angina, clinically at bedside, should take into consideration the following variables:

1. *Pre-test probability of disease (CAD)*: Based on prevalence of disease and presence of risk factors.
2. *Characteristics of ischaemic manifestations*: Angina and its equivalent location, duration, intensity, precipitating factors, relieving factors and associated features. These ischaemic manifestations generally do not last for 10–15 minutes in stable coronary artery disease, but may last longer (greater than 20 minutes), are more frequent at lower threshold (of angina) in acute coronary syndromes.

New onset of these ischaemic symptoms and change in character of manifestations are the hallmarks of ACS. These changes in clinical manifestations are due to sudden and severe decreases in coronary blood flow due to a decrease in coronary artery lumen, consequent to thrombus over underlying atherosclerotic plaque, with or without superadded spasms.

The three principal presentations of ACS are:

1. *Rest angina*: Angina at rest lasting more than 20 minutes
2. *New onset angina*: New onset angina at least Canadian Cardiovascular Society (CCS) class III severity
3. *Crescendo angina*: Worsening of pre-existing angina frequency, duration and lower threshold (1 or more CCS class to at least class III)

In the diagnosis of ACS, not only should one evaluate symptom characteristics but also search/investigate for objective evidence of ischaemia.

The most commonly used investigation for ischaemia is ECG (electrocardiogram), especially for ST segments and T wave abnormalities. Dynamic ECG changes are more reliable than pre-existing changes, and ST segment deviations are better predictors than changes in T waves. The magnitude of ST changes and number of leads showing similar changes are more reliable. Recent occurrence of deep T wave inversions and new onset LBBB are equally important and indicate ischaemic origin (a detailed description of ECG in ACS is described in a subsequent chapter).

The gold standard for diagnosis of coronary ischaemia is increasing levels of metabolic products of ischaemia, importantly lactic acid in the coronary sinus. Equally diagnostic are the perfusion defects on MPI, with corresponding regional wall motion abnormalities, during ischaemia (spontaneous or induced).

CONCLUSION

ACS represents a spectrum of clinical manifestations, due to acute decreased coronary blood flow. This acute decrease is secondary to luminal thrombus occurring over a ruptured/eroded atherosclerotic plaque, with a variable component of coronary spasm.

Diagnostic confirmation of ACS includes symptoms of myocardial ischaemia coupled with objective evidence of ischaemia. These investigations for ischaemia include non-invasive (ECG, 2D echocardiography, MPI) and invasive catheter-based coronary angiography showing significant coronary obstruction, generally coupled with super-added overlying thrombus. The evaluation of the severity of angina by CCS is useful in decision-making, for urgency of therapy and impact of intervention.

REFERENCES

1. Obrastzow WP, Straschesko ND. Zur Kenntnis der Thrombose der Koronararterien des Herzens. *Z Klin Med.* 1910;71:116–132.
2. Wood P. Therapeutic applications of anticoagulants. *Trans Med Soc London.* 1948;13:80–85.
3. Heberden W. Some account of disorder of the breast. *Med Trans Coll Physcian Lond.* 1772;2:59.
4. Simmons J. *Rudolph Virchow and the Cell Doctrine. The Scientific 100—A Ranking of the Most Influential Scientists, Past and Present.* Secaucus, NJ: Carol Publishing Group. 1996; 88–92.
5. Sampson JJ, Eliaser M Jr. The diagnosis of impending acute coronary artery occlusion. *Am Heart J.* 1937;13:675–686.
6. Feil H. Preliminary pain in coronary thrombosis. *Am J Med Sci.* 1937;193:42–48.
7. Constantinides P. Plaque fissuring in human coronary thrombosis. *J Atheroscler Res.* 1966;6:1.
8. Davies MJ, Thomas AEC. Plaque fissuring: The cause of acute myocardial infarction, sudden ischemic death, and crescendo angina. *Br Heart J.* 1985;53:363.
9. Vakil RJ. Intermediate coronary syndrome. *Circulation.* 1961;24:557–571.
10. Graybiel A. *United States Armed Forces Medical Journal,* 1955;6:1.
11. Vakil RJ. Preinfarction syndrome: Management and followup. *Am J Cardiol.* 1964;14:55–63.
12. Fowler NO. 'Preinfarctional' angina: A need for an objective definition and for a controlled clinical trial of its management. *Circulation.* 1971;44:755–758.
13. Arbustini E, Dal Bello B, Morbini P et al. Plaque erosion is a major substrate for coronary thrombosis in acute myocardial infarction. *Heart.* 1999;82(3):269–272.
14. Buckberg GD, Fixler DE, Archie JP, Hoffman JI. Experimental subendocardial ischemia in dogs with normal coronary arteries. *Circ Res.* 1972;30:67–81.
15. Braunwald E. Unstable angina A classification: *Circulation.* 1989;80:410–414.
16. American Heart Association. *Heart Disease and Stroke Statistics–2005 Update.* Dallas, TX: American Heart Association. 2004.
17. McCaig L, Burt C. National hospital ambulatory medical care survey: 2002 emergency department summary. *Adv Data.* 2004;340:1–34.
18. Coronado BE, Pope JH, Griffith JL et al. Clinical features, triage, and outcome of patients presenting to the ED with suspected acute coronary syndrome but without pain: A multicenter study. *Am J Emerg Med.* 2004;22:568–574.
19. Short D. Diagnosis of slight and subacute coronary attacks in the community. *Br Heart J.* 1981;45:299–310.
20. Lee T, Cook E, Weisberg M et al. Acute chest pain in the emergency room: Identification and examination of low-risk patients. *Arch Intern Med.* 1985;145:65–69.
21. Kinlen L. Incidence and presentation of myocardial infarction in an English community. *Br Heart J.* 1973;35:616–622.
22. Sawe U. Pain in acute myocardial infarction. A study of 137 patients in a coronary care unit. *Acta Med Scand.* 1971;190:79–81.
23. Uretsky B, Farquhar D, Berezin A et al. Symptomatic myocardial infarction without chest pain: Prevalence and clinical course. *Am J Cardiol.* 1977;40:498–503.
24. Pope J, Ruthazer R, Beshansky J et al. Clinical features of emergency department patients presenting with symptoms of acute cardiac ischemia: A multicenter study. *J Thromb Thrombolysis.* 1998;6:63–74.
25. . Areskog M, Tibbling L, Wranne B. Oesophageal dysfunction in non-infarction coronary care unit patients. *Acta Med Scand.* 1979;205:279–282.
26. Tierney W, Roth B, Psaty B et al. Predictors of myocardial infarction in emergency room patients. *Crit Care Med.* 1985;13:526–531.
27. Wasson J, Sox H, Neff R et al. Clinical prediction rules: Applications and methodological standards. *N Engl J Med.* 1985;313:793–799.
28. Alonzo A, Simon A, Feilieb M. Prodromata of myocardial infarction and sudden death. *Circulation.* 1975;52:1056–1062.

5

ECG spectrum in acute coronary syndrome

ANKIT BANSAL AND VIVEK CHATURVEDI

ECG SPECTRUM IN ACUTE CORONARY SYNDROMES

The spectrum of ACS includes ST-segment elevation myocardial infarction (STEMI), and the non-ST-elevation acute coronary syndromes (NSTE-ACS). The latter consists of non-ST- elevation myocardial infarction (NSTEMI) and unstable angina (UA), a distinction based on cardiac biomarkers. ECG is integral to the diagnostic work-up of patients with suspected ACS and subsequent management. An ECG should be obtained within 10 minutes after arrival for individuals with suspected ACS. Acute myocardial ischaemia is often associated with dynamic changes in ECG waveform and serial ECG acquisition can provide critical information, particularly if the ECG at initial presentation is non-diagnostic (Figure 5.1a and b).

ECG CHANGES IN ST-ELEVATION MYOCARDIAL INFARCTION (STEMI)

Prolonged new convex ST-segment elevation, particularly when associated with reciprocal ST-segment depression, usually reflects acute coronary occlusion and ensuing myocardial injury with necrosis (Figure 5.2). Reciprocal changes in opposite facing leads can help to differentiate STEMI from pericarditis or early repolarisation changes.

Box 5.1 lists ST-segment–T wave (ST-T) criteria suggestive of acute myocardial ischaemia [1]. The J-point (junction of QRS termination and ST-segment onset) is used to determine the magnitude of the ST-segment shift with the onset of the QRS serving as the reference point. In patients with a stable baseline, the TP segment (isoelectric interval) is a more accurate method to assess the magnitude of ST-segment shift and in distinguishing pericarditis from acute myocardial ischaemia. Tachycardia and baseline shift are common in the acute setting and can make this determination difficult. Therefore, QRS onset is recommended as the reference point for J-point determination.

Importantly, lesser degrees of ST displacement or T wave inversion than those described can also represent an acute myocardial ischaemic response. In patients with known or a high likelihood of coronary artery disease (CAD), the clinical presentation is critical to enhance the specificity of these findings.

An ECG not only helps in establishing the diagnosis of STEMI but also provides valuable information on infarct location, success or failure of reperfusion, as well as prognosis. Arterial occlusion at particular anatomical sites is associated with specific ECG patterns as shown in Table 5.1. It is important to remember that in extensive multi-vessel disease and with previous infarctions, the ECG criteria described lose accuracy and discriminating ability.

ECG changes in the distribution of the left circumflex (LCx) artery are very subtle and often overlooked. ST-segment depression in leads V1–V3 may be suggestive of inferobasal myocardial ischaemia (previously termed posterior infarction), especially when the terminal T wave is positive (ST-elevation equivalent). These ECG changes may indicate left circumflex occlusion and can be best demonstrated by using posterior leads at the fifth intercostal space (V7 at the left posterior axillary line, V8 at the left mid-scapular line, and V9 at the left paraspinal border). A cut-off point of 0.5 mm ST-elevation is recommended in leads V7–V9; specificity is increased at a cut-off point $\geq$ 1 mm ST-elevation.

In patients with inferior and suspected right ventricular myocardial infarction (RVMI), leads aVR or V1 may exhibit ST-segment elevation $\geq$ 1 mm. The early recording of right precordial leads V3R and V4R should be performed, as ST-elevation $\geq$ 0.5 mm

(a)　　　　　　　　　　　　　　　　　　　　　　　　(b)

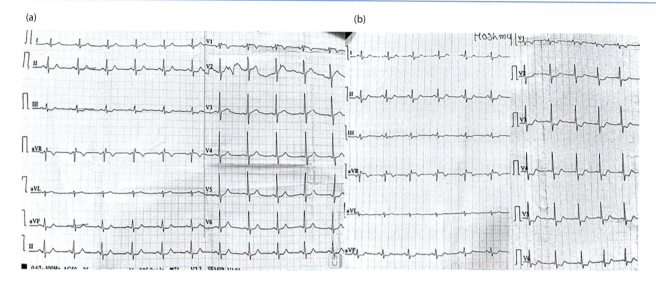

Figure 5.1 (a) Patient with suspected ACS, first ECG has no alarming changes. (b) ECG repeated after 30 minutes, ST depression in multiple leads along with ST elevation in aVR. Patient had ostial LAD critical stenosis on angiogram.

(≥1 mm in men <30 years old) provides supportive criteria for the diagnosis.

The ECG also can suggest specific information about the location of an acute occlusion within the coronary system (the *culprit lesion*). Each artery contributes its blood supply to specific regional areas in the heart.

The left anterior descending (LAD) artery supplies the anterior, anteroseptal or anterolateral wall of the LV (leads V1-V6, I, and aVL).

The right coronary artery (RCA) supplies the inferior wall (leads II, III and aVF) and often the posterolateral wall of the LV (special leads V7-V9). The right coronary artery is the only artery that supplies the right ventricular free wall (special leads V3R to V6R).

The left circumflex (LCx) artery supplies the anterolateral (leads I, aVL, V5 and V6) and the posterolateral (leads V7-V9) walls of the LV. In 10%–15% of patients, it supplies the inferior wall of the LV also.

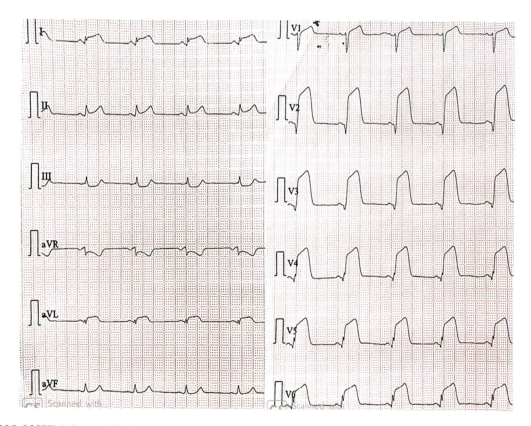

Figure 5.2 ECG Of STEMI showing ST elevation in precordial and lateral leads with reciprocal depression in leads III and aVF.

BOX 5.1: Electrocardiographic manifestations suggestive of acute myocardial ischaemia (in the absence of left ventricular hypertrophy and bundle branch block)

ST-ELEVATION

New ST-elevation at the J-point in two contiguous leads with the cut-point

$\geq$1 mm in all leads other than leads V2–V3 where the following cut-points apply

$\geq$2 mm in men $\geq$40 years; $\geq$2.5 mm in men <40 years, or $\geq$1.5 mm in women regardless of age

ST-DEPRESSION AND T WAVE CHANGES

New horizontal or downsloping ST-depression

$\geq$ 0.5 mm in two contiguous leads and/or T inversion

>1 mm in two contiguous leads with prominent R wave or R/S ratio > 1

When the magnitudes of J-point elevation in leads V2 and V3 are registered from a prior electrocardiogram, new J-point elevation $\geq$1 mm (as compared with the earlier electrocardiogram) should be considered an ischaemic response

Table 5.1 Localization of ST elevation infarction

Location of infarct	ECG Leads showing ST elevation or Q Waves	Epicardial coronary artery involved
Septal	V1, V2	LAD
Anterior	V3, V4	LAD
Lateral	V5, V6	LAD or LCx
Anteroseptal	V1-V4	LAD
Anterolateral	V3-V6	LAD
Extensive anterior	V1-V6	LAD
Inferior	II, III, aVF	RCA or LCx
High lateral	I, aVL	LCx
Posterior	Tall R wave and ST depression in V1-V2	LCx

Abbreviations: LAD: Left anterior descending; LCx: Left circumflex; RCA: Right coronary artery.

INFERIOR WALL MI

Inferior wall MI (IWMI) may be caused by occlusion in the course of either the RCA (in 80% of the cases) or the LCx artery and this may determine the clinical and hemodynamic course. Patients with LCx artery occlusion are prone to develop mitral valve

regurgitation, whereas patients with RCA occlusion may present with right ventricular infarction, bradyarrhythmia and conduction disturbances. Table 5.2 and Figures 5.3 to 5.6 list the criteria to differentiate the culprit artery in IWMI.

Recently a new three-step criteria has been proposed for electrocardiographic distinction of LCx and RCA occlusion in patients with IWMI [4], based on findings from 230 non-selected cases of IWMI undergoing primary percutaneous intervention (111 with LCx occlusion). Initially, RCA occlusion is confirmed by ST depression $\geq$0.1 mV in lead I and aVL. In its absence, the presence of ST elevation $\geq$0.1 mV in lead V6 or ST elevation in V6 greater than III identifies MI due to LCx occlusion. In the absence of both of these criteria, the ratio of ST depression in V3/ST-elevation in III >1.2 identifies LCx occlusion. The algorithm had a sensitivity of 77%, specificity of 86% and accuracy of 82%.

After localising the culprit artery to the RCA, we can further narrow the site of occlusion within the RCA based on the ECG criteria noted in Table 5.3.

Importantly, inferior lead ST-segment elevation accompanying acute anterior wall infarction suggests either occlusion of the LAD artery that extends onto the inferior wall of the left ventricle (the wrap-around vessel) or multivessel disease with jeopardised collaterals (Figure 5.7).

Table 5.2 Localisation of culprit artery in inferior wall myocardial infarction [2,3]

ECG Criteria	Favours RCA	Favours LCx
ST-segment elevation in lead III > in lead II	Present	Absent
ST depression in aVL > ST depression in lead I	Present	Absent
Ratio of sum of ST depression in V1-V3 divided by sum of ST elevation in II, III, aVF	<1	>1
ST elevation in V1 or V4R	Present	Absent
Lead V4R	T wave upright	T wave inverted
ST elevation in lead aVL and I	Absent	Present
ST depression in V1 and V2	Absent (can be seen in occlusion of dominant RCA causing posterior wall MI)	Present

Abbreviations: LCx: Left circumflex; RCA: Right coronary artery.

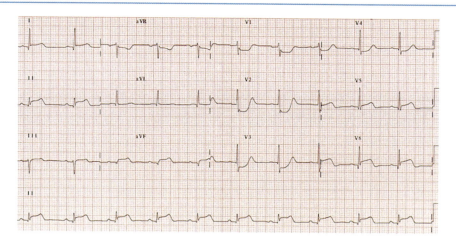

Figure 5.3 Acute Inferior wall ST elevation MI. Note the ST-segment elevation in leads II > III, ST elevation in lead V6 >1 mm, consistent with occlusion of the left circumflex artery. Features of posterior extension like horizontal ST depression in V1-V3, Tall R waves in V2-V3, and upright T waves in V2-V3 are also present.

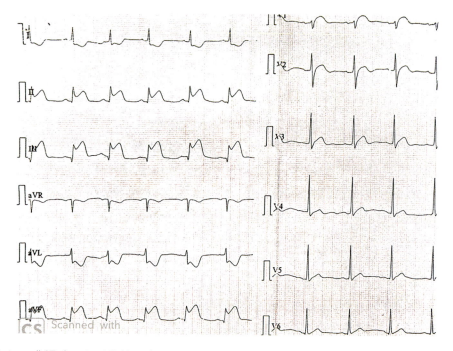

Figure 5.4 Acute Inferior wall ST elevation MI. Note the ST-segment elevation in leads II, III, and aVF, with reciprocal changes in leads I and aVL. ST-segment elevation in lead III greater than in lead II and there is ST segment elevation in lead aVR and V1, consistent with proximal occlusion of the right coronary artery.

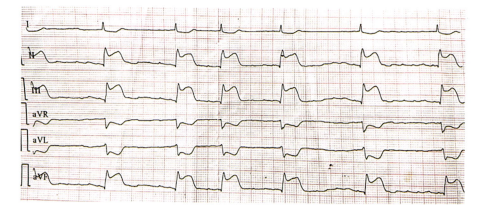

Figure 5.5 Another ECG of acute Inferior wall ST elevation MI. Note the underlying atrial fibrillation along with ST-segment elevation in leads II, III and aVF.

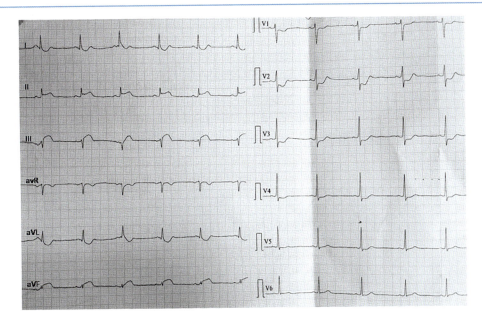

Figure 5.6 Acute inferior wall ST elevation MI. Note the ST-segment elevation in leads II, III and aVF, with reciprocal changes in leads I and aVL. ST-segment elevation in lead III greater than in lead II but there is no ST segment elevation in lead aVR or V1, consistent with distal occlusion of the right coronary artery.

Table 5.3 ECG Distinction of proximal versus distal occlusion of right coronary artery in inferior wall myocardial infarction

ECG Criteria	Occlusion of proximal RCA	Occlusion of distal RCA
ST elevation in lead V4R	Present	Absent
ST elevation in lead V1	Present	Absent
ST elevation in aVR > ST elevation in V1-V3	Present	Absent
Ratio of Sum of ST depression in V1-V3 divided by sum of ST elevation in II, III, aVF	<0.5	>0.5 but <1

Abbreviation: RCA: Right coronary artery

ANTERIOR WALL MYOCARDIAL INFARCTION (AWMI)

In AWMI, the site of occlusion in the LAD determines the myocardium at risk and also predicts the prognosis and further plan of action. Table 5.4 and Figures 5.8 to 5.10 discuss the various criteria for the characterisation of the site of occlusion in AWMI.

POSTERIOR WALL MYOCARDIAL INFARCTION

None of the standard 12 leads face the posterior wall of LV, hence standard ECG is a relatively insensitive tool for detecting posterior wall MI (PWMI).

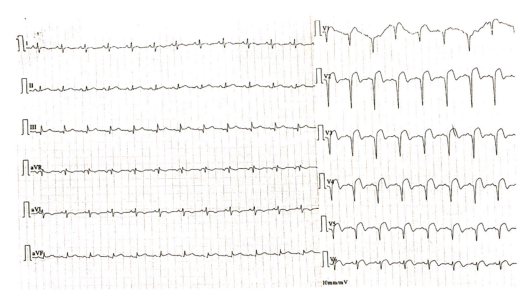

Figure 5.7 Acute anterior wall ST elevation MI. Note the ST segment elevation in leads II, III and aVF, consistent with occlusion of the wrap around left anterior descending artery.

Table 5.4 ECG Distinction for site of occlusion in left anterior descending artery in anterior wall myocardial infarction

ECG Criteria	Site of occlusion in LAD
Acquired RBBB	Proximal to 1st septal
ST elevation V1 > 2.5 mm	
ST elevation in lead aVR	
ST depression in lead V5	
New onset LAHB	
ST depression in leads II, III, aVF	
Sum of ST deviation in VR + V1 − V6	
≥0	Proximal to 1st septal
<0	Distal to 1st septal
Q in lead aVL	Proximal to 1st diagonal
ST depression in lead III> lead II	
ST depression in III + aVF ≥2 .5 mm	
ST segment in lead III and aVF, isoelectric or elevated	Distal to 1st diagonal

Abbreviations: LAD: Left anterior descending; RBBB: Right bundle branch block; LAHB: left anterior hemi-block.

During acute inferior infarction, PWMI can be indirectly recognised by reciprocal ST depression in precordial leads V1-V3, which can be confirmed by ST-segment elevation in the posterior chest leads V7-V9 (Figure 5.11). Patients with an abnormal R wave in V1 (0.04 in duration and/or R/S ratio ≥ 1 in the absence of pre-excitation or right ventricular hypertrophy), with inferior or lateral Q waves, have an increased incidence of isolated occlusion of a dominant LCx artery.

All these criteria will always be subject to limitations and exceptions based on interindividual variations in coronary anatomy, the dynamic nature of acute ECG changes, the presence of multivessel involvement, collateral flow, previous infarctions and the presence of ventricular conduction delays. Sometimes, however, partial normalisation can result from the cancellation of opposing vectoral forces.

ECG DIAGNOSIS OF MYOCARDIAL INFARCTION WITH BUNDLE BRANCH BLOCKS

The diagnosis of MI often is more difficult when the baseline ECG has a pre-existing bundle branch block pattern or when bundle branch block develops as a complication of the MI.

The criteria for the diagnosis of a Q wave infarct in a patient with right bundle branch block (RBBB) are the same as in patients with normal conduction.

Left bundle branch block (LBBB) alters both the early and the late phases of ventricular depolarisation and produces secondary ST-T changes which may mask and/or mimic MI findings. Thus, the diagnosis of infarction in the presence of LBBB is considerably more complicated and confusing.

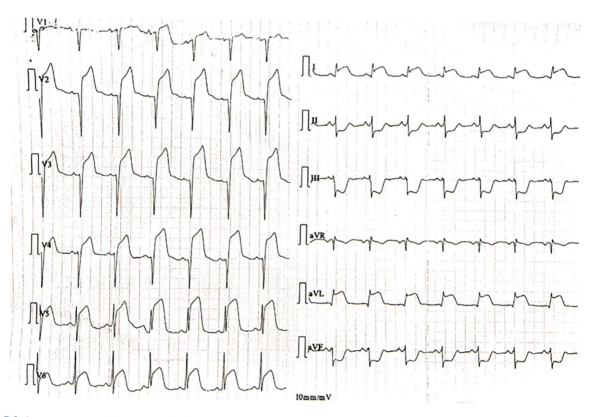

10mm/mV

Figure 5.8 Acute anterior wall ST elevation MI. Note the ST-segment elevation in leads V1-V6 and I, aVL with reciprocal changes in leads II, III and aVF. ST depression in lead III> lead II, but there is no ST segment elevation in lead aVR, consistent with occlusion of the left anterior descending artery proximal to 1st diagonal branch.

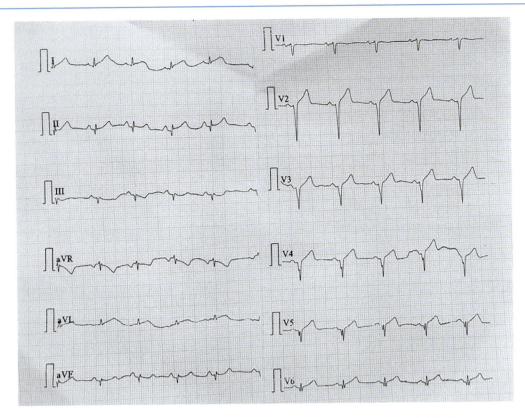

Figure 5.9 Acute anterior wall ST elevation MI. Note the ST segment in lead III and aVF, isoelectric or slightly elevated, consistent with occlusion of the left anterior descending artery distal to 1st diagonal branch.

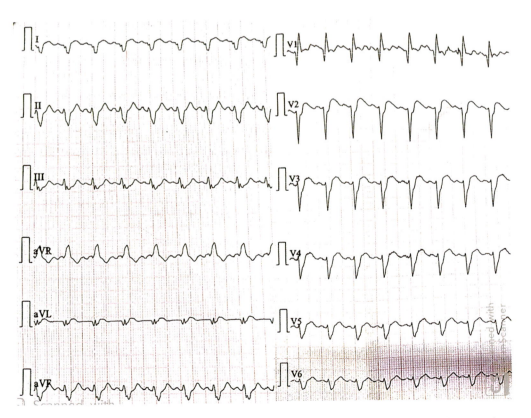

Figure 5.10 Acute anterior wall ST elevation MI with RBBB. Note the ST-segment elevation in leads V1-V6 and I, aVL with reciprocal changes in leads III and aVF. Coronary angiogram revealed complete occlusion of the left anterior descending artery from ostium.

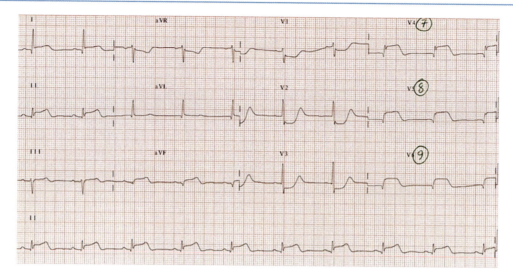

Figure 5.11 Posterior leads V7-V9 were recorded in case of suspected LCx occlusion, note the marked ST elevation in V7-9 confirming the involvement of the posterior wall.

The following points summarise the ECG signs of MI in LBBB:

1. *Sgarbossa rule:*

Sgarbossa rule	Points
ST-segment elevation ≥1 mm and concordant with the QRS complex	5
ST-segment depression ≥1 mm in lead V1, V2, or V3	3
ST-segment elevation ≥5 mm and discordant with the QRS complex	2
A score of ≥3 had a specificity of 98% for acute MI.	

2. *Modified Sgarbossa rule:* Use of the ratio of the absolute amplitude of the ST segment to S wave, determined in any relevant lead of greater than 0.25 has been proposed as having greater accuracy than that of the original criterion [5].
3. The presence of QR complexes in leads I, V5 or V6 or in II, III, and aVF with LBBB strongly suggests underlying MI.
4. Chronic MI also is suggested by notching of the ascending part of a wide S wave in the midprecordial leads or the ascending limb of a wide R wave in lead I, aVL, V5 or V6.

Similar findings can be useful in detecting ECG evidence for acute myocardial ischaemia in patients with right ventricular paced rhythms.

LEAD aVR IN ACUTE CORONARY SYNDROMES

Lead aVR may provide important diagnostic as well as prognostic information in ACS. Left main (or severe multivessel) involvement should be considered when leads aVR and V1 show ST-segment elevation (Figure 5.12), especially in association with diffuse prominent ST-segment depression in other leads [6,7].

In both STEMI and non-STEMI, the degree of ST-elevation in aVR correlates with worse disease and worse outcomes, independent of the clinical presentation; these patients must be treated aggressively with early angiography and revascularisation.

ABNORMAL Q WAVES

Abnormal Q waves were once considered as the hallmark of transmural MI, whereas subendocardial infarcts were considered as non-Q MI. ECG change associated with prior MI (including pathological Q Waves) are shown in Box 5.2. However, it has been proven that both the transmural and subendocardial MI can occur with or without Q waves. ST-elevations accompanying abnormal Q waves do not necessarily imply acute ischaemia and can be seen with LV aneurysms, e.g. after large infarcts (Figure 5.13).

POTENTIAL CONFOUNDERS IN ECG CHANGES IN ACS

1. A QS complex in lead V1 is normal.
2. A Q wave <0.03 s and <0.25 of the R wave amplitude in lead III is normal.
3. Pre-excitation, cardiomyopathy, Takotsubo syndrome, cardiac amyloidosis, LBBB, left anterior hemi-block, LVH, right ventricular hypertrophy, myocarditis, acute cor pulmonale or hyperkalaemia may be associated with Q waves or QS complexes in the absence of MI.

BOX 5.2: ECG changes associated with prior MI (in the absence of LVH and LBBB)

Any Q wave in leads V2–V3 > 0.02 s or QS complex in leads V2–V3.
Q wave ≥ 0.03 s and ≥ 1 mm deep or QS complex in leads I, II, aVL, aVF or V4–V6 in any two leads of a contiguous lead grouping (I, aVL; V1–V6; II, III, aVF).
R wave > 0.04 s in V1–V2 and R/S > 1 with a concordant positive T wave in absence of conduction defect.

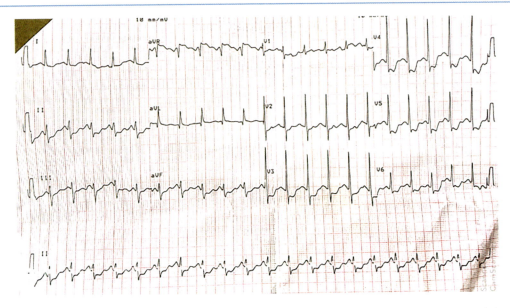

Figure 5.12 65-year-old diabetic lady presented with acute chest pain. Note the ST-segment depression in precordial as well as inferior leads with ST segment elevation in aVR, consistent with multi-vessel disease.

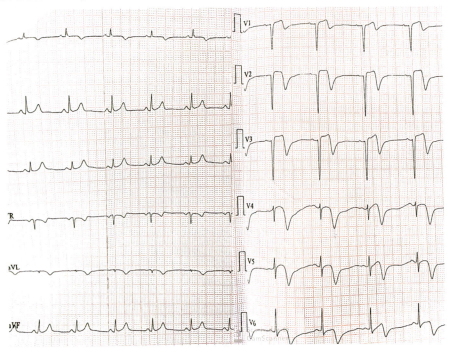

Figure 5.13 60-year-old male admitted with anterior wall ST elevation MI a week back. Current ECG is showing deep anteroseptal QS complexes with persistent ST elevation and inverted T waves. Note the absence of reciprocal ST depressions. This pattern is suggestive of LV aneurysm, which was later confirmed on echocardiography.

ANTERIOR WALL ST-ELEVATION MI EQUIVALENTS

Some patients with ACS have deep T wave inversion in multiple precordial leads (e.g. V1 through V4), with or without cardiac enzyme level elevations. This pattern is due to critical stenosis in the proximal LAD artery (referred to as the LAD–T wave or Wellens pattern) [8]. These T wave inversions may be preceded by transient ST-segment elevations and unfavourable prognosis with high incidence of recurrent angina and myocardial infarction (Figure 5.14).

There are two patterns of T wave abnormality in Wellens syndrome:

Type A: Biphasic, with initial positivity and terminal negativity (25% of cases)
Type B: Deeply and symmetrically inverted (75% of cases)

The two types of T waves found in Wellens syndrome exist on a spectrum of disease with type-A T waves evolving into type-B T waves.

In another pattern, there is 1–3 mm upsloping ST-segment depression at the J-point in leads V1 to V6 along with tall,

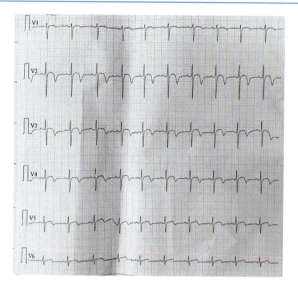

positive symmetrical T waves. This characteristic pattern called de Winters T waves can be seen in 2% of anterior MI [9]. The de Winter ECG pattern typically displays tall T waves, but the static nature and characteristic ST depression differentiates this pattern from hyperacute T waves.

MYOCARDIAL ISCHAEMIA AND REPOLARISATION CHANGES

It can be difficult to differentiate myocardial ischaemia and repolarization changes secondary to left ventricular hypertrophy, enlargement or use of medications like digoxin. Clinical context, imaging and biomarker estimation are helpful. Box 5.3 enumerates certain ECG changes that differentiate between left ventricular hypertrophy and acute ischaemia. The discriminating ability increases in the presence of multiple differentiating features on ECG (Figures 5.15 and 5.16).

Figure 5.14 54-year-old male admitted presented with typical angina but with negative cardiac enzymes. Note deep, symmetrical and inverted T waves in leads V2 and V3, extending up to V5 (type 2 Wellens pattern).

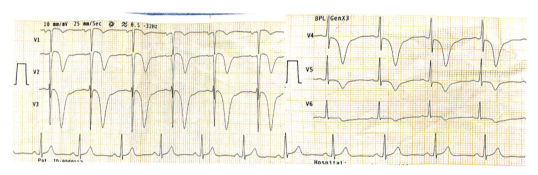

Figure 5.15 A 48-year male old who was a chronic smoker presented with acute chest pain. Note the T wave inversion in the precordial leads. T inversion in lead V6 is less than V3 and absence of voltage criteria for LVH.

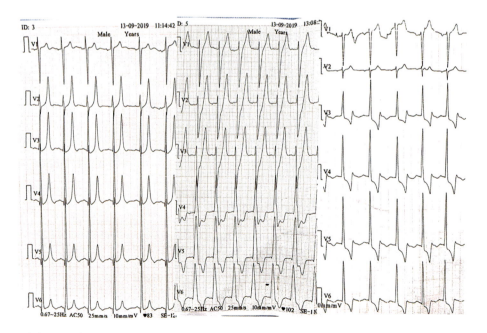

Figure 5.16 A 40-year diabetic male presented with typical angina. Note the hyperacute T waves in precordial leads (Panel A), appearance of ST depression and T wave inversion in leads V4 to V6 (Panel B) and biphasic T waves (Panel C) all suggestive of ACS.

BOX 5.3: ST depression and T wave inversion: Is it ischaemia or LVH?

	LVH	Ischaemia
Voltage Criteria for LVH	Present	If absent, ischaemia is likely
J-point depression	Present	Absent
T wave symmetry	Asymmetric	Symmetric
Ascending limb of T wave	Steep	Less steep
Terminal T positivity and overshoot	Overshoot	Do not overshoot the baseline
T inversion in V6	>3 mm	<3 mm
T inversion in V6 vs V3	V6 > V3	V6 ≤ V3

REFERENCES

1. Thygesen K, Alpert JS, Jaffe AS et al. ESC Scientific Document Group. Fourth universal definition of myocardial infarction (2018). *Eur Heart J.* 2019;40:237–269.
2. Fiol M, Cygankiewicz I, Carrillo A et al. Value of electrocardiographic algorithm based on "ups and downs" of ST in assessment of a culprit artery in evolving inferior wall acute myocardial infarction. *Am J Cardiol.* 2004;94:709–714.
3. Verouden NJ, Barwari K, Koch KT et al. Distinguishing the right coronary artery from the left circumflex coronary artery as the infarct-related artery in patients undergoing primary percutaneous coronary intervention for acute inferior myocardial infarction. *Europace.* 2009;11:1517–1521.
4. Vives-Borrás M, Maestro A, García-Hernando V et al. Electrocardiographic distinction of left circumflex and right coronary artery occlusion in patients with inferior acute myocardial infarction. *Am J Cardiol.* 2019;123:1019–1025.
5. Smith SW, Dodd KW, Henry TD et al. Diagnosis of ST-elevation myocardial infarction in the presence of left bundle branch block with the ST-elevation to S-wave ratio in a modified Sgarbossa rule. *Ann Emerg Med.* 2012;60:766.
6. Barrabés JA, Figueras J, Moure C et al. Prognostic value of lead aVR in patients with a first non–ST-segment elevation acute myocardial infarction. *Circulation.* 2003;108:814–819.
7. Nikus KC. Electrocardiographic presentations of acute total occlusion of the left main coronary artery. *J Electrocardiol.* 2012;45:491–493.
8. Rhinehardt J, Brady WJ, Perron AD, Mattu A. Electrocardiographic manifestations of Wellens' syndrome. *Am J Emerg Med.* 2002;20:638–643.
9. de Winter RJ, Verouden NJ, Wellens HJ et al. A new ECG sign of proximal LAD occlusion. *N Engl J Med.* 2008;359:2071–2073.

6

Arrhythmias in acute coronary syndrome

NISHAD CHITNIS AND B HYGRIV RAO

INTRODUCTION

Arrythmias are commonly seen in both treated and untreated patients with acute coronary syndrome (ACS). Tachyarrhythmias and bradyarrhythmias are both seen in patients with ACS. This chapter is confined to dealing with tachyarrhythmias. Serious arrythmias frequently occur and can be fatal before the patient reaches a hospital. In-hospital arrythmias are also a common cause of morbidity and mortality in these patients [1]. Underlying ischaemic heart disease is recognised to be the most common cause of sudden cardiac death (SCD) in India [2].

VENTRICULAR TACHYARRHYTHMIAS

Ventricular tachyarrhythmias are by far the most important arrhythmias seen in patients with ACS.

VENTRICULAR PREMATURE DEPOLARISATIONS

Ventricular premature complexes (VPCs) are common in patients with ACS and constitute the most common arrhythmias in this substrate. They may occur during the acute phase as well as during reperfusion. Before the advent of modern reperfusion therapy, certain configurations of VPCs were considered to predict ventricular fibrillation (VF) and sudden death, namely frequent VPCs, multiform VPCs, 'R-on-T' phenomenon, couplets and salvos. It was expected that suppression of these VPCs would reduce the risk of sudden death. However, the Cardiac Arrhythmia Suppression Trial (CAST) conclusively demonstrated increased mortality in patients prophylactically treated with class I anti-arrhythmic agents [3]. Current data shows that VPCs are very unreliable predictors of occurrence of significant ventricular arrhythmias [1].

Today, the only therapy used for VPCs is beta-blockers, which not only suppress VPCs, but also reduce the incidence of VF [1,4].

ACCELERATED IDIOVENTRICULAR RHYTHM

Accelerated idioventricular rhythm (AIVR) usually occurs in the first 48 hours after an infarction. The episodes are usually brief, relatively slow in rate (<100 beats per minute), and do not usually cause hemodynamic compromise. Though AIVR was previously believed to be a marker of successful reperfusion, it is now known to be an unreliable predictor. AIVR does not affect prognosis and does not need to be routinely treated [1].

VENTRICULAR TACHYCARDIA AND VENTRICULAR FIBRILLATION

Ventricular tachycardia (VT) and ventricular fibrillation (VF) are the most important causes of sudden cardiac death (SCD) following myocardial infarction. They are most prevalent in the first month following infarction, and this is unrelated to the presence of LV dysfunction [5]. With early revascularisation and evidence-based medications, their incidence is declining, but in India the SCD mortality following myocardial infarction still remains high [6] Interestingly, SCD has not declined even in populations which are showing a decline in coronary artery disease [7]. The rapidly fatal nature of these arrythmias makes VT/VF the most dreaded and most important arrhythmic complication of ACS.

PATHOPHYSIOLOGY OF VT/VF

The pathophysiology of VT/VF in ACS depends on the time since onset of ischaemia. While VT/VF occurring several days after an acute myocardial infarction is predominantly due to re-entrant circuits created by myocardial scarring, arrhythmias occurring in the acute setting have been shown in animal models to have two distinct mechanisms [8–10].

Phase I VT/VF occurs early when myocardial injury is still reversible and is associated with either ischaemia of large areas of the myocardium or with reperfusion injury where myocardial reperfusion results in cellular oedema and endothelial dysfunction. In contrast, phase II VT/VF occurs during the stage of infarct evolution. The damaged Purkinje fibre cells develop increased automaticity, resulting in re-entrant circuits within the ventricular myocardium [9].

While extrapolation from animal models to human beings has its limitations, this distinction is likely to be important from the therapeutic point of view. Hugh-Clements et al. [9] have proposed that the difference in mechanisms between the two phases may explain the disappointing results of the Survival With ORal D-sotalol (SWORD) trial [11]. They have proposed a definition for distinguishing between the two phases of VT/VF. Phase I VF is defined as VF occurring during the first 30 minutes after onset of ischaemia, while phase II VF is defined as occurring during the later phase, approximately 90 minutes after the onset of ischaemia. The two phases are not distinguishable by ECG characteristics but have distinct mechanisms. Work on rats suggests that drugs which are effective in suppressing phase I VT/VF may be ineffective in phase II VT/VF. Hugh-Clements et al. have suggested that any prophylactic approach should be effective in both phases to show a decrease in mortality [9].

MANAGEMENT OF VT/VF

As the first presentation of VT/VF can be sudden death or refractory VF, primary prophylaxis is highly desirable. The most important strategy to reduce occurrence of these arrhythmias is timely reperfusion and administration of beta-blockers. Antiarrhythmic drugs have not been shown to be safe and effective in preventing these arrhythmias. The CAST study was terminated early due to significantly higher mortality in the treatment arm compared to placebo [3]. Similarly, the SWORD trial showed a higher mortality with sotalol compared to placebo [11].

The only drugs shown to be effective prophylaxis against tachyarrhythmias in ACS are beta-blockers [1,4,12]. Beta-blockers not only reduce infarct size and incidence of arrhythmia but also reduce all-cause mortality and SCD in patients with ACS, both acutely and in the long term [12]. In fact, patients who have not received beta-blockers in the first 24 hours after ACS have a significantly higher risk of in-hospital VT/VF and associated mortality [13].

Intravenous beta-blocker use has now fallen out of favour after demonstration of increased mortality. Oral beta-blocker therapy, however, has shown a consistent decrease in mortality in the absence of contraindications [14–16]. The major contraindications for use of beta-blockers are acute cardiac failure as evidenced by low output state, pulmonary congestion or shock, significant bradyarrhythmias, and uncontrolled beta-blocker sensitive pulmonary disease [16].

Pharmacological therapy

Though anti-arrhythmic drugs (AADs) have not demonstrated a mortality benefit in primary and secondary prevention (except for beta-blockers), they are necessary in the acute therapy of VT/VF.

Beta-blockers form the first-line therapy and have been used both alone and as an adjunct with other agents. Beta-blockers enhance anti-arrhythmic efficacy when used in combination with membrane stabilising agents. They are the only drugs to conclusively demonstrate reduction in arrhythmic mortality in ACS [17].

Amiodarone, a class 3 AAD, has become the preferred drug for the treatment of VT/VF in virtually any scenario (except polymorphic VT). It is usually administered as an intravenous bolus followed by infusion which is followed by oral therapy. Amiodarone has shown some reduction in mortality in patients with out-of-hospital cardiac arrest, as a result of which the European Society of Cardiology (ESC) currently recommends it as the first choice AAD co-administered with beta-blockers for therapy of VT/VF in all cases without contraindications including ACS patients [18].

However, it should be remembered that long-term amiodarone administration has several serious side-effects including thyroid toxicity, lung toxicity and even increased heart failure mortality in patients with severe LV dysfunction [19]. Lidocaine has been used as an intravenous infusion for treatment of VT/VF for decades. However, when lidocaine was used prophylactically in patients of ACS, an increase in mortality was observed. This has resulted in concerns of using lidocaine as a therapeutic agent in ACS. This has been challenged recently by Piccini et al. who demonstrated an increase in 30-day mortality when amiodarone was used in VT/VF, while lidocaine was neutral, thereby highlighting the need for randomised control trials (RCT) in the ACS population [20].

Ranalozine, an anti-anginal drug, has shown some promise in reducing the incidence of VT in ACS patients. While the data is scant, ranalozine has been found to reduce the incidence of ICD shocks in patients with drug refractory VT/VF and to reduce the incidence of VT treated by anti-tachycardia pacing (ATP) [17].

Device therapy

Implantable cardiovertor-defibrillator (ICD) is the only therapy beside beta-blockers that has shown a reduction in mortality when used as primary and secondary prophylaxis for SCD. Patients who survive cardiac arrest or have a documented episode of hemodynamically unstable VT should receive ICD as a class I-B recommendation. Patients of ACS who have a left ventricular ejection fraction (LVEF) of less than 35% after 40 days of the index event should receive ICD for primary prevention of SCD (Class IA) [17].

These guidelines leave a period of around 35 days when the patient is discharged from hospital but is not a candidate for ICD. This was based on the results of the Defibrillation IN Acute Myocardial Infarction Trial (DINAMIT) which showed no mortality benefit of prophylactic ICD implantation in the first 40 days after an infarction [21]. However, the highest incidence of SCD is during the first month after an infarction and does not appear to be related to LVEF. Ventricular arrhythmias occurring 48 hours following MI may warrant ICD implantation (Class II B).

Wearable cardioverter-defibrillator

Wearable cardioverter-defibrillator is a vest-like device worn by the patient under the clothing. It should be worn continuously except while bathing. The US FDA has approved the use of this device for patients who are at risk for SCD but are not candidates for ICD or for those who have refused ICD. The device shows promise for patients in the first 40 days after an infarction. While large RCTs are lacking, smaller studies have shown a benefit in terms of mortality [17,22]. However, in a recent randomised trial involving 2302 patients with acute myocardial infarction and LVEF ≤ 35%, a wearable defibrillator did not reduce arrhythmic mortality in comparison to controls [23].

ELECTRICAL STORM

Electrical storm is usually defined as 'the occurrence of two or more VT/VF episodes within 24 hours' in patients without an ICD [24,25]. Most studies have found electrical storm to be an adverse prognostic factor. In the Antiarrhythmic Versus Implantable Defibrillators (AVID) trial, electrical storm was a predictor of death independent of other prognostic factors including LVEF [26]. It is still uncertain if electrical storm denotes adverse substrate or if the storm itself increases mortality by a combination of worsening heart failure and myocardial damage caused by recurrent shocks [24].

Arborisation of Purkinje fibres which cross the infarct border zones is now believed to be an important source of triggers for electrical storm. The Purkinje fibres survive transmural infarction by imbibing nutrients from intracavitary blood and demonstrate triggered activity, heightened automaticity, supernormal excitability and prolongation of the action potential duration. The result is a pro-arrhythmogenic milieu [27].

Management of electrical storm

Electrical storm is an emergency and should be treated aggressively. A protocol directed strategy for dealing with ES is recommended. Key steps involved in the protocol are adequate sedation, correction of ischaemia, hemodynamic support, elective mechanical ventilation, administration of maximum tolerated beta blockers, appropriate anti arrhythmic drugs, sympathetic ganglionectomy and catheter ablation. These have been detailed in a recent publication [28].

Pharmacological therapy

By controlling the sympathetic overdrive, beta-blockers increase the threshold for VF. Metoprolol, atenolol and carvedilol have been used [24]. Amiodarone is extensively used in combination with beta-blockers for controlling electrical storm. A combination of amiodarone or sotalol with beta-blockers has demonstrated a 56% reduction in mortality compared to beta-blockers alone. Intravenous amiodarone and beta-blockers can be used in patients already on oral amiodarone and beta-blockers [24].

Sotalol has been shown to reduce VT/VF, all-cause ICD shocks, and all-cause death compared to placebo. While the combination of sotalol and beta-blockers is superior compared to beta-blockers alone, sotalol alone has not shown superiority to metoprolol [24]. Azilimide is a new drug which has demonstrated reduction in shock recurrence, emergency department visits and hospital admissions. However, its role in electrical storm is still unclear [24].

Stellate ganglionectomy

Another strategy to counter electrical storm is to interrupt sympathetic inflow to the myocardium [29].

Suppressing the sympathetic outflow from the heart to higher brain centres reduces the propensity for VT recurrence and reduces the psychological and physiological trauma. The autonomic nervous system alters arrhythmogenesis based on the afferent inputs received from the heart. Cardiac function is regulated by the efferent sympathetic preganglionic neurons that reside within the intermediate zone at the level of T1–T4 of the thoracic spinal cord. Preganglionic axons synapse on neurons within the stellate ganglion formed by the fusion of inferior cervical and T1 ganglia and on the ganglia at spinal levels T2–T4. The postganglionic fibres to the heart arise from the left and right stellate ganglia. Thoracic epidural infusion of bupivicaine and surgical removal of the sympathetic chain including the stellate ganglion have been shown to reduce propensity for VT and electrical storm. Left cardiac sympathetic denervation (LCSD) interrupts the primary source of norepinephrine in the heart. Bilateral cardiac sympathetic denervation (BCSD) appears to be more effective than LCSD in achieving freedom from recurrent VT [29].

Catheter ablation (CA)

In ACS, catheter ablation should be considered only in an electrical storm unresponsive to medical therapy and revascularisation. Sometimes electrical storm may occur following revascularisation. VT/VF is often triggered by VPCs (called triggering VPCs) which are generated predominantly in ischaemic foci in the His-Purkinje system (Figure 6.1). Ablation of these foci has been shown to be an effective therapy of electrical storm in the acute phase of a myocardial infarction, with low recurrence (Figure 6.2) [27,30].

CA has shown promise in therapy of patients with scar VT caused by an old infarction. The targets are usually around the scar. CA is usually used in conjunction with ICD in these patients [30]. Presence of a thrombus in LV may be a concern for subjecting the patient to endocardial ablation but a recent series has demonstrated the safety of ablation in this clinical subset [31].

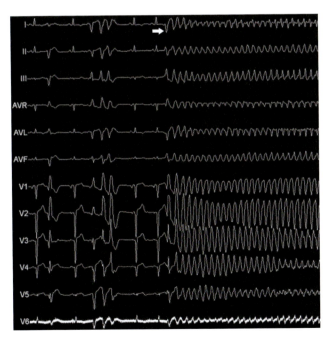

Figure 6.1 A monomorphic PVC triggering VF in a patient with acute MI in VT storm following revascularisation. This VPC (shown by arrow) is a target for ablation.

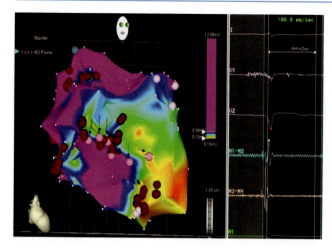

Figure 6.2 Electroanatomic bipolar voltage map of LV in RAO projection demonstrating a large scar in anterolateral LV. The voltage map delineates the region of scar border zone. The red tags represent the sites recording late diastolic potentials and pink tags (bold arrows) represents the sites recording discrete Purkinje potentials triggering the VT, which had survived the infarct (successful ablation sites). (Reused from Thoppil PS et al. *Indian Pacing Electrophysiol J.* 2008;8(4):298–303, under Creative Commons Attribution License.)

POLYMORPHIC VENTRICULAR TACHYCARDIA

Polymorphic VT is usually a marker of ongoing ischaemia in ACS (Figure 6.3a,b). Therapy of polymorphic VT requires reversing myocardial ischaemia using beta-blockers, intra-aortic balloon pump and emergency revascularisation (percutaneous intervention or bypass grafting). Maintenance of serum potassium above 4 mEq/L and serum magnesium above 2 mEq/L is recommended. Patients with bradycardia and long QTc interval may benefit from temporary pacing at a higher rate [16].

The key recommendations of the ACC/AHA guidelines for management of VT/VF in ACS are summarised in Table 6.1 [16,18].

SUPRAVENTRICULAR ARRHYTHMIAS

SINUS TACHYCARDIA

Sinus tachycardia is common in ACS. It is a secondary arrhythmia caused by increased sympathetic drive due to anxiety, pain, heart failure, fever, pericarditis, hypotension, hypovolemia, drugs, and occasionally, pulmonary embolism. While typically described in

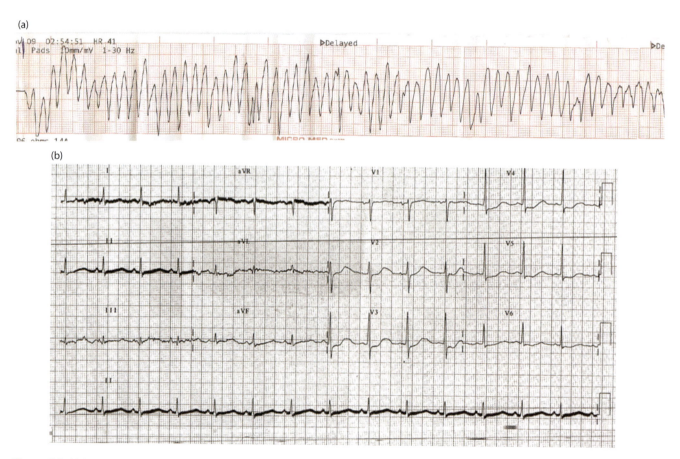

Figure 6.3 (a) Patient presenting with ACS, ECG showing prolonged QTc and ST–T changes in V4 to V6 leads. Prolonged QTc is a marker of ischaemia. Coronary angiogram showed severe triple vessel disease. (b) Patient had cardiac arrest due to polymorphic VT, which was DC verted.

Table 6.1 ACC/AHA guidelines for the management of ventricular arrythmias: Key recommendations

S. No	Arrhythmia/procedure	Recommendations	Class of recommendation and level of evidence
1	VF and pulseless VT	Unsynchronized DC shock of 200 J, followed by 300 J, followed by 360 J, as needed.	I-B
2	Refractory VF and pulseless VT	IV amiodarone 300 mg followed by repeat DC shock.	IIa-B
		Keep serum potassium >4 mEq/L and serum magnesium >2 mEq/L.	IIa-C
		IV Procainamide.	IIb-C
3	Sustained polymorphic VT	Unsynchronized DC shock of 200 J, followed by 300 J, followed by 360 J, as needed.	I-A
4	Refractory polymorphic VT	Anti-anginal therapy- Beta-blockers, IABP, revascularization.	IIa-B
		Keep serum potassium >4 mEq/L and serum magnesium >2 mEq/L.	IIa-C
		In patients with bradycardia, temporary pacing may be considered.	IIa-C
5	Sustained monomorphic VT with haemodynamic compromise	Synchronized electric shock of 100 J followed by increasing energies if required	I-B
6	Sustained stable monomorphic VT	Amiodarone 150 mg boluses or infusion	I-B
		Synchronized electrical cardioversion starting at 50 J and escalating as needed	I-B
		IV procainamide	IIb-C
7	VPCs	Treatment not recommended	III
8	AIVR	Treatment not recommended	III
9	Use of ICD	Patients with VF or haemodynamically significant VT >2 days after STEMI	I-A
		Patients with LVEF of 31% to 40% one month after STEMI and evidence of electrical instability and inducible VT/VF on EPS	I-B
		LVEF ≤ 30% one month post-STEMI or 3 months after revascularization	IIa-B
		Usefulness is not established in patients with LVEF 31% to 40% one month after STEMI without evidence of electrical instability or have electrical instability but no inducible VT/VF on EPS	IIb-B
10	Radiofrequency catheter ablation (ESC 2015 guidelines)	In patients with recurrent VT/VF or electrical storms despite revascularization and optimum medical therapy	IIa-C

Source: Antman EM et al. Circulation. 2004;110(5):588–636; Ibanez B et al. 2017 *Eur Heart J.* 2018;39(2):119–177.

Note: Class of Recommendation—I- Strong, benefit >>> risk, IIa- Moderate, benefit >> risk, IIb- Weak, benefit ≥ risk, III- No benefit (benefit = risk) or harm (risk > benefit). Level of Evidence—A- High quality evidence from >1 RCT or meta-analysis, B-R- Moderate quality evidence from ≥1 RCT or meta-analysis, B-NR- Moderate quality evidence from ≥1 well-designed, non-randomised or observational study or registry, C-LR- Evidence of limited designed study or registry, C-EO- based on expert opinion.
As the ACC/AHA guidelines do not mention any recommendations regarding catheter ablation in ACS, the ESC guidelines have been mentioned.

Abbreviations: VT, ventricular tachycardia; VF, ventricular fibrillation; IV, intravenous; DC, direct current; IABP, intra-aortic balloon pump; AIVR, accelerated idioventricular rhythm; VPC, ventricular premature complex; ICD, implantable cardioverter-defibrillator; EPS, electrophysiology study.

patients with anterior wall infarction, sinus tachycardia is rarely caused by atrial infarction.

This rhythm is a poor prognostic marker as it may denote heart failure, persistent angina or hypotension. It can precipitate heart failure by increasing myocardial oxygen demand. The treatment is correction of primary causes which lead to sinus tachycardia. Beta-blockers are the most effective drugs. In patients with contraindications to beta-blockers, ivabradine may be useful for persisting sinus tachycardia despite correction of primary causes.

ATRIAL FLUTTER AND FIBRILLATION

Atrial flutter and fibrillation are common in patients of ACS. Atrial fibrillation (AF) is the one of the most common arrhythmias in ACS, affecting up to 21% of patients [18]. It is caused mainly by increased atrial pressure and augmented sympathetic stimulation due to LV dysfunction. The loss of atrial contribution to cardiac output and increased ventricular rate can cause haemodynamic deterioration in these patients. Persistent and recurrent AF can result in thromboembolic episodes and increased risk of stroke [1].

MANAGEMENT OF ATRIAL FIBRILLATION

The treatment of AF in ACS follows the usual recommendations for this rhythm. Beta-blockers are used for rate control in most patients. Those with hypotension or acute heart failure should receive oral or intravenous digoxin. Amiodarone may be used to restore rhythm. In cases with inadequate ventricular rate control by beta-blockers or digoxin, combination with amiodarone may help even if the rhythm does not change [18]. In patients with acute haemodynamic compromise cardioversion may be necessary. Recurrence is common, however [18]. Patients with persistent and recurrent AF should receive long-term anti-coagulation to manage the high stroke risk [1]. Ibutilide can be safely used if there is no prolonged QTc.

CONCLUSION

Arrhythmias remain a major concern in patients with ACS. Timely reperfusion and administration of standard evidence-based medications are the principal strategy in treating them. Ventricular tachycardia and fibrillation, at times presenting as electrical storm, are the major causes of sudden death in ACS. Protocol directed therapy which includes catheter ablation and stellate ganglion excision is helpful in treating these arrhythmias. Further risk stratification tools are needed to identify suitable candidates to prevent SCD early post-ACS period. Atrial arrhythmia indicates large areas of ischaemia and may be associated with heart failure.

REFERENCES

1. Zipes DPA, Libby PA, Bonow ROA, Mann DLA, Tomaselli GFA, Braunwald EHD. *Braunwald's Heart Disease: A Textbook of Cardiovascular Medicine.* 11th ed. Philadelphia: Elsevier/Saunders, 2012.

2. Rao BH, Sastry BK, Chugh SS et al. Contribution of sudden cardiac death to total mortality in India - a population based study. *Int J Cardiol.* 2012;154(2):163–167.

3. Echt DS, Liebson PR, Mitchell LB et al. Mortality and morbidity in patients receiving encainide, flecainide, or placebo. The cardiac arrhythmia suppression trial. *N Engl J Med.* 1991;324(12):781–788.

4. Roolvink V, Ibáñez B, Ottervanger JP et al. Early intravenous beta-blockers in patients with ST-segment elevation myocardial infarction before primary percutaneous coronary intervention. *J Am Coll Cardiol.* 2016;67(23):2705–2715.

5. Chitnis N, Vooturi S, Hygriv Rao B. Sudden cardiac death early after ST elevation myocardial infarction with and without severe left ventricular dysfunction. *Indian Heart J.* 2014;66(6):569–573.

6. Rao HB, Sastry BK, Korabathina R, Raju KP. Sudden cardiac death after acute ST elevation myocardial infarction: Insight from a developing country. *Heart Asia.* 2012;4(1):83–89.

7. Zheng ZJ, Croft JB, Giles WH, Mensah GA. Sudden cardiac death in the United States, 1989–1998. *Circulation.* 2001;104(18):2158–2163.

8. Curtis MJ. Characterisation, utilisation and clinical relevance of isolated perfused heart models of ischaemia-induced ventricular fibrillation. *Cardiovasc Res.* 1998;39(1):194–215.

9. Clements-Jewery H, Hearse DJ, Curtis MJ. Phase 2 ventricular arrhythmias in acute myocardial infarction: A neglected target for therapeutic antiarrhythmic drug development and for safety pharmacology evaluation. *Br J Pharmacol.* 2005;145(5):551–564.

10. Johnston KM, MacLeod BA, Walker MJ. Responses to ligation of a coronary artery in conscious rats and the actions of antiarrhythmics. *Can J Physiol Pharmacol.* 1983;61(11):1340–1353.

11. Pratt CM, Camm AJ, Cooper W et al. Mortality in the Survival With ORal D-sotalol (SWORD) trial: Why did patients die? *Am J Cardiol.* 1998;81(7):869–876.

12. Gielen SE, Backer GDDE, Piepoli MFE, Wood DE. *The ESC Textbook of Preventive Cardiology.* Oxford: Oxford University Press; 2015.

13. Piccini JP, Hranitzky PM, Kilaru R et al. Relation of mortality to failure to prescribe beta blockers acutely in patients with sustained ventricular tachycardia and ventricular fibrillation following acute myocardial infarction (from the VALsartan In Acute myocardial iNfarcTion trial [VALIANT] Registry). *Am J Cardiol.* 2008;102(11):1427–1432.

14. Park KL, Goldberg RJ, Anderson FA et al. Beta-blocker use in ST-segment elevation myocardial infarction in the reperfusion era (GRACE). *Am J Med.* 2014;127(6):503–511.

15. Otterstad JE, Ford I. The effect of carvedilol in patients with impaired left ventricular systolic function following an acute myocardial infarction. How do the treatment effects on total mortality and recurrent myocardial infarction in CAPRICORN compare with previous beta-blocker trials? *Eur J Heart Fail.* 2002;4(4):501–506.

16. Antman EM, Anbe DT, Armstrong PW et al. ACC/AHA guidelines for the management of patients with ST-elevation myocardial infarction--executive summary: A report of

the American College of Cardiology/American Heart Association Task Force on Practice Guidelines (Writing Committee to Revise the 1999 guidelines for the management of patients with acute myocardial infarction). *Circulation*. 2004;110(5):588–636.

17. Al-Khatib SM, Stevenson WG, Ackerman MJ et al. 2017 AHA/ACC/HRS guideline for management of patients with ventricular arrhythmias and the prevention of sudden cardiac death: A report of the American College of Cardiology/American Heart Association Task Force on Clinical Practice Guidelines and the Heart Rhythm Society. *Heart Rhythm*. 2018;15(10):e73–e189.

18. Ibanez B, James S, Agewall S et al. 2017 ESC Guidelines for the management of acute myocardial infarction in patients presenting with ST-segment elevation: The Task Force for the Management of Acute Myocardial Infarction in patients presenting with ST-segment elevation of the European Society of Cardiology (ESC). *Eur Heart J*. 2018;39(2):119–177.

19. Gorenek B, Lundqvist CB, Terradellas JB et al. Cardiac arrhythmias in acute coronary syndromes: Position paper from the Joint EHRA, ACCA, and EAPCI Task Force. *Eur Heart J Acute Cardiovasc Care* 2015;4(4):386.

20. Piccini JP, Schulte PJ, Pieper KS et al. Antiarrhythmic drug therapy for sustained ventricular arrhythmias complicating acute myocardial infarction. *Crit Care Med*. 2011;39(1):78–83.

21. Dorian P, Hohnloser SH, Thorpe KE et al. Mechanisms underlying the lack of effect of implantable cardioverter-defibrillator therapy on mortality in high-risk patients with recent myocardial infarction: Insights from the Defibrillation IN Acute Myocardial Infarction Trial (DINAMIT). *Circulation*. 2010;122(25):2645–2652.

22. Kao AC, Krause SW, Handa R et al. Wearable defibrillator use in heart failure (WIF): Results of a prospective registry. *BMC Cardiovasc Disord*. 2012;12:123.

23. Olgin JE, Pletcher MJ, Vittinghoff E et al. Wearable cardioverter-defibrillator after myocardial infarction. *N Engl J Med*. 2018;379(13):1205–1215.

24. Gao D, Sapp JL. Electrical storm: Definitions, clinical importance, and treatment. *Curr Opin Cardiol*. 2013;28(1):72–79.

25. Proietti R, Sagone A. Electrical storm: Incidence, prognosis and therapy. *Indian Pacing Electrophysiol J*. 2011;11(2):34–342.

26. Exner DV, Pinski SL, Wyse DG et al. Electrical storm presages nonsudden death: The Antiarrhythmics Versus Implantable Defibrillators (AVID) trial. *Circulation*. 2001;103(16):2066–2071.

27. Thoppil PS, Rao BH, Jaishankar S, Narasimhan C. Successful catheter ablation of persistent electrical storm late post myocardial infarction by targeting Purkinje arborization triggers. *Indian Pacing Electrophysiol J*. 2008;8(4):298–303.

28. Rao BH, Azam MS, Manik G. Management of electrical storm of unstable ventricular tachycardia in post myocardial infarction patients: A single centre experience. *Indian Heart J*. 2018;70(2):289–295.

29. Meng L, Tseng CH, Shivkumar K, Ajijola O. Efficacy of stellate ganglion blockade in managing electrical storm: A systematic review. *JACC Clin Electrophysiol*. 2017;3(9):942–949.

30. Tan VH, Yap J, Hsu LF, Liew R. Catheter ablation of ventricular fibrillation triggers and electrical storm. *Europace*. 2012;14(12):1687–1695.

31. Rao HB, Yu R, Chitnis N et al. Ventricular tachycardia ablation in the presence of left ventricular thrombus: Safety and efficacy. *J Cardiovasc Electrophysiol*. 2016;27(4):453–459.

7

Intravascular imaging in acute coronary syndrome

VIJAYAKUMAR SUBBAN AND SUMA M VICTOR

INTRODUCTION

Acute coronary syndrome (ACS) refers to a gamut of clinical presentations ranging from ST-segment elevation myocardial infarction (STEMI) to non-ST-segment elevation myocardial infarction (NSTEMI) or unstable angina, and usually results from occlusive/non-occlusive thrombus in coronary arteries. Clinical outcomes can be optimised by swift revascularisation with percutaneous coronary intervention (PCI) coupled with aggressive medical therapy. Large thrombus burden and disruption of underlying lipid/necrotic core plaques may result in significant distal embolisation and no-reflow during balloon dilatation and stent implantation that may curb the efficacy of PCI. In addition, ACS results from a range of other pathological abnormalities that may require personalised treatment and is also known to be a major predictor of failure of drug-eluting stent (DES) [1].

Coronary angiography (CAG) is the gold standard for invasive evaluation of coronary artery disease (CAD). However, it is handicapped by its inferior resolution, angle dependency, vessel foreshortening, vessel overlap and significant inter- as well as intra-observer variability in assessing the severity of coronary stenoses. Moreover, CAG is a luminogram and does not reveal the details of the vessel wall and plaque composition. Intravascular imaging (IVI) modalities, with their capacity to produce histology like cross-sectional images of the coronary arteries and tissue characterisation proficiencies, complement angiography in the qualitative and quantitative evaluation of CAD [2].

INTRAVASCULAR IMAGING MODALITIES

Although there is a plethora of IVI modalities, only intravascular ultrasound (IVUS) and optical coherence tomography (OCT) are commonly used in clinical practice and further discussion is limited to these two technologies.

IVUS is an ultrasound-based intravascular imaging modality and its operating principle is similar to any other ultrasound-based imaging tool. The IVUS system has a console, a transducer with piezo-electric crystals and a pullback device. The console serves as the electrical source for the transducer in addition to the image display, analysis and storage functions. The electrical stimulation of piezo-electric crystals in the transducer produces high-frequency ultrasound waves. These ultrasound waves are reflected from interface of tissues in the vessel wall. The transducer receives the reflected waves and converts them back to electrical signals. The console decodes these electrical signals to greyscale tomographic images based on the time delay (depth) and intensity (brightness) of the reflected signals. The operating frequency varies between 20 and 60 MHz and resolution ranges between 40 and 200 μ. The enhanced depth penetration (10 mm) of IVUS enables the assessment of plaque burden accurately [2].

OCT is an optical equivalent of IVUS that uses near infra-red light in place of ultrasound to create high resolution images of the coronary artery. Similar to IVUS, OCT images are also constructed by measuring the echo time delay (depth) and intensity (brightness) of the backscattered optical signals from the different interfaces of the vessel wall. In contrast to IVUS, the speed of light (3×10^8 m/s) necessitates the use of an interferometer to measure the echo time delays of the reflected light waves. The ultra-high frequency of the light enables 10–15 μ resolution, but on the other hand, restricts tissue penetration to 1–2 mm. Red blood cells scatter light intensely, hence contrast injection to clear blood from the coronary artery is essential for good quality imaging by OCT [2].

INTRAVASCULAR IMAGING: TISSUE CHARACTERISATION

A normal adult coronary artery has a three layered structure: echogenic intima, echolucent media and echogenic adventitia (bright-dark-bright pattern) (Figure 7.1a,b). Tissue characterisation by greyscale IVUS is based on the echo reflectivity of intimal plaque with reference to that of adventitia: (1) *fibrocalcific plaque*: a structure which is hyperechoic to adventitia with acoustic shadowing and reverberations, (2) *fibrous plaque*: a structure which is isoechoic to adventitia, and (3) *soft plaque*: a structure which is hypoechoic to adventitia [3] (Figure 7.1c–e). OCT tissue characterisation is based on the intensity of backscatter, signal attenuation, tissue texture and delineation of plaque borders: (1) *fibrous plaque*: a homogeneous structure with high backscatter and low attenuation; (2) *fibro-calcific plaque*: heterogeneous structure with low backscatter, low attenuation with well-defined borders; and (3) *lipidic plaque*: a homogeneous structure with low backscatter, high attenuation with ill-defined borders [4] (Figure 7.1f–h).

INTRAVASCULAR IMAGING IN ACS

IVI plays an important role in the evaluation of patients with ACS. Although both IVUS and OCT are used for the assessment of these lesions, the superior resolution of OCT makes it better suited for this purpose. The various roles of IVI in patients with ACS are as follows: (1) assessment of plaque vulnerability, (2) evaluation of thrombus, (3) identification of underlying pathology, (4) prediction of no-reflow and (5) sizing and optimisation of stent.

ASSESSMENT OF PLAQUE VULNERABILITY

Vulnerable plaque is one which predisposes the patient to clinical events by rapid progression or thrombosis. It is characterised by expansive remodelling, large lipid content/necrotic core, thin fibrous cap (<65 μ), inflammation, spotty calcification, neoangiogenesis and intraplaque haemorrhage. Detection of such plaques may help in implementing treatment strategies that reduce progression to ACS [5].

IVI modalities help in the identification of these high-risk features *in vivo* and also monitor their response to treatment. The greyscale IVUS features of vulnerability are positive remodelling, large eccentric plaque, spotty calcification, signal attenuation (attenuated plaque) and intraplaque echolucency (echolucent plaque) (Figure 7.2a,b). However, lower resolution of greyscale IVUS limits its precision to detect thin cap fibrous atheroma (TCFA), neovascularisation and inflammation [5].

Addition of radiofrequency data to the greyscale IVUS (virtual histology, VH) improves its sensitivity to detect plaque vulnerability accurately. VH defined TCFA (confluent necrotic core abutting to >30% of luminal border) is an important predictor of future adverse events (Figure 7.2c). In the PROSPECT (Providing Regional Observations to Study Predictors of Events in the Coronary Tree) study, VH-TCFA along with a lumen area ≤4 mm^2 and a plaque burden of ≥70% predicted non-culprit lesion related adverse events during follow-up [6].

With its high resolution, OCT detects features of plaque vulnerability with greater accuracy. OCT features such as large lipid content (lipid involving >180° of circumference), thin fibrous cap (cap thickness <65 μ), microchannels (intraplaque signal voids of 50–200 μ diameter), macrophages (signal rich spots with shadowing), spotty calcification (calcium with an arc of <90°), and

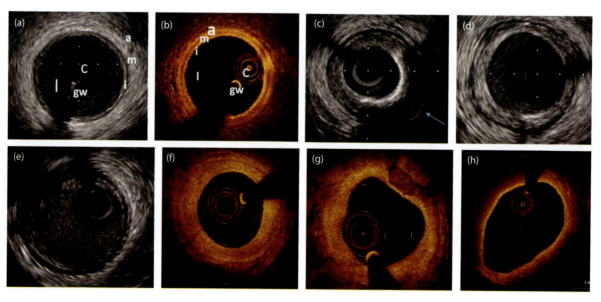

Figure 7.1 Normal coronary artery on IVUS (a) and OCT (b). c - Imaging catheter, gw - Guide wire, l - lumen, i - intima, m - media, a - adventitia. (c) IVUS fibrocalcific plaque – plaque between 2 o'clock and 7 o'clock is hyperechoic to adventitia with acoustic shadowing and reverberations (blue arrow). (d) IVUS fibrous plaque – concentric plaque which is isoechoic to adventitia. (e) IVUS soft plaque – plaque between 8 o'clock and 11 o'clock is hypoechoic to adventitia. (f) OCT fibrous plaque – concentric plaque which is homogeneous with high backscatter and low attenuation. (g) OCT fibro-calcific plaque: heterogeneous structure with low backscatter, low attenuation with well-defined borders between 1 o'clock and 3 o'clock. (h) OCT lipidic plaque: a homogeneous structure with low backscatter, high attenuation with ill-defined borders.

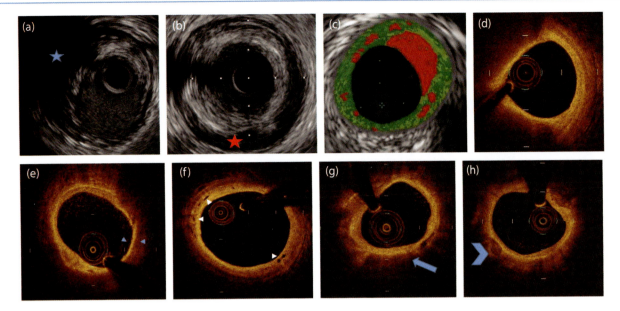

Figure 7.2 Features of plaque vulnerability for rupture. (a) Attenuated plaque (blue star). (b) Echolucent plaque (red star). Attenuated plaque indicates large lipid/necrotic core content. Echolucent plaque indicates smaller lipid/necrotic core content. (c) VH thin-cap fibroatheroma. (d–h) OCT features of plaque vulnerability. (d) Lipid-rich plaque. (e) Thin-cap fibroatheroma (arrow heads indicate thin-fibrous cap). (f) Microvessels (white arrow heads). (g) Macrophage accumulation (arrow). (h) Spotty calcification (arrow head).

intraluminal thrombi have been associated with rapid progression of plaque during follow-up examinations (Figure 7.2d–h) [7].

It is important to understand that the natural history of vulnerable plaque is difficult to predict as some of the TCFAs detected by IVI stabilise over a period of time, and some of the fibroatheromas with thick fibrous cap may transform into TCFA. Thus, the treatment should be tailored to address the risk profile of the patient as a whole instead of basing it solely on the IVI finding of vulnerable plaque [8].

EVALUATION OF THROMBUS

Intracoronary thrombus is the most common underlying mechanism of sudden lumen narrowing in patients presenting with ACS. Both the quality and quantity of thrombus at the culprit site determines the outcome of PCI in this subset of patients. Although CAG remains the common modality for invasive evaluation of coronary anatomy, it has a very limited role in the detection and quantification of intracoronary thrombus. Similarly, the sensitivity of IVUS for identification of thrombus is low and, in addition, it cannot differentiate between white and red thrombus [2].

In contrast, OCT can detect intracoronary thrombus with high sensitivity and the light reflective properties of the red blood cells allow exact differentiation of white from red thrombus. OCT also enables quantitative assessment of thrombus.

Thrombus usually appears as an intraluminal lobulated or pedunculated mass with a clear interface from the underlying intima (Figure 7.3a) when imaged by IVUS. On OCT imaging, red thrombus has a high backscattering surface and a high attenuating deeper part (Figure 7.3b), whereas white thrombus has a high backscatter on the surface and low attenuation in the deeper part (Figure 7.3c). A mixed thrombus has properties of both white and red thrombi. Recanalised thrombus has a lotus root or Swiss cheese appearance (Figure 7.3d,e) [2].

The clinical utility of OCT in the evaluation of thrombus is three-fold: (1) identification of angiographically occult culprit lesion, (2) quantification of intracoronary thrombus burden and (3) evaluation of response to treatment [9].

1. *Identification of angiographically occult culprit lesion:* It is not uncommon for patients presenting with ACS to have multiple complex lesions on angiography. Presence of thrombus indicates recent activation of the atherosclerotic plaque and that separates the culprit lesion from bystander non-culprit lesions. OCT with its higher resolution clearly

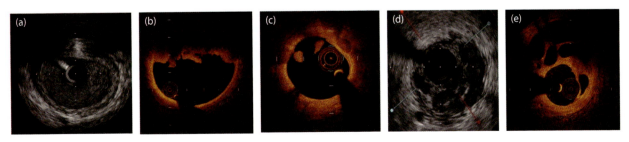

Figure 7.3 IVI examples of thrombi: (a) IVUS thrombus (intraluminal mass at 3 o'clock position). (b) Red thrombus (intraluminal mass between 9 o'clock and 3 o'clock). (c) White thrombus (11 o'clock and 1 o'clock positions). (d) IVUS and (e) OCT Recanalized thrombus: showing Swiss cheese appearance.

identifies thrombus in culprit lesions, thus avoiding over-treatment of stable non-culprit lesions [9].

2. *Quantification of intracoronary thrombus burden and guiding treatment strategy:* OCT enables quantitative evaluation of intracoronary thrombus with high accuracy. Various quantitative parameters, based on area, volume and the quadrants of cross-sectional area occupied by thrombus, have been proposed in different studies. This additional information helps in selecting different treatment strategies such as direct stenting in case of small thrombus burden, and manual/mechanical thrombus aspiration versus establishment of flow followed by pharmacotherapy [9].

3. *Assessment of response to treatment:* OCT evaluation following treatment can identify residual thrombus burden, which enables decisions regarding further thrombus aspiration, stenting or no stenting. Similarly, in patients with large intra-stent thrombus, OCT helps in assessing response to thrombus aspiration and prolonged balloon dilatation [9].

ACS PATHOLOGY AND RESPONSE TO TREATMENT

Coronary thrombosis in ACS commonly results from three basic pathologies: plaque rupture (PR), plaque erosion (PE) and calcified nodule (CN). PR results from disruption of the fibrous cap overlying a TCFA and accounts for 65% of all ACS cases. Fibrous cap damage directly exposes highly thrombogenic necrotic core to the circulating elements of blood promoting thrombosis. PE results from disruption of the endothelial layer covering the plaque and constitutes up to one-third of ACS cases. CN accounts for the remaining cases and results from fibrous cap disruption

Table 7.1 IVI definition ACS pathologies

1. *Plaque rupture:* Intraplaque cavity communicating with the lumen and fibrous cap remnants (Figure 7.4a,b).
2. *Plaque erosion:* Definite erosion – thrombus attached to a visualised intact fibrous cap (Figure 7.4c). *Probable erosion* – irregular lumen surface with no thrombus or luminal thrombus in the absence of adjacent superficial calcium or lipid/necrotic core when the underlying plaque is not visible (Figure 7.4d).
3. *Calcified nodules:* Protruding nodular calcification with dorsal shadowing (Figure 7.4e,f).

Source: Subban V et al. *Indian Heart J Interv.* 2018;1:71–94.

by protruding nodular calcification [10]. IVI definitions of ACS pathologies are summarised in Table 7.1.

Two recent studies analysed the morphological characteristics of culprit plaques in ACS and compared their post-procedure outcomes [11,12].

Saia et al. [11] evaluated 140 STEMI patients with OCT imaging before and after placement of stent and at 9-months postprocedure. Culprit lesion morphology was clearly identified in 97 patients: PR in 63 (64.9%), PE in 32 (33.0%) and spontaneous coronary dissection (SCAD) in 2 (2.1%). PE was more often associated with a patent infarct related artery (IRA), and a lower peak creatinine kinase myocardial band levels. In addition, PE patients had smaller volumes of both red and white thrombi before PCI, more fibrotic areas and fewer lipid areas at the lesion site, a lower number of TCFA along the IRA, and similar lumen areas. There

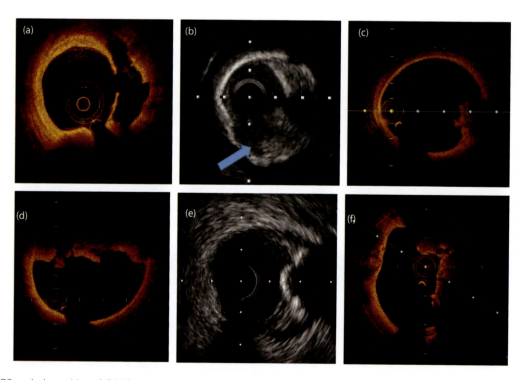

Figure 7.4 ACS pathology. (a) and (b) Plaque rupture. (a) OCT image showing evidence of fibrous cap rupture with underlying cavity at 3 o'clock position. (b) IVUS image showing plaque rupture with underlying cavity containing thrombus (arrow). (c) OCT definitive erosion (intact fibrous cap with attached red thrombus). (d) OCT probable erosion (large red thrombus with no adjacent necrotic core/lipid or superficial calcium [not shown in the figure]). (e) and (f) Calcified nodules (2 to 5 o'clock position).

was no difference in the mean stent area, stent expansion index, malapposition area and volume of tissue protrusion at the time of index procedure and strut coverage and percentage volume obstruction at 9-month follow-up. The clinical outcomes were not different between the groups up to 2 years follow-up.

In another study, Higuma et al. [12] assessed 112 STEMI patients following thrombus aspiration with both IVUS and OCT imaging. Culprit lesion pathology was PR in 72 (64.3%), PE in 30 (26.8%), CN in 9 (8.0%) and SCAD in the remaining patient (0.9%). IVUS detected only 17 (23.6%) PR identified with OCT. Compared with PR, the prevalence of fibrous plaque was significantly higher, and lipid plaque and TCFA were lower in both PE and CN. Microchannels were less prevalent with PE compared to PR. Although there was no difference in the prevalence and arc of calcium between the groups, the location was deeper in PE. In CN, the calcium was more often located superficially and the arc was larger than the other groups. Compared with PR, PE was associated with smaller plaque burden, larger lumen cross-sectional area and greater eccentricity index. Positive remodelling was noted more often with PR and negative remodelling with CN. PE was associated with lower incidence of no reflow compared to PR.

PATHOLOGY-TARGETED THERAPY IN ACS

PR is the most common mechanism of ACS and the therapeutic strategies for the treatment of ACS are focussed on the pathophysiology of it. PR is associated with gross changes in the vessel architecture with positive remodelling, large PB, TCFA, fibrous cap rupture, intraplaque cavity and importantly a small residual lumen area. Further, the thrombus burden is large and the necrotic core elements serve as a persistent stimulus for thrombus formation at the lesion site. This results in high re-occlusion rates in the thrombolytic trials. Thus, stent implantation along with potent antithrombotic therapy is the standard of care in ACS patients with PR [13,14].

In contrast, in PE, the vessel wall architecture is mostly preserved and once the thrombus resolves, a non-flow limiting plaque with low vulnerability remains. In addition, the fibrous cap is intact and the plaque core is not exposed. The thrombotic stimulus is limited to the disrupted endothelium that can be readily controlled with antithrombotic treatment. Thus, a large proportion of patients with PE may be treated with just antithrombotic and secondary prevention strategies. Given the risk of stent thrombosis (ST), instent-restenosis (ISR) and dual anti-platelet therapy (DAPT) related bleeding, this strategy may improve the long-term outcome of this subgroup of patients. This novel approach was evaluated in three registries: two retrospective and one prospective.

In a study by Prati et al. [15], 31 patients with OCT identified PE were treated either with thrombectomy alone (no stent group, n = 12) or thrombectomy and stenting (stent group, n = 19). Four patients in either group were treated with GP IIb-IIIa inhibitor. All patients received DAPT (aspirin + clopidogrel or prasugrel). The median follow-up period was 753 days. One patient in the stent group underwent repeat revascularisation and there was no death, myocardial infarction (MI) or heart failure admission in either group.

Hu et al. [16] retrospectively analysed the treatment strategies and clinical outcomes of 141 ACS patients evaluated with preprocedure OCT imaging. The mechanism of ACS was PR in 79 (56%) and PE in 62 (44%). Patients with PE were younger and more often presented with non-ST-segment elevation myocardial infarction (NSTEMI) compared to patients with PR. PE was associated with larger mean lumen diameter, smaller diameter stenosis and lower incidence of multi-vessel disease. Seventy-seven (97.5%) in the PR group and 49 (79%) patients in the PE received stenting (p < 0.001). PR patients had significantly higher incidence of malapposition, thrombus and tissue prolapse. PE was associated with lower incidence of distal embolisation and no-reflow. The 1-year event rate was not different between the groups and none of the patients treated without stenting suffered adverse events.

The EROSION (effective antithrombotic therapy without stenting: intravascular optical coherence tomography-based management in plaque erosion) study [17] evaluated prospectively the strategy of antithrombotic treatment alone in patients with OCT-detected PE and non-critical angiographic stenosis (<70%) at the culprit site. Fifty-five patients met the inclusion criteria and were included in the final analysis. Thrombus aspiration was performed in 85% of the patients and 63.3% received GP IIb/IIIa inhibitor. At 1 month OCT follow-up, the primary end point (>50% reduction in thrombus volume) was met in 47 patients and 22 of them did not have any visible thrombus. In addition, there was a reduction in thrombus volume (3.7 mm^3 to 0.2 mm^3) and improvement in minimal flow area (1.7 mm^2 to 2.1 mm^2). One patient received repeat PCI and the remaining were asymptomatic. Forty-nine patients underwent repeat OCT imaging at 1-year follow-up. Although further thrombus reduction was observed between 1 month and 1 year (0.3 mm^3 vs. 0.1 mm^3, p = 0.001), there was no improvement in the minimal effective flow area (2.1 mm^2 vs. 2.1 mm^2, p = 0.152). The clinical end point of MACE (a composite of cardiac death, recurrent MI, ischaemia-driven target lesion revascularisation [TLR], stroke and major bleeding) developed in four patients (three revascularisations and one major bleed) [18].

Although OCT-guided pathology targeted therapy appears promising, we need more clarity on some aspects of this strategy: (1) PE constitutes one-third of patients with ACS and a proportion of them have flow limiting disease and need stenting. Hence, only a small fraction of ACS patients qualify for this conservative strategy. It is not cost effective to evaluate all the patients with ACS by OCT imaging to identify this small proportion of patients. Selective application of OCT imaging to patients with angiographically non-flow limiting stenosis needs further evaluation. (2) While thrombus in PE is predominantly platelet rich and responds well to anti-platelet treatment, the need for additional oral anti-coagulant therapy especially in the presence of predominantly red thrombus and a large thrombus burden is not known (Figure 7.5). (3) In the EROSION study, the final mean residual flow area at 1 year was 2.1 mm^2. Although this is similar to OCT cut off value for non-flow limiting stenoses in patients with stable angina whether these patients need to be evaluated with non-invasive stress test or intravascular physiology is not clear. (4) The OCT definition of PE is based on the exclusion of PR or CN. This makes the identification of PE difficult in clinical practice. (5) The current generation DES are associated with excellent long-term outcomes. So, the real advantage of antithrombotic-alone strategy needs to be evaluated against this gold standard treatment in large randomised trials [14,19].

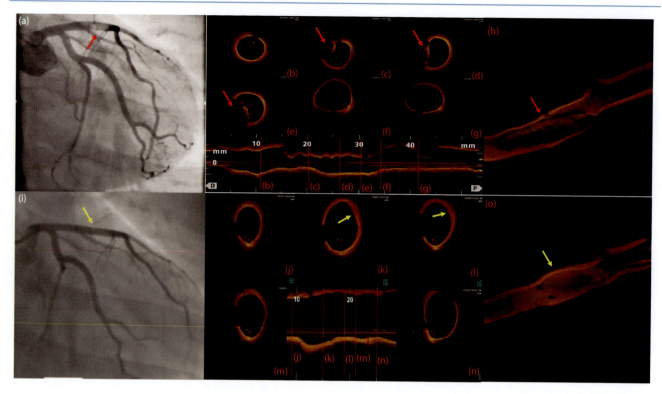

Figure 7.5 OCT guided treatment in ACS. (a) CAG showing a thrombotic lesion in proximal LAD (red arrow). OCT images (b – g) showing large red thrombus burden (red arrows) in proximal LAD with adequate residual lumen area. Patient was treated with a course of oral anti-coagulant therapy. Follow-up angiogram (I) revealed disappearance of haziness in the proximal LAD (yellow arrow). Follow-up OCT images (j – n) showed complete thrombus resolution with intimal thickening suggestive of plaque erosion (yellow arrows). (h&o) 3D OCT images baseline and post oral anti-coagulant therapy.

CALCIFIED NODULE

Calcified nodule (CN) is a less frequent cause of ACS with an overall prevalence of 2%–8% [20] that increases to 30% in ACS lesions associated with severe calcification [21]. It is most frequently observed in elderly patients and those with renal failure on haemodialysis. It is proposed to evolve from the fragmentation of the calcium sheets due to mechanical stress and thus more often observed in the mid-right coronary artery [20,21]. On IVI, it appears as a protruding calcific nodular mass with shadowing on the dorsal side. The exact treatment strategy for CN is not known. In ACS lesions with CN, thrombus burden is usually small and TCFA occurs less often and thus the treatment strategy is similar to that of calcified lesions [14]. Although stent under-expansion is commonly observed in calcified lesions, in a study by Lee et al. [21], stent expansion was similar in patients with or without CN. This was attributed to natural fractures observed in calcium sheets in lesions with CN. IVI helps in the treatment of CN by assessing its response to balloon dilatation/debulking strategies and confirming stent expansion (Figure 7.6). As with PE, patients with CN and large flow area on IVI may be left alone safely without stenting [22].

SPONTANEOUS CORONARY DISSECTION

SCAD indicates non-atherosclerotic/non-traumatic dissection of an epicardial coronary artery and accounts for 1%–4% of all ACS. Correct diagnosis of SCAD is important as the treatment is drastically different from that of atherosclerotic CAD [23,24].

CAG is the initial imaging modality for the assessment of patients suspected with SCAD. However, angiographic diagnosis is challenging as the typical appearance of multiple lumens and arterial wall staining occurs only in one-third of the patients. Thus, the guidelines recommend additional diagnostic imaging evaluation (IVUS or OCT) when there is high clinical suspicion of SCAD [24].

Diagnosis of SCAD on IVI is based on the identification of the intimo-medial membrane with a dual lumen or intramural hae-matoma (IMH, accumulation of blood in the medial space). OCT, with its higher resolution, clearly delineates lumen-intimal interface, intimal rupture and intraluminal thrombi. However, its poor depth penetration prevents evaluation of the full extent of the false lumen and haematoma. In addition, contrast flushing may further extend the dissection or haematoma. Although IVUS imaging fails to identify the intimal ruptures in most of the cases, it can visualise the full extent of IMH and false lumen even in large vessels. Moreover, it does not need contrast clearance and is possible to image through thrombus (Figure 7.7) [25].

Management of SCAD is mainly conservative as spontaneous healing occurs in most of the patients. Revascularisation is indicated only in the presence of persistent ischaemia, hemodynamic instability or severe left main coronary artery involvement. IVI provides important information on the position of wire in true versus false lumen, entry and exit tears, length of the haematoma, severity of the lumen narrowing, intraluminal thrombus, side branch involvement and reference vessel luminal dimensions. Treatment strategy is based on the presence and extent of the IMH. In the absence of IMH, a short stent is implanted at the site of maximum separation of the layers to tack down the dissection

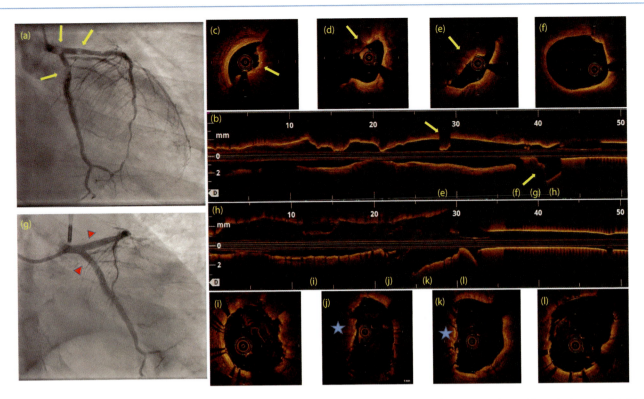

Figure 7.6 Calcified nodule. 60-year-old male, S/P renal transplant presented with ACS. (a) Angiogram showed hazy lesions in distal left main, proximal LAD, proximal LCX (yellow arrows). There was no change in the appearance after thrombus aspiration. (b – f) OCT imaging showed calcified nodules involving above areas (yellow arrows). (g) Lesion was prepared with cutting balloon and two drug eluting stents were implanted using double-kiss crush technique with good angiographic result (red arrow heads). (h – l) Post-stenting OCT imaging showed eccentrically expanded stent with tissue prolapse (blue star). (Courtesy: Dr Rony Mathew.)

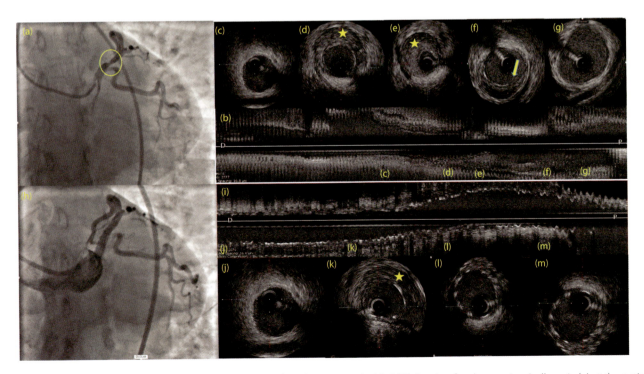

Figure 7.7 IVUS imaging in SCAD. (a) CAG in a 45-year-old female presented with ACS showing focal narrowing (yellow circle) at the ostio-proximal LAD. (b – g) IVUS longitudinal (b) and cross-sectional images (c – g) showing intramural hematoma extending from distal part of left main to mid LAD. (e) severe lumen narrowing at ostial LAD (stars indicate IMH). (f) Entry tear in left main (yellow arrow). In view of significant lumen narrowing and ischemic symptoms, patient underwent PCI with stent place from ostial left main to mid-LAD well beyond the distal extend of the hematoma (h). (i – m) longitudinal (l) and cross-sectional IVUS images (j – m) post-stenting.

plane. In the presence of haematoma and an entry only tear, the stent should be placed from distal to proximal, and in case of exit only tear, from proximal to distal to avoid haematoma propagation in the other direction [26]. In the absence of entry or exit tears, the ends of the haematoma may be stented first before tackling the middle part or a cutting balloon may be used to decompress the haematoma [27]. Further, IVI also helps in confirming full lesion coverage and stent optimisation [26].

CORONARY VASOSPASM

Coronary vasospasm is an important cause of ACS and should be considered in patients presenting with ACS and non-obstructive CAD. The prevalence of vasospasm in this population varies between 20% and 48.8% in different studies [28]. Coronary spasm may occur at sites with or without atheroma. The main role of OCT in patients with suspected spasm are to exclude other causes of ACS such as plaque erosion or SCAD and to identify angiographically invisible thrombus. The typical OCT appearances of coronary spasm are thickened media and intimal bumps (smooth intimal projections that disappear with nitroglycerine) in the resting state and intimal gathering (multiple intimal kinks or folds that resolve with nitroglycerine) in the spasmodic state [29]. In addition, there is higher prevalence of features of erosion (intact fibrous cap, lumen irregularity and thrombus) at the spasmodic sites compared to the normal segments [30]. In contrast, patients with chronic stable vasospastic angina less often demonstrate intimal tear, erosion or intraluminal thrombi and significantly lesser maximal intimal thickness in the spastic segment [31].

INTRAVASCULAR IMAGING-GUIDED INTERVENTION TO PREVENT NO-REFLOW

No-reflow during PCI adversely impacts both acute and long term outcomes [32]. Distal embolisation is an important predictor of no-reflow during PCI in ACS patients. Although embolic protection is expected to shield the distal circulation from embolisation, its routine use during primary PCI was not associated with reduction in the incidence of no-reflow [33,34]. The various predictors of no-reflow in ACS patients are attenuated plaque, positive remodelling (IVUS), TCFA, large lipid core, and thrombus (OCT) [35]. Thus, identification of these markers by IVI may enable selective use of embolic protection in high-risk patients.

The VAMPIRE 3 (Vacuum Aspiration Thrombus Removal 3) trial randomised 200 ACS patients with IVUS detected attenuated plaque ($\geq$5 mm in length) to either PCI with distal protection filter (Filtrap, Nipro, Tokyo, Japan) or standard care. Distal protection was associated with lower incidence of no-reflow (26.5% vs. 41.7%; p = 0.026), better TIMI frame count (23.0 vs. 30.5; p = 0.0003) and fewer in-hospital adverse events. However, myocardial blush grade or cardiac enzyme elevation were similar between the groups [36]. Although this imaging guided selective use of embolic protection is promising, its impact on hard end points and cost effectiveness needs to be evaluated in large clinical trials.

Table 7.2 IVI Stent sizing and optimisation criteria

Stent sizing

Diameter: Mean distal lumen diameter up-rounding to the nearest 0.25 mm stent diameter or mean EEL diameter down-rounding to the nearest 0.25 mm stent diameter

Landing zone: Plaque burden <50%, absence of lipid-rich plaque

Length: Distance between the two landing zones

Stent optimisation targets

Expansion: MSA > 80% of the average reference lumen area or >5.5 mm² (IVUS)/>4.5 mm² (OCT)

Apposition: Malapposition axial distance <400 µ and <1 mm length

Dissection: <60° Vessel circumference, flap limited to intima and <2 mm in length and no intramural or extramural haematoma

Landing zone: Plaque burden <50%, absence of lipid-rich plaque

Tissue protrusion: <10% of stent area

IMAGING-GUIDED STENT IMPLANTATION

The most important role of IVI during PCI is stent sizing and optimisation. The stent sizing may be based either on the mean lumen or external elastic membrane diameters of the distal reference vessel. Post-stenting, IVI identifies parameters of suboptimal deployment such as underexpansion, malapposition, geographic miss, edge dissection, haematoma, and tissue prolapse [37]. Table 7.2 summarises the commonly used stent sizing and optimisation criteria.

CONCLUSION

ACS represents a spectrum with various underlying pathologic abnormalities. IVI helps in precise delineation of the underlying abnormality that enables individualised pathology focussed management of ACS and avoids unnecessary stenting in a significant proportion of patients. In addition, IVI also provides valuable information on risk of no-reflow and thrombus burden and its response to treatment. Importantly, it helps in stent selection and optimisation. Though IVI shows lots of promise in the evaluation of patients presenting with ACS, we need large randomised studies before widespread application of this technology.

REFERENCES

1. Amabile N, Hammas S, Fradi S et al. Intra-coronary thrombus evolution during acute coronary syndrome: Regression assessment by serial optical coherence tomography analyses. *Eur Heart J Cardiovasc Imaging.* 2015;16:433–440.
2. Subban V, Raffel OC, Victor SM, Vasu N, Ajit MS. Intravascular ultrasound and optical coherence tomography for the assessment of coronary artery disease and percutaneous coronary intervention optimization—The basics. *Indian Heart J Interv.* 2018;1:71–94.

3. Mintz GS, Nissen SE, Anderson WD et al. American College of Cardiology clinical expert consensus document on standards for acquisition, measurement and reporting of IntraVascular Ultrasound Studies (IVUS). A report of the American College of Cardiology Task Force on clinical expert consensus documents. *J Am Coll Cardiol.* 2001;37:1478–1492.

4. Tearney GJ, Regar E, Akasaka T et al. International Working Group for Intravascular Optical Coherence Tomography (IWG-IVOCT). Consensus standards for acquisition, measurement, and reporting of intravascular optical coherence tomography studies: A report from the International Working Group for Intravascular Optical Coherence Tomography standardization and validation. *J Am Coll Cardiol.* 2012;59:1058–1072.

5. Vancraeynest D, Pasquet A, Roelants V, Gerber BL, Vanoverschelde JL. Imaging the vulnerable plaque. *J Am Coll Cardiol.* 2011;57:1961–1979.

6. Stone GW, Maehara A, Lansky AJ et al.; PROSPECT Investigators. A prospective natural-history study of coronary atherosclerosis. *N Engl J Med.* 2011;364:226–235.

7. Uemura S, Ishigami K, Soeda T et al. Thin-cap fibroatheroma and microchannel findings in optical coherence tomography correlate with subsequent progression of coronary atheromatous plaques. *Eur Heart J.* 2012;33:78–85.

8. Narula J, Kovacic JC. Putting TCFA in clinical perspective. *J Am Coll Cardiol.* 2014;64:681–683.

9. Porto I, Mattesini A, Valente S, Prati F, Crea F, Bolognese L. Optical coherence tomography assessment and quantification of intracoronary thrombus: Status and perspectives. *Cardiovasc Revasc Med.* 2015;16:172–178.

10. Yahagi K, Kolodgie FD, Otsuka F et al. Pathophysiology of native coronary, vein graft, and in-stent atherosclerosis. *Nat Rev Cardiol.* 2016;13:79–98.

11. Saia F, Komukai K, Capodanno D et al. Eroded versus ruptured plaques at the culprit site of STEMI: In vivo pathophysiological features and response to primary PCI. *JACC Cardiovasc Imaging.* 2015;8:566–575.

12. Higuma T, Soeda T, Abe N et al. A combined optical coherence tomography and intravascular ultrasound study on plaque rupture, plaque erosion, and calcified nodule in patients with ST-segment elevation myocardial infarction: Incidence, morphologic characteristics, and outcomes after percutaneous coronary intervention. *JACC Cardiovasc Interv.* 2015;8:1166–1176.

13. Stone GW, Narula J. Emergence of plaque erosion as an important clinical entity. *JACC Cardiovasc Imaging.* 2015; 8:623–625.

14. Holmes DR Jr, Lerman A, Moreno PR, King SB 3rd, Sharma SK. Diagnosis and management of STEMI arising from plaque erosion. *JACC Cardiovasc Imaging.* 2013;6:290–296.

15. Prati F, Uemura S, Souteyrand G et al. OCT-based diagnosis and management of STEMI associated with intact fibrous cap. *JACC Cardiovasc Imaging.* 2013;6:283–287.

16. Hu S, Zhu Y, Zhang Y et al. Management and outcome of patients with acute coronary syndrome caused by plaque rupture versus plaque erosion: An intravascular optical coherence tomography study. *J Am Heart Assoc.* 2017;6:e004730.

17. Jia H, Dai J, Hou J et al. Effective anti-thrombotic therapy without stenting: Intravascular optical coherence tomography-based management in plaque erosion (the EROSION study). *Eur Heart J.* 2017;38:792–800.

18. Xing L, Yamamoto E, Sugiyama T et al. EROSION study (Effective Anti-Thrombotic Therapy Without Stenting: Intravascular Optical Coherence Tomography-Based Management in Plaque Erosion): A 1-year follow-up report. *Circ Cardiovasc Interv.* 2017 Dec;10. pii: e005860.

19. Alfonso F, Rivero F. Antithrombotic therapy alone for plaque erosion: Ready for a paradigm shift in acute coronary syndromes? *Circ Cardiovasc Interv.* 2017;10. pii: e006143.

20. Otsuka F, Joner M, Prati F, Virmani R, Narula J. Clinical classification of plaque morphology in coronary disease. *Nat Rev Cardiol.* 2014;11:379–389.

21. Lee T, Mintz GS, Matsumura M et al. Prevalence, predictors, and clinical presentation of a calcified nodule as assessed by optical coherence tomography. *JACC Cardiovasc Imaging.* 2017;10:883–891.

22. Xu Y, Mintz GS, Tam A et al. Prevalence, distribution, predictors, and outcomes of patients with calcified nodules in native coronary arteries: A 3-vessel intravascular ultrasound analysis from Providing Regional Observations to Study Predictors of Events in the Coronary Tree (PROSPECT). *Circulation.* 2012;126:537–545.

23. Alfonso F, García-Guimaraes M, Bastante T et al. Spontaneous coronary artery dissection: From expert consensus statements to evidence-based medicine. *J Thorac Dis.* 2018;10:4602–4608.

24. Hayes SN, Kim ESH, Saw J et al. Spontaneous Coronary Artery Dissection: Current state of the science: A scientific statement from the American Heart Association. *Circulation.* 2018;137:e523–e557.

25. Paulo M, Sandoval J, Lennie V et al. Combined use of OCT and IVUS in spontaneous coronary artery dissection. *JACC Cardiovasc Imaging.* 2013;6:830–832.

26. Poon K. Spontaneous coronary artery dissection. In: Jang IK, Editor. *Cadiovascular OCT Imaging.* 1st ed. Switzerland: Springer International Publishing. 2015; 119–128.

27. Yumoto K, Sasaki H, Aoki H, Kato K. Successful treatment of spontaneous coronary artery dissection with cutting balloon angioplasty as evaluated with optical coherence tomography. *JACC Cardiovasc Interv.* 2014;7:817–819.

28. Kanwar SS, Stone GW, Singh M, Virmani R, Olin J, Akasaka T, Narula J. Acute coronary syndromes without coronary plaque rupture. *Nat Rev Cardiol.* 2016;13:257–265.

29. Tanaka A, Shimada K, Tearney GJ et al. Conformational change in coronary artery structure assessed by optical coherence tomography in patients with vasospastic angina. *J Am Coll Cardiol.* 2011;58:1608–1613.

30. Shin ES, Ann SH, Singh GB et al. OCT-defined morphological characteristics of coronary artery spasmsites in vasospastic angina. *JACC Cardiovasc Imaging.* 2015;8:1059–1067.

31. Park HC, Shin JH, Jeong WK, Choi SI, Kim SG. Comparison of morphologic findings obtained by optical coherence tomography in acute coronary syndrome caused by vasospasm and chronic stable variant angina. *Int J Cardiovasc Imaging.* 2015;31:229–237.

32. Chan W, Stub D, Clark DJ et al. Usefulness of transient and persistent no reflow to predict adverse clinical outcomes following percutaneous coronary intervention. *Am J Cardiol.* 2012;109:478–485.

33. Jang JS, Jin HY, Seo JS et al. Meta-analysis of plaque composition by intravascular ultrasound and its relation to distal embolization after percutaneous coronary intervention. *Am J Cardiol*. 2013;111:968–972.

34. Kelbaek H, Terkelsen CJ, Helqvist S et al. Randomized comparison of distal protection versus conventional treatment in primary percutaneous coronary intervention: The drug elution and distal protection in ST-elevation myocardial infarction (DEDICATION) trial. *J Am Coll Cardiol*. 2008;51:899–905.

35. Claessen BE, Maehara A, Fahy M, Xu K, Stone GW, Mintz GS. Plaque composition by intravascular ultrasound and distal embolization after percutaneous coronary intervention. *JACC Cardiovasc Imaging*. 2012;5:S111–S118.

36. Hibi K, Kozuma K, Sonoda S et al. A randomized study of distal filter protection versus conventional treatment during percutaneous coronary intervention in patients with attenuated plaque identified by intravascular ultrasound. *JACC Cardiovasc Interv*. 2018;11:1545–1555.

37. Räber L, Mintz GS, Koskinas KC et al. Clinical use of intracoronary imaging. Part 1: Guidance and optimization of coronary interventions. An expert consensus document of the European Association of Percutaneous Cardiovascular Interventions. *Eur Heart J*. 2018;39:3281–3300.

8

Cardiac biomarkers in acute coronary syndrome

RK JAIN AND GEETESH MANIK

INTRODUCTION

Acute coronary syndrome (ACS) is a broad term which encompasses thrombotic coronary artery diseases, including unstable angina (UA) and both ST-segment elevation (STEMI) and non-ST-segment elevation myocardial infarction (NSTEMI). Approximately 15–20 million patients per year present to the emergency department (ED) with acute chest pain or other symptoms suggestive of ACS in Europe and the United States. India has the highest burden of ACS in the world. The CREATE Registry has provided contemporary data on 20,468 patients from 89 centres from 10 regions and 50 cities in India [1]. The risk of death and the benefit from early revascularisation are highest within the first hours; therefore, early diagnosis is critical. As about two-thirds of these patients will be found not to have ACS, rule-in and rule-out seem to be equally important [2,4].

It is evident that the epidemiological importance of the phenomenon, the potentially lethal consequences for the patient, and the economical and legal implications for clinicians create the need of an adequate strategy of diagnostic and therapeutic management, including risk stratification and prevention of possible new events.

Cardiac markers are used in the diagnosis and risk stratification of patients with chest pain and suspected acute coronary syndrome (ACS). The cardiac troponins, in particular, have become the cardiac markers of choice for patients with ACS. Indeed, cardiac troponin is central to the definition of acute myocardial infarction (MI) in the consensus guidelines from the European Society of Cardiology (ESC) and the American College of Cardiology (ACC): These guidelines recommend that cardiac biomarkers should be measured at presentation in patients with suspected MI, and that the only biomarker that is recommended to be used for the diagnosis of acute MI at this time is cardiac troponin due to its superior sensitivity and accuracy [5–7].

TRADITIONAL CARDIAC BIOMARKERS

CREATINE KINASE (CK) AND CREATINE KINASE-MB (CK-MB)

CK-MB is a CK isoenzyme, predominantly found in the myocardium. Its elevation occurs 4–6 hours after the onset of myocardial necrosis and remains for 24–48 hours. CK-MB sensitivity and specificity in detecting myocardial injury can be increased by serial testing. CK-MB is relatively sensitive, but its specificity is affected by the presence of this marker in skeletal muscle. Elevation in CK-MB, in fact, may occur as a result of occasional analytical interferences and in patients with trauma, rhabdomyolysis, myopathies, renal failure or during the peripartum period. To improve its specificity, it was proposed to use CK-MB relative index (CK-MB/total CK). Ratios greater than 2.5% are considered suggestive of myocardial damage. CK-MB mass, CK-MB activity and total CK are more specific than myoglobin, but may not be detectable for 4–6 hours in the bloodstream following myocardial injury. The sensitivity of CK-MB mass for AMI is only 50% when measured early at the time of presentation. In clinical practice, peak levels of markers of necrosis and area under the time release curve of CK-MB from repetitive serial samplings are used to estimate infarct size [8,9].

CARDIAC TROPONIN T (cTnT) AND I (cTnI)

Cardiac troponin T (cTnT) and cardiac troponin I (cTnI) are more sensitive and specific markers than CK-MB in detecting myocardial necrosis and have become the preferred biomarkers for the diagnosis of AMI. Troponin is a complex of three proteins that is integral to muscle contraction in skeletal and cardiac muscle, regulating the calcium-mediated interaction between actin and myosin. Its three subunits are TnC, TnI and TnT. Troponin C binds to calcium ions in order to produce movement; troponin T binds to tropomyosin, interlocking it to form a troponin-tropomyosin complex; troponin I binds to actin in thin myofilaments to hold the troponin-tropomyosin complex in place. Troponin C has an identical amino-acid sequence in both skeletal and cardiac tissues and, thus, it has no potential as a cardiac specific marker. However, troponin T and troponin I have different isoforms in cardiac and skeletal muscle, encoded by separated genes, and consequently, have different amino-acid sequences. The respective cardiac isoforms of TnT (cTnT) and TnI (cTnI) allow production of antibodies that exclusively recognize these myocardial-specific proteins. Higher diagnostic sensitivity and specificity require specimen collection at patient presentation, 6–9 hours later and at 12–24 hours if clinical suspicion is high and earlier results are negative. Indeed, troponin is not considered as an early biomarker of myocardial necrosis: cardiac troponins need 4–10 hours after symptoms onset to appear in serum, and peak at 12–48 hours, remaining then abnormal for several days to two weeks [10–12].

Increase in troponin levels represents a powerful marker of high short-term risk of death or non-fatal myocardial infarction in patients with non-ST-elevation acute coronary syndromes (NSTE-ACS); it is one of the indicators for an early invasive strategy, according to the American College of Cardiology/American Heart Association guidelines (ACC/AHA). There is also a relationship between the severity of the infarct and the duration of the elevated serum cardiac troponins. The new global definition of myocardial infarction receives and organizes these observations defining any amount of cardiac troponin >99th percentile (10% coefficient of variation method) as myocardial infarction. Although cardiac troponins are specific of cardiac damage, they cannot be considered as the definitive marker of myocardial ischaemic injury [13]. Troponin release occurs due to non-ischaemic cardiac damage, too, causing 'false positive' elevations: myopericarditis, aortic dissection, aortic valve disease, hypertrophic cardiomyopathy, cardiac contusion or other trauma, tachy- or bradyarrhythmias, apical ballooning syndrome, and congestive heart failure. Furthermore, elevation of cardiac troponin can also occur in non-primary cardiac pathologies, such as acute neurological diseases, including stroke or sub-arachnoid haemorrhage, infiltrative diseases, drug toxicity or toxins, or burns affecting >30% of body surface area. Another important clinical challenge is the significance of elevated concentrations of cTnT commonly found in patients with renal failure but no clinical signs of recent myocardial damage; even in this setting, however, raised levels of troponin are associated with adverse cardiac prognosis [11,15].

There are a few methodological problems, in particular the lack of standardisation of assays for cTnI. More than 15 companies presently market assays for cTnI employing different standard materials and antibodies with different epitope specificities. Consequently, different results from different cTnI systems and assay generations may be obtained and this problem may cloud the interpretations of reported data, creating a substantial problem for the clinical and laboratory communities [16].

B-TYPE NATRIURETIC PEPTIDE (BNP)

The predominant stimulus controlling the synthesis and release of BNP from cardiac atria and ventricles is wall stretch. In general,

the plasma concentrations of these peptides are increased in diseases characterised by an expanded fluid volume, such as renal failure, primary aldosteronism and congestive heart failure (CHF), or by stimulation of peptide production caused by ventricular hypertrophy or strain, thyroid disease, excessive circulating glucocorticoids or hypoxia. Natriuretic peptides inhibit renin-angiotensin-aldosterone axis, increasing diuresis and reducing ventricular preload and arterial blood pressure, and inhibit central sympathetic outflow and catecholamine release from peripheral sympathetic neurons. The clinical usefulness of cardiac natriuretic peptides (especially BNP and NT-proBNP) in the evaluation of patients with suspected heart failure, in prognostic stratification of patients with CHF, in detecting LV systolic or diastolic dysfunction and in the differential diagnosis of dyspnoea was confirmed [17,18]. In general, heart failure is unlikely at BNP values <100 pg/mL and is very likely at BNP values >500 pg/mL and, similarly, unlikely at NT-proBNP values <300 pg/mL and very likely at NT-proBNP values >450 pg/mL (>900 pg/mL in patients above 50 years of age) [19]. Although originally BNP and NT-proBNP were considered biomarkers for heart failure only, now they are also considered biomarkers of myocardial ischaemia. Elevated BNP and NT-pro-BNP levels have been observed in patients with stable coronary artery disease (CAD), in patients with UA and during and after percutaneous coronary intervention (PCI) [20]. Recent studies suggest that the augmented release of BNP following brief periods of ischaemia occurs without concomitant change in LV end diastolic pressure, suggesting that ischaemia per se is the stimulus for BNP release. This association was observed across the spectrum of ACS, including patients with STEMI, NSTEMI and UA, those with and without elevated cardiac troponins, and those with and without clinical evidence of heart failure. In a recent analysis made by the group of Sabatine in 450 patients of the OPUS-TIMI 14 and in 1635 patients of the TACTICS-TIMI18 in which was investigated an approach with multiple markers in ACS without ST elevation, BNP, C-reactive protein (CRP) and cTnI were all independent predictors of adverse outcome. The incidence of the adverse events not only correlated with the positivity of each marker but also with the number of positive markers. Although patients with the worse prognosis (with a relative risk of death to 30 days between 6.0 and 13.0) were those with combined increase of levels of cTnI (marker of thrombosis and myocardial necrosis), of CRP (expression of inflammatory status) and of BNP (marker of myocardial dysfunction). Similar results were reported for the predictive value of BNP and NT-proBNP after STEMI [21–23].

C-REACTIVE PROTEIN (CRP)

CRP is the most widely studied inflammation marker. CRP is a pentraxin, synthesized by the liver after stimulation by cytokines, especially IL-6, IL-1β and TNF-α, in response to tissue injury or infection. The advantages of CRP as an inflammatory biomarker are related in part to analytic properties (such as the availability of low-cost, accurate high-sensitivity assay) and in part to its biological profile, including a long half-life (19 hours). Liuzzo et al. showed that patients presenting with unstable angina and elevated plasma concentrations of CRP had a higher rate of death, AMI and need for revascularisation compared with patients without elevated concentrations [24,25].

A variety of cut-off points have been used in clinical studies of CRP in ACS, leaving some uncertainty about the optimal decision limits. In primary prevention studies, the relationship is graded with a very low risk reported for CRP levels <1.0 mg/L, intermediate risk between 1 and 3 and high risk above 3 mg/L [26]. Liuzzo et al. used a cut-off of 3 mg/L based on the 90th percentile of a normal distribution. Dichotomised at this cut-off point, CRP identified patients at increased risk of in-hospital recurrent ischaemic events. Biasucci et al. observed that levels of CRP >3 mg/L at discharge distinguished those patients at higher risk of cardiovascular events. However, the majority of studies with CRP assessed at entry for ACS have found 10 mg/L as an optimal cut-off point for future events, in particular death. Mueller et al. found that a serum CRP >10 mg/L was associated with a higher risk of death in patients with NSTE-ACS despite aggressive management with early invasive therapy [27].

The American Heart Association/Centers for Disease Control and Prevention (AHA/CDC) have defined specific cut-off points for clinical interpretation: CRP concentrations <1 mg/L are considered low, 1–3 mg/L are average and >3 mg/L indicate high relative risk. A CRP concentration >10 mg/L appears to be the optimal cut-off point (when applied during hospitalisation) for prediction of new AMI and death in secondary prevention [28].

MARKER OF PLAQUE DESTABILISATION AND RUPTURE

PLACENTAL GROWTH FACTOR

Placental growth factor (PlGF), a member of the vascular endothelial growth factor (VEGF) family, was shown to be profoundly upregulated in early and advanced atherosclerotic lesions. PlGF is a 50 kDa platelet-derived protein consisting of 149 aminoacids. It might have a role in the first phases of the inflammatory process through stimulation of vascular smooth muscle growth, recruitment of macrophages into atherosclerotic lesions, upregulation of tumour necrosis factor-α (TNF-α) and monocyte chemoattractant protein-1 production by macrophages. Besides, it enhances production of tissue factor and stimulates pathological angiogenesis [29,30]. Interestingly, experimental PlGF inhibition, by blocking its receptor Flt-1, suppresses both atherosclerotic plaque growth and vulnerability via inhibition of inflammatory cell infiltration. In 2004, Heeschen et al. investigated the potential role of PlGF for assessing risk of death or non-fatal myocardial infarction in the 30 days after index presentation. They studied 1173 patients divided into two cohorts: one having angiographically confirmed ACS (n = 547 enrolled in the CAPTURE trial) and the other presenting to the emergency department (ED) with chest pain (n = 626 enrolled in Germany). In order to avoid the possibly confounding effect of anti-platelet therapy, only patients of the CAPTURE placebo arm were included in the assessment of PlGF. In the CAPTURE cohort, 40.8% patients were found to have increased PlGF concentrations and were found to have a markedly increased risk of adverse events at 30 days; also in the other cohort, PlGF was a predictor of increase in risk. These data suggest that PlGF blood levels may represent a novel, powerful, independent, prognostic determinant of clinical outcome in patients with ACS [31].

In summary, although large trials are still needed to obtain PlGF validation and commercialization, it appears to have great potential as an independent biomarker for plaque disruption, ischaemia and thrombosis and also as a novel anti-inflammatory therapeutic target in patients with CAD.

MYELOPEROXIDASE

Myeloperoxidase (MPO) is a hemoprotein (molecular mass ~140 kDa) composed of a pair of heavy and light chains. It is an enzyme that catalyzes the conversion of chloride and hydrogen peroxide to hypo-chlorite and has the optimum of activity at acid pH. It is stored in azurophilic granules of polymorpho-nuclear neutrophils and macrophages and is released into extracellular fluid in the setting of inflammatory process. The observation that MPO is involved in oxidative stress and inflammation has been a leading factor to study MPO as a possible marker of plaque instability. Oxidative stress and inflammation play a pivotal role in the pathogenesis of the destabilisation of CAD leading to ACS: macrophages and neutrophils are implicated in the transformation of stable coronary artery plaques to unstable lesions and are found in high levels in the culprit lesions of patients with ACS. In 2001, Zhang et al. showed that blood and leukocyte myeloperoxidase activities were higher in patients with CAD than angiographically verified normal controls, and that these increased activities were significantly associated with the presence of CAD (odds ratio, 11.9; 95% confidence interval, 5.5–25.5). Results were independent of patient's age, sex, hypertension, smoking, diabetes status, LDL concentration, leukocyte count and Framingham Global Risk Score [32,33].

Brennan et al. enrolled 604 patients admitted to the ED with chest pain. They investigated the correlation between risk of major cardiac events at 30 days and 6 months and increase in MPO concentration. The result was a progressive increase in odds ratios for major cardiac events with each quartile of MPO concentration. In the CAPTURE trial, MPO mass concentration was measured in 1090 patients with diagnosis of ACS and the death and MI were determined at 6 months of follow-up. The result was that MPO and the other markers studied (cTnT, soluble cd40L, CRP and vascular endothelial growth factor) were independent predictors of adverse cardiac events. Using a cut-off of 350 µg/L for MPO in patients with ACS, the adjusted hazard ratio was 2.25 (95% CI 1.32–3.82) and considering only patients with undetectable cardiac troponin the hazard ratio was 7.48 (95% CI 1.98–28.29). In summary, observations from studies that have investigated MPO activity, demonstrated MPO is more than a marker of oxidative stress and not only a marker of plaque instability [34,35].

PREGNANCY-ASSOCIATED PLASMA PROTEIN

Pregnancy-associated plasma protein (PAPP-A) is a high molecular mass (~200 kDa) glycoprotein typically measured during pregnancy for screening of Down syndrome. PAPP-A has also been implicated in coronary plaque disruption [36]. It is released during atherosclerotic plaque disruption in a homodimeric active form, uncomplexed with the inhibitor proform of eosinophil major basic protein (proMBP) contrary to the form present during pregnancy. Bayes-Genis et al. found abundant PAPP-A expression in unstable plaques but not in stable plaques from patients who died of sudden cardiac death, mostly in the inflammatory shoulder region. They also described increased PAPP-A concentrations in the serum of patients with both UA and AMI, with PAPP-A levels >10 mIU/L identifying ACS patients with a sensitivity of 89% and a specificity of 81%. Lund J et al. found that PAPP-A plasma levels >2.9 mUI/L were associated with a risk of MI, death, or revascularisation 4.6-fold higher versus PAPP-A plasma levels <2.9 mUI/L. Similar results were obtained by Heeschen et al. They demonstrated the role of PAPP-A as an independent marker of future cardiac events in ACS patients [37–39].

Although preliminary studies suggest that PAPP-A may be useful to evaluate patients with ACS, additional investigations will be necessary for better acceptance of PAPP-A as an independent biomarker for cardiovascular risk in ACS. Because preliminary findings showed that serum PAPP-A concentrations sensitively reflect changes in renal function and correlate with serum creatinine, the possible influence of renal function on PAPP-A concentrations should be also clarified [40].

METALLOPROTEINASE-9

Metalloproteinases (MMPs) are a class of 24 endopeptidases that are physiologic regulators of the extracellular matrix. They are an expanding group of proteolytic enzymes that participate in numerous physiological and pathological processes including embryogenesis, connective tissue turn-over, healing, and angiogenesis. Inflammatory stimuli augment the production of the interstitial collagenases MMP-1, MMP-13, and MMP-8 from several cell types found in atherosclerotic plaques. Human atherosclerotic plaque also contains elevated levels of the MMP-9 active form, an enzyme with gelatinolytic activity that can continue the catabolism of collagen cleaved by interstitial collagenases [41].

Recently, Fiotti et al. studied patients with stable angina and patients with ACS undergoing PCI and have assessed MMP-2, MMP-9, and TIMP-1 expressions. They have found that MMP-9, but not TIMP-1 or MMP-2 expression, is increased in plaques causing ACS. MMP-9 is localized in the plaque shoulder, the thinner area prone to rupture. So MMP-9 may be the most promising, among MMP, as a marker. The potential role of MMP-9 as a marker for risk stratification of patients with ACS was examined by Blankenberg et al. They studied 1127 patients with stable (n = 795) and unstable (n = 332) angina and found that MMP-9 values were related to future cardiovascular death. Its prognostic value was also maintained after correction for CRP, fibrinogen, IL-6, and IL-18 [42,43].

MARKERS OF ISCHAEMIA-NECROSIS

FATTY ACID BINDING PROTEINS

Fatty acid binding proteins (FABPs) are low molecular mass proteins that are abundant in the cytoplasm of tissues having active fatty acid metabolism, including the heart, striated muscle, liver, and intestine.

H-FABP appears in the blood soon after the onset of infarction, so it has been proposed as an early marker for the MI diagnosis.

Its plasma concentration increases within 2–3 hours after MI and returns to the normal range within 12–24 hours in individuals without renal impairment [44].

In general, H-FABP was found to perform better than or similar to myoglobin in diagnosis of ACS, probably due to the higher cardiac tissue content of H-FABP compared with myoglobin. Seino et al. compared a blood rapid test for H-FABP with a rapid cTnT test regarding diagnostic accuracy in cardiac ischaemia: rapid H-FABP assay seemed to effectively exclude non-AMI patients within 3 hours of onset. Therefore, H-FABP may be useful in the diagnostic assessment of ACS patients in ED, in combination with troponin, along with the electrocardiographic and clinical evaluation [45,46].

Nakata et al. have shown that H-FABP has greater diagnostic value and sensitivity than cTnT, CK-MB, and myoglobin in patients with suspected ACS within 6 hours from acute chest pain onset and an early or sustained elevation in H-FABP could indicate unfavourable clinical outcome [47].

Because H-FABP rapidly returns to the normal range within 24 hours after AMI, it can also be used to assess a recurrent infarction within 10 hours after first AMI, possibly missed by CK-MB, cTnT, and cTnI evaluation because plasma concentration of these markers returns more slowly to reference values. H-FABP has a renal clearance, therefore impaired renal function potentially impact its clinical utility; however, data from de Groot et al. indicate that H-FABP, after correction for estimated renal function, can be applied successfully for infarct size estimation. Although H-FABP is generally considered a marker of myocardial necrosis, a recent study has indicated its additional potential utility as a marker of ischaemia, also in absence of myocardial necrosis, therefore it could be useful for early identification of ACS in patients with chest pain of uncertain origin [48,49].

FREE FATTY ACIDS UNBOUND TO ALBUMIN

Free fatty acids unbound to albumin (FFAu) were also evaluated for early identification of cardiac ischaemia. FFAs are localised in the cytoplasm, bound to fatty acid binding protein (FABP), and represent the primary metabolic sources for the myocardium.

In the TIMI II trial, FFAu concentration was measured in 458 patients on admission and 50 minutes, 5 hours and 8 hours after the initiation of tissue Plasminogen Activator (tPA) treatment. Sensitivity of FFA was 91% at admission and 98% at 50 minutes after tPA (cut-off 5 nmol/L); specificity, compared with healthy individuals and patients with non-cardiovascular disease, was 93%. FFAu were increased in 100% of MI patients on admission, whereas only 22% of these patients had increased cTnI at presentation, indicative of earlier appearance of this analyte in the circulation before traditional markers of myocyte necrosis [50].

Current data, although limited, suggest that monitoring FFAu concentrations in patients presenting with ischaemia symptoms may provide an early indication of cardiac ischaemia. Additional studies are needed to fully evaluate the true potential of this biomarker.

ISCHAEMIA MODIFIED ALBUMIN

Ischaemia modified albumin (IMA), measured by the albumin cobalt binding test (ACB), has been shown to be a marker of myocardial ischaemia. A multicentre study, involving 224 patients, who arrived at the ED within 3 hours after symptoms onset, examined the ability of the ACB test to predict a positive or negative cTnI result within 6–24 hours after presentation. All patients had a negative cTnI result at presentation. At the optimum cut-off for the ACB test, sensitivity and specificity were 70% and 80%, respectively, with a negative predictive value of 96% [51].

Peacock et al. have performed a meta-analysis of IMA in ACS risk stratification. In the presence of a triple negative prediction test (non-diagnostic electrocardiogram, negative troponin, and negative IMA), they found that sensitivity and negative predictive value for ACS were 94.4% and 97.1% and, for long-term outcomes, were 89.2% and 94.5%, respectively. IMA appears to be indicative of oxidative stress and, therefore, might not be specific for cardiac ischaemia. Increased IMA values are also found in patients with cancer, infections, end-stage renal disease, liver disease, and brain ischaemia.

CONCLUSION

Several biomarkers have been proposed as useful candidates to contribute to cTn as relevant tools for the diagnosis and risk stratification of myocardial infarction. The ideal biomarker should provide increased sensitivity, especially over the first 3 hours after onset of symptoms, greater precision regarding mechanisms of cardiomyocyte injury, and sufficient prognostic information as to guide clinicians to the best management strategy. However, no available biomarker offers ideal properties such as very early raise, very high sensitivity and specificity, and easy and cheap assay. Hence a multi-marker strategy, employing pathobiologically different biomarkers, might help significantly in the identification of the 'vulnerable' patient at risk for myocardial Infarction.

REFERENCES

1. Xavier D, Pais P, Devereaux PJ et al. Treatment and outcomes of acute coronary syndromes in India (CREATE): a prospective analysis of registry data. *Lancet* 2008;371(9622):1435–1442.
2. Thygesen K, Mair J, Giannitsis E, Mueller C, Lindahl B, Blankenberg S, Huber K, Plebani M, Biasucci LM, Tubaro M, Collinson P, Venge P, Hasin Y, Galvani M, Koenig W, Hamm C, Alpert JS, Katus H, Jaffe AS, the Study Group on Biomarkers in Cardiology of the ESCWGoACC. How to use high-sensitivity cardiac troponins in acute cardiac care. *Eur Heart J.* 2012;33:2252–2257.
3. Wu AH. The ischemia-modified albumin biomarker for myocardial ischemia. *MLO Med Lab Obs.* 2003;6:36–40.
4. Safford MM, Parmar G, Barasch CS, Halanych JH, Glasser SP, Goff DC, Prineas RJ, Brown TM. Hospital laboratory reporting may be a barrier to detection of 'microsize' myocardial infarction in the US: An observational study. *BMC Health Serv Res.* 2013;13:162.
5. [Guideline] Amsterdam EA, Wenger NK, Brindis RG et al., for the ACC/AHA Task Force Members. 2014 AHA/ACC guideline for the management of patients with non-ST-elevation acute coronary syndromes: A report of the American College of Cardiology/American Heart Association Task Force on Practice Guidelines. *Circulation* 2014;130(25):e344–e426.
6. [Guideline] O'Gara PT, Kushner FG, Ascheim DD et al., for the American College of Cardiology Foundation/American Heart Association Task Force on Practice Guidelines. 2013 ACCF/AHA guideline for the management of ST-elevation myocardial infarction: A report of the American College of Cardiology Foundation/American Heart Association Task Force on Practice Guidelines. *Circulation* 2013;127(4):e362–e425.
7. [Guideline] Roffi M, Patrono C, Collet JP et al. 2015 ESC Guidelines for the management of acute coronary syndromes in patients presenting without persistent ST-segment elevation: Task Force for the Management of Acute Coronary Syndromes in Patients Presenting without Persistent ST-Segment Elevation of the European Society of Cardiology (ESC). *Eur Heart J.* 2016;37(3):267–315.
8. Gibler WB, Lewis LM, Erb RE et al. Early detection of acute myocardial infarction in patients presenting with chest pain and nondiagnostic electrocardiograms: Serial CK-MB. Sampling in the emergency department. *Ann Emerg Med.* 1990;19:1359–1366.
9. Pearson JR, Carrea F. Evaluation of the clinical usefulness of a chemiluminometric method for measuring creatine kinase MB. *Clin Chem.* 1990;36:1809.
10. Jaffe AS, Ravkilde J, Roberts R et al. It's time for a change to a troponin standard. *Circulation* 2000;102:1216–1220.
11. Thygesen K, Alpert JS, Harvey D, White October. Universal definition of myocardial infarction. *Circulation* 2007;116:2634–2653.
12. Gillis TE, Marshall CR, Tibbis GF. Functional and evolutionary relationships of Troponin C. Physiol. *Genomic* 2007;32(1):16–27.
13. Anderson JL, Adams CD, Antman EM et al. ACC/AHA 2007 Guidelines for the Management of Patients with Unstable Angina/Non–ST-Elevation Myocardial Infarction. *J Am Coll Cardiol.* 2007;50:1–157.
14. Peacock F, Morris DL, Anwaruddin S et al. Meta-analysis of ischemia-modified albumin to rule out acute coronary syndromes in the emergency department. *Am Heart J.* 2006;152:253–262.
15. Freda BJ, Tang WH, van Lente F et al. Cardiac troponins in renal insufficiency. Review and clinical implications. *J Am Coll Card.* 2002;40:2065–2071.
16. Apple FS. Clinical and analytical standardization issues confronting cardiac troponin I. *Clin Chem.* 1999;45(2):18–20.
17. Clerico A, Iervasi G, Mariani G. Pathophysiologic relevance of measuring the plasma levels of cardiac natriuretic peptide hormones in humans. *Horm Metab Res.* 1999;31(9):487–498.
18. Cowie MR, Jourdain P, Maisel A et al. Clinical applications of B-type natriuretic peptide (BNP) testing. *Eur Heart J.* 2003;24:1710–1718.
19. Kay JD, Trichon BH, Kisslo M et al. Serum brain natriuretic peptide levels cannot differentiate pulmonary disease from left-heart failure if the right ventricle is dilated. *Circulation.* 2003;108:IV–397.

20. Tateishi J, Masutani M, Ohyanagi M et al. Transient increase in plasma brain (B-type) natriuretic peptide after percutaneous transluminal coronary angioplasty. *Clin Cardiol.* 2000;23(10):776–780.

21. Sabatine MS, Morrow DA, de Lemos JA et al. Multimarker approach to risk stratification in non-ST elevation acute coronary syndromes: Simultaneous assessment of troponin I, C-reactive protein, and B-type natriuretic peptide. *Circulation* 2002;105(15):1760–1763.

22. de Lemos JA, Morrow DA. Brain natriuretic peptide measurement in acute coronary syndromes. Ready for clinical application? *Circulation* 2002;106:2868–2870.

23. Wang TJ, Larson MG, Levy D et al. Plasma natriuretic peptide levels and the risk of cardiovascular events and death. *N Engl J Med.* 2004;350(7):655–663.

24. Volanakis JE. Human C-reactive protein: expression, structure, and function. *Mol Immunol.* 2001;38(2–3):189–197.

25. Liuzzo G, Biasucci LM, Gallimore JR et al. The prognostic value of C-reactive protein and serum amyloid A protein in severe unstable angina. *N Engl J Med.* 1994;331:417–424.

26. James SK, Armstrong P, Barnathan E et al. Troponin T and C-reactive protein have a different relation to subsequent mortality and myocardial infarction after acute coronary syndrome: A GUSTO-IV substudy. *J Am Coll Cardiol.* 2003;41:916–924.

27. Mueller C, Buettner HJ, Hodgson JM et al. Inflammation and long-term mortality after non-ST elevation acute coronary syndrome treated with a very early invasive strategy in 1042 consecutive patients. *Circulation* 2002;105:1412–1415.

28. Pearson TA, Mensah GA, Alexander RW et al. Markers of inflammation and cardiovascular disease: Application to clinical and public health practice: A statement for healthcare professionals from the Centers for Disease Control and Prevention and the American Heart Association. *Circulation* 2003;107:499–511.

29. Luttun A, Tjwa M, Moons L et al. Revascularization of ischemic tissues by PIGF treatment, and inhibition of tumor angiogenesis, arthritis and atherosclerosis by anti-Flt1. *Nat Med.* 2002;8(8):831–840.

30. Autiero M, Luttun A, Tjwa M et al. Placental growth factor and its receptor, vascular endothelial growth factor receptor-1: Novel target for stimulation of ischemic tissue revascularization and inhibition of angiogenic and inflammatory disorders. *J Thromb Haemost.* 2003;1:1356–1370.

31. Heeschen C, Dimmeler S, Hamm CW et al. CAPTURE Study Investigators. Soluble CD40L in acute coronary syndromes. *N Engl J Med.* 2003;348:1104–1111.

32. Takahiko N, Ueda M, Haze K et al. Neutrophil infiltration of culprit lesions in acute coronary syndromes. *Circulation* 2002;106:2894–2900.

33. Zhang R, Brennan ML, Fu X et al. Association between myeloperoxidase levels and risk of coronary artery disease. *JAMA* 2001;286:2136–2142.

34. Brennan ML, Penn MS, Van Lente F et al. Prognostic value of myeloperoxidase in patients with chest pain. *N Engl J Med.* 2003;349:1595–1604.

35. Baldus S, Heeschen C, Meinertz T et al. Myeloperoxidase serum levels predict risk in patients with acute coronary syndromes. *Circulation* 2003;108:1440–1445.

36. Lawrence JB, Oxvig C, Overgaard MT et al. The insulin-like growth factor (IGF)-dependent IGF binding protein-4 protease secreted by human fibroblasts is pregnancy-associated plasma protein A. *Proc Natl Acad Sci USA.* 1999;96:3149–3153.

37. Bayes-Genis A, Con Over CA, Overgaard MT et al. Pregnancy-associated PAPP-A as a marker of acute coronary syndromes. *N Engl J Med.* 2001;345:1022–1029.

38. Lund J, Qin QP, Ilva T et al. Circulating pregnancy-associated plasma protein A predicts outcome in patients with acute coronary syndromes. *Circulation* 2003;108:1924–1926.

39. Heeschen C, Fichtlscherer S, Hamm CW. Pregnancy associated plasma protein A (PAPP-A) plasma level independently predicted outcome in patients with acute coronary syndrome. *Circulation* 2003;108(suppl IV):470.

40. Fialova L, Kalousova M, Soukupova J et al. Relationship of pregnancy associated plasma protein A (PAPP-A to renal function and dialysis modalities. *Kidney Blood Press Res.* 2004;27:88–95.

41. Galis Z, Sukhova G, Lark M et al. Increased expression of matrix metalloproteinases and matrix degrading activity in vulnerable regions of human atherosclerotic plaques. *J Clin Invest.* 1994;94:2493–2503.

42. Fiotti N, Altamura N, Orlando C et al. Metalloproteinases-2, -9 and TIMP-1 expression in stable and unstable coronary plaques undergoing PCI. *Int J Cardiol.* 2008 Jul 21;127(3):350–357.

43. Blankenberg S, Rupprecht HJ, Poirier O et al. Plasma concentrations and genetic and genetic variation of matrix metalloproteinase 9 and prognosis of patients with cardiovascular disease. *Circulation* 2003;107:1579–1585.

44. Kleine AH, Glatz JF, Van Nieuwenhoven FA et al. Release of heart free fatty acid-binding protein into plasma after acute myocardial infarction in man. *Mol Cell Biochem.* 1992;116(1–2):155–162.

45. Okamoto F, Sohmiya K, Ohkaru Y et al. Human heart-type cytoplasmic fatty acid-binding protein (H-FABP) for the diagnosis of acute myocardial infarction. Clinical evaluation of H-FABP in comparison with myoglobin and creatinine chinase isoenzyme MB. *Clin Chem Lab Med.* 2000;38(3):231–238.

46. Seino Y, Tomita Y, Takano T et al. Tokyo Rapid-Test Office Cardiologists (Tokyo-ROC) Study. Office cardiologists cooperative study on whole blood rapid panel tests in patients with suspicious acute myocardial infarction: Comparison between heart-type fatty acid-binding protein and troponin T tests. *Circ J.* 2004;68(2):144–148.

47. Nakata T, Hashimoto A, Hase M et al. Human heart-type fatty acid-binding protein as an early diagnostic and prognostic marker in acute coronary syndrome. *Cardiology* 2003;99(2):96–104.

48. de Groot MJ, Wodzig KW, Simoons ML et al. Measurement of myocardial infarct size from plasma fatty acid-binding protein or myoglobin, using individually estimated clearance rates. *Cardiovasc Res.* 1999;44(2):315–324.

49. Tambara K, Fujita M, Miyamoto S et al. Pericardial fluid level of heart-type cytoplasmatic fatty acid-binding protein (H-FABP) is an indicator of severe myocardial ischemia. *Int J Cardiol.* 2004;93(1–2):281–284.

50. Kleinfeld AM, Kleinfeld KJ, Adams JE. Serum levels of unbound free fatty acids reveal high sensitivity for early detection of acute coronary syndrome in patient samples from the TIMI II trial. *J Am Coll Cardiol.* 2002;39:312A.

51. Christenson RH, Hong DS, Sanhai WR et al. Characteristics of an Albumin Cobalt Binding Test for assessment of acute coronary syndrome patients: A multicenter study. *Clin Chem.* 2001;47:464–470.

9

Risk stratification in acute coronary syndromes

AVANTI GURRAM REDDY, GIANLUCA RIGATELLI AND RAMESH DAGGUBATI

INTRODUCTION

Acute coronary syndrome (ACS) remains the most severe form of cardiovascular disease and accounts for one third of all global deaths. It also represents the most important basis of chronic heart failure – one of the most problematic and the most frequent chronic diseases, which causes perpetual debility. All-cause mortality at 2 years amounted to 6.2% among patients with AMI, and rates of rehospitalisation due to ACS and revascularisation were 6.8% and 4.1%, respectively [1]. CAD epidemiology in India is characterised by premature occurrence in the young and low-/middle-income group, high mortality and high prevalence of diabetes compared to the west. In the spectrum of ACS, 30 days in-hospital mortality of STEMI patients is higher in the first 2 hours after onset before patients reach the hospital compared to stable ischaemic heart disease post-PCI mostly due to arrythmias, hemodynamic instability and/or lack of early reperfusion procedures. Hence, it is noteworthy to develop strategies to prevent/reduce MACE (major adverse cardiac events) and complications. There is a lack of availability of satisfactory diagnostic markers and appropriate treatment for high-risk versus low-risk patients. In order to manage the potential complications of ACS, considering limited invasive facilities and high recurrence of events, risk stratification is clinically reasonable. The most widely validated risk models for patients with ACS are TIMI (Thrombolysis in Myocardial Infarction), dynamic TIMI, APEX AMI (Assessment of Pexelizumab in Acute Myocardial Infarction), CADILLAC (Controlled Abciximab and Device Investigation to Lower Late Angioplasty Complications) and GRACE (Global Registry of Acute Cardiac Events) algorithms.

DETERMINATION OF RISK FACTORS AND PRE-TEST ASSESSMENT

Risk assessment is a dynamic process and risk determinants may vary with time, new arrythmias, mechanical complications and heart failure. It is essential to evaluate risks for early appropriate management. The three major determinants of prognosis in ACS include: (1) the extent of myocardial injury; (2) the extent of coronary artery disease; and (3) the instability of the disease and its refractoriness to management. Various non-invasive tests need to be taken into consideration before the patient is discharged as the maximum event rate occurs within 30–60 days post-ACS. Other than the basis of detailed history and a physical exam, EKG is a primary modality for diagnosis followed by 2D ECHO, myocardial perfusion imaging and NST. Over-reliance on troponins can lead to misdiagnosis and inappropriate treatment and must always be taken as supportive evidence in the fitting clinical situation. Risk stratification can be made based on biochemical results and therapeutic management can be guided after the risk assessment for secondary prevention. Patients are classified into three risk categories: low, intermediate or high to guide therapeutic management.

Factors like advanced age (over 70 years), clinical parameters (BP, heart rate), lipid profile, BMI, psychomotor agitation, biochemical results (CPK-troponin, BNP, CRP, HbA1C, Cr, etc.), paraclinical profile (O2 sat, blood glucose), bleeding risk, clinical comorbidities, ventricular function, arrythmias, residual ischaemia like ongoing chest pain and ST segment changes, stress test and coronary angiography results justify a cumulative impact for increase in the mortality of the pre-hospital and in-hospital population. V-Fib accounts for more than 80% of out of hospital deaths which is a major risk determinant.

Currently, it is imperative to identify coronary artery disease in early forms, before clinical manifestation in patients with low to intermediate risks, in order to guide therapy. Patient characteristics, type of coronary disease and impact of ongoing treatment need to be integrated to individualise therapy based on valid scores versus personalised scores for a positive result. Patients requiring revascularisation and additional tests for refining risk status due to comorbidities, especially heart failure, need appropriate follow-up, making risk stratification an incremental process and superior prognostic value.

Several studies have revealed various theoretical conclusions using complex methods such as cluster analysis and tree structured analysis or neural networks [2]. Even though risk models show appropriate theoretical and statistical performance, it needs to be simple and clinically accessible to guide treatment in order to be useful to predict event-free survival on one hand and potentially life-threatening cardiac events on the other hand. Several risk scores have been published: INTERHEART study (2004), Framingham (1948), HEART (2007), PROCAM (1979) and Reynolds (2008). They use classic modifiable and non-modifiable risk factors while patients with intermediate risk require more precise estimation by using parameters like coronary calcium score, where <100 is low risk and >400 is high risk [HNR (Heinz Nixdorf Recall) study] [3], and homocysteine levels, while CRP as an independent additional biomarker may be used for intermediate risk groups but may not provide long term prognostic value (RISCA study) [4]. TIMI score is simple and applied more widely to identify high-risk patients who benefit from aggressive therapy, while the dynamic TIMI risk model is an upgrade of the classic TIMI risk score, using in-hospital events for an easy reassessment of the risk of patients discharged from hospital. The Zwolle score was created for the prediction of 30-day mortality to identify low-risk patients suitable for an early discharge from hospital.

Initially, a functional assessment using patient history and a physical exam is of the utmost importance. Certain classification systems like the Canadian Cardiovascular Society and the Killip classification system are used widely, and others like the Duke Activity Specific Index, the Braunwald Classification of Unstable Angina or the Seattle Angina Questionnaire may provide additional prognostic value but are hardly used in clinical practice.

ECG ASPECT

ECG changes like ST-elevation amplitude (>1 mm for inferior), Q waves and QRS duration, especially anterior location of MI (>1.5 mm) and signal gated ECG, are significant prognostic markers. Presentations like anterior T wave inversions should necessitate suspicion of possible critical LAD stenosis (Wellens syndrome) which would require urgent cardiac catheterisation. Rescue angioplasty might be essential for failed reperfusion/ coronary occlusion when recurrent ST-elevations and left bundle branch blocks complicate the condition, subsequently leading to extensive myocardial injury. False STEMI activation has been identified in close to 15%–20% STEMI ECGs based on various studies all over the world. The triggers that cause false STEMI are yet to be identified, and they are even more difficult to identify in the presence of LBBB. Partly this problem can be overcome by comparing old ECGs, recognising early repolarisation changes, LVH, RBBB and Brugada pattern. Nevertheless, the adjusted short-term mortality was similar for patients with confirmed STEMI and those with a false-positive STEMI diagnosis making it vital to risk a needless activation rather than to ignore a possible STEMI and not initiate the treatment protocol. Non-sustained ventricular tachycardia, sustained monomorphic ventricular tachycardia and V-fib within the first 48 hours of ACS increase in-hospital mortality while post-admission arrythmias with stage C and D heart failure are at increased risk of death in the first year. Holter monitoring can record silent ischaemia, electrical instability and identify uncomplicated early recovery cases who remain at high risk. Pre-discharge ST changes account for 20% increased risk of reinfarction and an added prognostic value for risk stratification [5]. Further studies are required to define its role to guide appropriate therapy.

STRESS TEST

Stress testing is crucial to predict recurrent ischaemic events and revascularisation protocol for uncomplicated MI as it adds value for pre-discharge risk stratification. ST depression, higher exertional intolerance, arrhythmias and failure of BP to rise during exercise are the usual abnormalities. A normal stress test usually would not require additional investigations, but an abnormal test has a more negative predictive value for post-MI mortality in the first year [6]. A stress test corresponds to reversible thallium perfusion defects and is cost effective.

INTERVENTIONAL ASPECT

There are several risk stratification scores (SYNTAX, TOPOL) based on angiographic results with varying study limitations (e.g. number of patients with fitting clinical criteria, cardiogenic shock, cardiac arrest) but are currently clinically applicable in stable CAD and ACS. In patients with higher risk of reinfarction, it is important to note the details of the infarct size, LV function and myocardial viability in the first 24–48 hours post-PCI, while myocardial scintigraphy, stress ECHO and cardiac MRI/PET give complimentary information. Ejection fraction <40% with symptomatic LV dysfunction classifies patients as a high-risk group who would need ACE inhibitors and may require stress testing to rule out residual ischaemia and possible cardiac catheterisation. CABG may be mostly beneficial when left ventricular dysfunction is associated with multi-vessel CAD. Unlike ECHO, PET and SPECT, MRI has the unique ability to provide quantitative information on cardiac function, perfusion and viability. Grading coronary flow (TIMI) and myocardial blush (MBG) are important prognostic markers, ≤3 TIMI and 0–1 MBG can be seen in 10%–40% patients post-angioplasty which increases the risk of arrythmias, mechanical complications and hemodynamic instability [7].

PAMI (Primary Angioplasty in Myocardial Infarction) and CADILLAC were based on individuals treated by invasive procedures that are used to estimate short-term mortality (6 months) as opposed to GRACE which is a good predictor for long-term mortality (6–12 months) in STEMI [8]. The GRACE score is a well-validated and is simple to apply as it not only predicts the outcomes but also confirms an ACS diagnosis and length of hospital stay. The FRISC (Fast Revascularisation in Instability in Coronary Disease) score is the only score that has a high capacity to identify patients who have a long-term benefit from an early invasive treatment strategy [9]; it is quite comparable to the TIMI score. A 2011 meta-analysis validates early revascularisation for NSTEMI ACS patients is safe and can decrease the incidence of recurrent ischaemia with lower major bleeding events [10]. The Global Use of Strategies To Open occluded arteries in acute coronary syndromes (GUSTO-IIb) study describes the clinical pattern of myocardial (re)infarction after discontinuation of antithrombin therapy in a large cohort (8943 patients), concluding that patients who suffered reinfarction post-heparin therapy discontinuation had a longer hospital stay and 10 times higher 30-day in-hospital mortality and significantly increased mortality at 6 months and 1-yr follow-up compared to patients who did not suffer reinfarction.

OBSERVATIONAL STUDIES AND USING ADDITIONAL PREDICTORS

Based on some observational databases and small cohort studies that evaluated clinical predictors of mortality using multivariable models in patients with ACS, simpler risk models had comparable performance to more complex risk models. These investigations varied from a single-centre experience to data from clinical trials and observational registries. With advances in interventional approach, risk models need to be upgraded for quality improvement. Many independent parameters and scoring systems in the developmental stage seem to have a potential of a new approach to risk stratification in ACS based on their results. For example, the KorMI system (Korea Working Group in Myocardial Infarction) added bare metal stent and regional wall motion score to its model compared with current models [11]. Comorbidity assessment in the elderly (75–85 yrs) using Charlson Comorbidity Index, biochemical parameters like high sensitivity cardiac troponin assays, white blood cell (WBC) to mean platelet volume ratio (WMR), beta 2-microglobulin, thrombomodulin, soluble Fms-Like Tyrosine kinase-1 (sFlt-1), high sensitive CRP and NT pro BNP have been studied but need further analysis and standardisation to appropriately interpret them across different medical systems. Electrocardiographic features like negative T waves post-acute MI after thrombolysis had improved 30-day survival rate [12], presence of late potentials (LP) in 24-h high resolution ambulatory ECG post-PCI. LP-positive populations had significantly higher incidences of ischaemic events as well as overall rehospitalisation compared to LP-negative populations, but the predictive power of LP was decreased when it was combined with other variables [13], and the therapeutic implications are yet to be defined.

Clinicians may use more of an instinctive method of identifying patterns and applying guidelines using their personal clinical experience, pathophysiologic reasoning and research meta-analysis

which could possibly lead to improper use of tools of risk stratifications and inappropriate use of treatment approaches and procedures. There is a need to assess cardiovascular risk on an individual basis in order to guide therapy even though aggressive management like usage of more potent anti-platelet and antithrombotic therapies are shown to be effective, particularly in high-risk patients. A better understanding of the pathophysiologic implication of each prognostic factor is needed to quantify its forte and evaluate its relative importance in different subgroups of patients. Hereafter, more large-scale studies and clinical trials are needed to develop better risk scores with upgraded performance to influence short- and long-term mortality in ACS.

REFERENCES

1. Pilgrim T, Vranckx P, Valgimigli M et al. Risk and timing of recurrent ischemic events among patients with stable ischemic heart disease, non-ST-segment elevation acute coronary syndrome, and ST-segment elevation myocardial infarction. *Am Heart J*. 2016;175:56–65.
2. Cooney MT, Dudina AL, Graham IM. Value and limitations of existing scores for the assessment of cardiovascular risk: A review for clinicians. *JACC*. 2009;54:1209–1227.
3. Erbel R, Möhlenkamp S, Moebus S et al.; Heinz Nixdorf Recall Study Investigative Group. Coronary risk stratification, discrimination, and reclassification improvement based on quantification of subclinical coronary atherosclerosis: The Heinz Nixdorf Recall Study. *JACC* 2010; 56:1397–1406.
4. Bogaty P, Boyer L, Simard S et al. Clinical utility of reactive protein measured at admission, hospital discharge, and 1 month later to predict outcome in patients with acute coronary disease: The RISCA (Recurrence and Inflammation in the Acute Coronary Syndromes) study. *J Am Coll Cardiol*. 17 Jun 2008;51(24):2339–2346.
5. Stevenson R, Ranjadayalan K, Wilkinson P et al. Assessment of Holter ST monitoring for risk stratification in patients with acute myocardial infarction treated by thrombolysis. *Br Heart J*. 1993;70:233–240.
6. Shaw LJ, Peterson ED, Kesler K et al. A meta-analysis of predischarge risk stratification after acute myocardial infarction with stress electrocardiographic, myocardial perfusion, and ventricular function imaging. *Am J Cardiol*. 1996;78:1327–1337, State of the art meta-analysis of non-invasive testing for predischarge risk stratification.
7. Van de Werf F, Bax J, Betriu A et al. Management of acute myocardial infarction in patients presenting with persistent ST-segment elevation. Full text. The Task Force on the management of ST-segment elevation acute myocardial infarction of the European Society of Cardiology. *Eur Heart J*. 2008;29:2909–2945.
8. Simona L, Petr K, Jiri J et al. GRACE score among six risk scoring systems (CADILLAC, PAMI, TIMI, Dynamic TIMI, Zwolle) demonstrated the best predictive value for prediction of long-term mortality in patients with ST-elevation myocardial infarction. *PLOS ONE*. 2015;10(4):e0123215.

9. Lagerqvist B, Husted S, Kontny F et al. 5year outcomes in the FRISC-II randomised trial of an invasive versus a non-invasive strategy in non-ST-elevation acute coronary syndrome: A follow-up study. *Lancet* 2006;368:998–1004.

10. Zhang S, Ge J, Yao K, Qian J. Meta-analysis of early versus deferred revascularization for non-ST-segment elevation acute coronary syndrome. *Am J Cardiol.* 1 Nov 2011;108(9):1207–1213.

11. Song PS, Ryu DR, Kim MJ et al.; Korea Acute Myocardial Infarction Registry Investigators. Risk scoring system to assess outcomes in patients treated with contemporary guideline-adherent optimal therapies after acute myocardial infarction. *Korean Circ J.* Jun 2018;48(6):492–504.

12. Sgarbossa EB, Meyer PM, Pinski SL et al. Negative T waves shortly after ST-elevation acute myocardial infarction are a powerful marker for improved survival rate. *Am Heart J.* Sep 2000;140(3):385–394.

13. Amino M, Yoshioka K, Ichikawa T et al. The presence of late potentials after percutaneous coronary intervention for the treatment of acute coronary syndrome as a predictor for future significant cardiac events resulting in re-hospitalization. *J Electrocardiol.* 2 Jan 2019;53:71–78.

10

Initial therapy and when to transfer at non-PCI centres

THOMAS ALEXANDER

India is in the midst of an epidemic of coronary artery disease and the prevalence of STEMI is rising. The mortality remains high despite the increase in number of cardiac catheterisation laboratories and Primary Percutaneous Interventions (PPCI). The primary reason for this is the inability of large numbers of patients to access timely and appropriate reperfusion [1].

The lack of a STEMI system of care or ambulance network in large parts of this country results in patients transporting themselves to the closest medical facility for treatment of chest pain. These could often be a doctor's private clinic or a primary health centre where even an ECG facility is not available. Emergency treatment and a clear transfer pathway is a paramount requirement for these patients.

When considering non-PCI centres, there are three scenarios that must be considered for management of the patient presenting with chest pain:

1. Doctor's clinic or a primary health centre (PHC)
2. A secondary care centre or a community health centre (CHC) with ECG facility
3. A district hospital/secondary care centre where thrombolysis is possible

DOCTOR'S CLINIC OR PHC

Most patients present to a general practitioner, a family physician or in rural areas to a PHC with symptoms that are perceived usually as due to acid peptic disease. Often, these medical facilities do not even have an ECG. Management of chest pain suggestive of ACS in these locations should include:

1. Do an ECG immediately, if available.
2. If the symptoms are suggestive of ACS, give
   – Soluble or chewable aspirin 300 mg
   – Atorvastatin 80 mg

3. If the patient is stable, move the patient to the closest centre where a 12-lead ECG can be done and ACS can be confirmed
4. If the patient is hemodynamically or electrically unstable, move the patient directly to a reperfusion centre

A SECONDARY CARE CENTRE OR A COMMUNITY HEALTH CENTRE (CHC) WITH AN ECG FACILITY

Management of chest pain, suggestive of ACS, in a patient presenting to a centre with an ECG facility should include the following:

1. Do an ECG and report it within 10 minutes of arrival to the emergency room. In certain hospitals it may be feasible to do an ECG on arrival but there may not be anyone who is able to make a confident diagnosis. In these circumstances there should be facilities to transmit the ECG directly to a physician who can read the ECG. There are multiple smartphone applications that can be used for this purpose if a dedicated ECG machine with transmittable capability is not available.
2. If the ECG confirms a STEMI, give the patient the following medications immediately:
   – Soluble or chewable aspirin 300 mg
   – Clopidogrel 300 mg
   – Atorvastatin 80 mg
3. Shift the patient immediately to the closest reperfusion centre. This could be a thrombolytic or PPCI centre.
4. Ensure that one or two IV lines are placed.
5. Supplemental oxygen when oxygen saturation is below 90% while awaiting and during transportation.
6. Ensure the time of drug administration, dosage of medications and the ECG are carried with the patient to the transferred reperfusion centre.
7. Transport the patient, preferably using an advanced ACLS ambulance with monitoring capability.

A DISTRICT HOSPITAL/SECONDARY CARE CENTRE WHERE THROMBOLYSIS IS POSSIBLE

Pharmaco-invasive reperfusion strategy in ST-elevation MI (STEMI) involves early fibrinolysis in a non-PCI centre, followed by transfer to a PCI centre within 2–24 hours for routine and systematic angiogram followed by PCI, if indicated. Immediate transfer to a PCI centre and rescue PCI may be required in a subset of thrombolysed patients who have clinical and/or ECG evidence of unsuccessful reperfusion.

Although rapid reperfusion with PPCI is widespread in the United States and Europe, limited resources and lack of infrastructure means that patients with STEMI in low- and middle-income countries (LMICs) receive significantly less reperfusion therapy. When they do, these patients are more likely to receive thrombolytic agents rather than PPCI. Data from multiple studies who receive fibrin-specific thrombolytics show that early catheterisation and definitive revascularisation is the preferred option based on trials supporting clinical equivalence of a pharmaco-invasive approach with PPCI [2]. Recent data from the TN STEMI programme has shown that this is also true in low and moderate risk patients who have undergone thrombolysis using streptokinase [3].

PPCI remains inaccessible to the majority of patients in a country like India due to demographical and financial constraints. Capital AMI [4] and CARESS-in-AMI [5] were the initial studies that demonstrated the superiority of pharmaco-invasive over stand-alone thrombolysis. A meta-analysis published in the *European Journal of Cardiology* demonstrated a significant reduction in death, reinfarction and refractory ischaemia at 30 days and at 1 year [6].

The STREAM study [7] was one of the pivotal trials that compared the pharmaco-invasive strategy using tenecteplase with primary PCI in STEMI patients. The primary end point, a composite of any death, shock, reinfarction or congestive heart failure, was similar between both groups at 30 days. Previous clinical trials comparing the efficacy of both the reperfusion modalities in STEMI have shown a time dependent benefit of thrombolysis up to 3 hours.

The FAST-MI Registry [8] evaluated the 'real world' management of 1492 patients with STEMI in France who sought medical treatment within 12 h of symptom onset. Ninety-six percent of the patients treated with fibrinolysis underwent coronary angiography within 3–24 h and 84% among them underwent subsequent PCI. Survival at 5 years was 88% in the fibrinolysis plus group and 84% for those in the PPCI group (HR = 0.73; CI: 0.50–1.06; p = 0.1). However, pre-hospital fibrinolysis resulted in lower 5-year mortality (HR = 0.57; CI: 0.36–0.88), whereas in-hospital fibrinolysis was associated with a tendency toward increased 5-year mortality (HR = 1.19; CI: 0.72–1.96) when compared to primary PCI.

The STEP-PAMI trial [9] in India using tenecteplase as the thrombolytic agent showed results comparable to PPCI without an increase in bleeding risk. However, the three studies used third-generation lytics which may not be available to the large majority of patients in India.

The non-fibrin-specific thrombolytic agent streptokinase is less effective in opening the infarct-related artery (IRA), especially in late presenters with a perceived increase in bleeding risk. Its use as a lytic in pharmaco-invasive treatment has not been elucidated until recently. A recent subgroup analysis from the TN STEMI programme [3] has shown that in low and moderate risk subsets of STEMI patients, it is comparable to PPCI with no increased risk of bleeding complications. However, the use of radial access and delayed invasive procedure (18 hours from time of lysis) were probably important factors that contributed to safety in this group of patients.

Thus, current evidence supports the following course of action in patients with STEMI presenting to a thrombolytic centre:

1. Do an ECG within 10 minutes of arrival to the hospital emergency room and have it read within 10 minutes.
2. If the ECG confirms a STEMI, give the patient the following medications immediately:
   - Soluble or chewable aspirin 300 mg
   - Clopidogrel 300 mg
   - Atorvastatin 80 mg
3. Within 30 minutes of arrival, a thrombolysis contraindication checklist must be completed and thrombolysis instituted.
4. Thrombolysis with a third-generation lytic is preferred, however, if not available or not affordable to the patient, then streptokinase is to be used.
5. Do a 90-minute ECG to assess for successful reperfusion.

The decision to transfer to a PCI centre should be based on the following criteria:

1. Any patient in cardiogenic shock or contraindication to thrombolysis should be shifted, as soon as a diagnosis of STEMI is made, to a PCI centre for primary PCI.
2. If the 90-minute ECG shows evidence of failed lysis – if more than 50% reduction of the sum of ST segment elevation in all the leads showing ST elevation is not demonstrable – or if the patient is electrically or hemodynamically unstable, then the patient should be immediately shifted to a PCI centre.
3. If the patient is clinically stable and the ECG shows evidence of successful lysis, then the patient can be shifted to a PCI centre for pharmaco-invasive treatment within a broad time window of 2–24 hours.

Stand-alone thrombolysis has been shown to have a much higher incidence of re-MI and recurrent ischaemia and should not be recommended. However, in geographies where access to PCI centres is limited or unaffordable, early thrombolysis will certainly benefit a STEMI patient.

CONCLUSION

Early reperfusion in STEMI patients is of paramount importance. Transfer to a reperfusion centre of a patient with chest pain or after a diagnosis of STEMI should be a priority. Patients who are thrombolysed should undergo pharmaco-invasive treatment and should be shifted to a PCI centre. The evidence showing superiority in outcomes for patients with pharmaco-invasive treatment over stand-alone thrombolysis is unequivocal.

REFERENCES

1. Xavier D, Pais P, Devereaux PJ et al.; for the CREATE Registry Investigators. Treatment and outcomes of acute coronary syndromes in India (CREATE): A prospective analysis of registry data. *Lancet*. 2008;371:1435–1442.

2. O'Gara PT, Kushner FG, Ascheim DD et al. ACCF/AHA guideline for the management of ST-elevation myocardial infarction: Executive summary: A report of the American College of Cardiology Foundation/American Heart Association Task Force on Practice Guidelines. *J Am Coll Cardiol*. 2013;61:485–510.

3. Kumbhani DJ, Alexander T, Nallamothu BK et al.; for the TN-STEMI Investigators. Pharmacoinvasive Approach with Streptokinase in Low to Intermediate Risk ST Elevation Myocardial Infarction Patients: Insights from the Tamil Nadu STEMI Initiative. *Am J Cardiovasc Drugs*. 2019;19(5):517–519.

4. Le May MR, Wells GA, Labinaz M et al. Combined angioplasty and pharmacological intervention versus thrombolysis alone in acute myocardial infarction (CAPITAL AMI study). *J Am Coll Cardiol*. 2005;46:417–424.

5. Di Mario C, Dudek D, Piscione F et al. Immediate angioplasty versus standard therapy with rescue angioplasty after thrombolysis in the Combined Abciximab REteplase Stent Study in Acute Myocardial Infarction (CARESS-in-AMI): An open, prospective, randomised, multicentre trial. *Lancet*. 2008;371:559–568.

6. Borgia F, Goodman SG, Halvorsen S et al. Early routine percutaneous coronary intervention after fibrinolysis vs. standard therapy in ST segment elevation myocardial infarction: A meta-analysis. *Eur Heart J*. 2010;31:2156–2169.

7. Armstrong PW, Gershlick AH, Goldstein P et al. Fibrinolysis or primary PCI in ST-segment elevation myocardial infarction. *N Engl J Med*. 2013;368:1379–1387.

8. Danchin N, Puymirat E, Steg PG et al. Five-year survival in patients with ST-segment-elevation myocardial infarction according to modalities of reperfusion therapy: The French Registry on Acute ST-Elevation and Non-ST-Elevation Myocardial Infarction (FAST-MI) 2005 Cohort. *Circulation*. 2014;129:1629–1636.

9. Victor SM, Subban V, Alexander T et al. A prospective, observational, multicentre study comparing tenecteplase facilitated PCI versus primary PCI in Indian patients with STEMI (STEPP-AMI). *Open Heart*. 2014;1:e000133.

11

Anti-platelet therapy in acute coronary syndrome
What is current and new?

KUNAL MAHAJAN, YASHASVI RAJEEV AND K SARAT CHANDRA

Vulnerable atherosclerotic plaques in the coronary arteries form the pathologic substrate for acute coronary syndromes (ACS) to develop. Following rupture, fissure, or erosion of an atherosclerotic plaque, there occurs adhesion, activation, and aggregation of platelets which are fundamental to the initiation of thrombus formation. This is a key pathological step in the development of ACS [1]. Because atherothrombotic events are essentially platelet-driven processes, anti-platelet agents are a mainstay of the treatment in the setting of ACS. Currently, three different classes of anti-platelet drugs are approved for treatment and prevention of ischaemic events in ACS: (1) Cycloxygenase-1(COX-1) inhibitor: aspirin; (2) Adenosine diphosphate (ADP) P2Y12 receptor antagonists: clopidogrel, prasugrel, ticagrelor, and cangrelor; and (3) Glycoprotein IIb/IIIa inhibitors (GPI): abciximab, eptifibatide, and tirofiban [2]. In a significant number of patients with ACS, recurrent ischaemic events continue to occur, despite them being treated adequately with dual anti-platelet therapy (DAPT) in the form of aspirin and clopidogrel. This has led to continuous research on developing newer and more potent anti-platelet agents [2].

CURRENTLY APPROVED ORAL ANTI-PLATELET AGENTS IN ACS

CYCLOXYGENASE-1 (COX-1) INHIBITOR: ASPIRIN

In addition to its analgesic and antipyretic effects, aspirin is also a very potent inhibitor of platelet function and has the distinction of being the most commonly used anti-platelet agent worldwide [3]. It causes irreversible blockade of COX-1, which catalyses the synthesis of thromboxane A2 (TXA2) from arachidonic acid. TXA2 renders changes in platelet shape and augments recruitment and aggregation of platelets through its binding to thromboxane and prostaglandin-endoperoxide receptors. Aspirin, therefore, decreases platelet activation and aggregation [2]. Data from a large-scale

randomised controlled study assessing the effectiveness of aspirin as an antithrombotic agent published in 1983, involving 1,266 men with unstable angina (UA) who received treatment with either aspirin or placebo, showed a significant reduction in progression to myocardial infarction (MI) among those taking aspirin [4]. The beneficial effects of aspirin on morbidity and mortality in patients with ACS have subsequently been confirmed in randomised trials and meta-analysis [5,6]. These benefits were observed at a dose of 75–100 mg daily. A dose-dependent risk for bleeding, particularly upper gastrointestinal bleeding without an increase in efficacy, has been observed with dose >100 mg daily [2]. A large multicentric, international trial, 'CURRENT-OASIS 7', randomised 25,086 patients with ACS treated with an early invasive strategy into two groups based on the dose of aspirin (lower-dose 75–100 mg daily vs. higher-dose 300–325 mg daily). No difference was noted in the composite of cardiovascular death, myocardial infarction, and stroke at 30 days (4.4% vs. 4.2%, respectively). Overall bleeding events were also the same (2.3%) for both aspirin doses. However, an increase in the rate of gastrointestinal bleeds in the higher-dose group (0.4% vs. 0.2%; P1/4.04) was observed [7]. It is still controversial whether aspirin resistance is clinically relevant or not, and whether patients deemed to be 'poor responders' to aspirin should be switched to an alternative anti-platelet agent or not [8]. The available data does demonstrate variable results on platelet function assays, suggesting the presence of aspirin resistance. However, platelet COX-1 activity, which is suggested by the levels of TXA2, is persistently and uniformly suppressed by low-dose aspirin [9] and therefore it is now mostly accepted that the true pharmacological resistance to aspirin is rare and clinically irrelevant.

ADENOSINE DIPHOSPHATE (ADP) P2Y12 RECEPTOR ANTAGONISTS

Adenosine diphosphate (ADP), an important platelet agonist, has P2Y1 and P2Y12 receptors on the platelet plasma membrane through which it exerts its effects. Out of these two, it is the P2Y12 pathway

Table 11.1 Comparison of various P2Y12 receptor antagonists

	Clopidogrel	Prasugrel	Ticagrelor	Cangrelor
Chemical class	Thienopyridine	Thienopyridine	Cyclopentyl-triazolopyrimidine	Stabilized ATP analogue
Administration	Oral	Oral	Oral	Intravenous
Dose	300–600 mg orally then 75 mg a day	60 mg orally then 10 mg a day	180 mg orally then 90 mg twice a day	30 μg/kg bolus and 4 μg/kg/min infusion
Dosing in CKD				
• Stage 3 (eGFR 30–59 mL/min/1.73 m^2)	No dose adjustment	No dose adjustment	No dose adjustment	No dose adjustment
• Stage 4 (eGFR 15–29 mL/min/1.73 m^2)	No dose adjustment	No dose adjustment	No dose adjustment	No dose adjustment
• Stage 5 (eGFR <15 mL/min/1.73 m^2)	Use only for selected indications (e.g. stent thrombosis prevention)	Not recommended	Not recommended	No dose adjustment
Binding reversibility	Irreversible	Irreversible	Reversible	Reversible
Activation	Prodrug, with variable liver metabolism	Prodrug, with predictable liver metabolism	Active drug, with additional active metabolite	Active drug
Onset of loading dose effect	2–6 hrs	30 min	30 min	2 min
Duration of effect	3–10 days	7–10 days	3–5 days	1–2 hrs
Withdrawal before surgery	5 days	7 days	3 days	1 hr
Plasma half-life of active P2Y12 inhibitor	30–60 min	30–60 min	6–12 hrs	5–10 min
Inhibition of adenosine reuptake	No	No	Yes	Yes ('inactive' metabolite only)

Source: Reprinted (adapted) from Roffi M et al. 2015. *Eur Heart J.* 2016;37:267–315.

that plays a major contribution in sustaining and stabilising the aggregation of platelets [10]. P2Y12 receptor antagonists are therefore recommended to prevent ischaemic events both in the acute and long-term treatment of ACS. The thienopyridine, ticlopidine, which was the first P2Y12 receptor inhibitor, is seldom prescribed now following the reports of serious adverse reactions with its use, particularly neutropenia and thrombotic thrombocytopenic purpura [11]. Three oral ADP P2Y12 receptors inhibiting drugs that are currently approved for clinical use include clopidogrel, prasugrel (irreversible inhibition), and ticagrelor (reversible inhibition) (Table 11.1).

CLOPIDOGREL

It is the most commonly prescribed P2Y12 receptor antagonist worldwide. It is an orally administered drug, up to 85% of which undergoes hepatic metabolism by carboxylesterases to form an inactive derivative, clopidogrelic acid. The remaining 15% of the absorbed drug is metabolised into an active thiol product by the cytochrome P450 isoenzymes [12]. Although clopidogrel has a short half-life of 6 hours, the thiol metabolite binds covalently to the P2Y12 receptor, thereby inducing an irreversible conformational change in the P2Y12 receptor and thus inhibiting the thrombotic function of the affected platelet for its remaining lifespan (7–10 days) [2,12]. The recommendation of using DAPT with aspirin and clopidogrel in ACS is based on various studies (Table 11.2) indicating a clear benefit of adding clopidogrel with aspirin in preventing atherothrombotic events [13–16]. However, with the increasing recognition of inter-patient unpredictability in

clopidogrel responsiveness due to genetic polymorphisms in the cytochrome P450 enzymes CYP2C19 and CYP2C9, and the proven weaker and delayed platelet inhibition in comparison to the newer P2Y12 antagonists, there has been an advocacy in favour of prasugrel and ticagrelor as the preferred agents in ACS [2,3].

PRASUGREL

It is an oral thienopyridine prodrug that needs hepatic biotransformation into an active metabolite, which then blocks the P2Y12 receptor irreversibly. Since prasugrel is metabolised via esterases and has less dependence upon the CYP enzymes, it has a more potent, quick, and consistent platelet inhibition in comparison to clopidogrel [[3]17]. TRITON-TIMI 38, a phase III study involving 13,608 patients, revealed that in patients with ACS undergoing PCI, prasugrel in a 60 mg loading dose followed by 10 mg daily was more effective in reducing death, ischaemic stroke, myocardial infarction, stent thrombosis, and urgent revascularization in comparison to clopidogrel, albeit with a higher risk of major bleeding [18]. In certain subgroups, such as diabetes and STEMI, benefits were more marked with a significantly greater ischaemic benefit without any appreciable increase in the major bleeding [19,20]. Prasugrel further led to a significant reduction in the recurrent events, including mortality, compared to clopidogrel at a median follow-up of 14.8 months [21]. Post-hoc analysis identified three subgroups that either did not derive any benefit (patients aged >75 years or those with weighing <60 kg) or had harm with the use of prasugrel (patients with prior transient ischaemic attack [TIA] or stroke). If these three features

Table 11.2 Selected landmark trials of currently used ADP P2Y12 receptor antagonists

Study/Trial	Study aim	Study population	Sample size	Principal efficacy outcomes (treatment vs. control)	Principal safety outcomes (treatment vs. control)
CURE [13]	To compare the efficacy and safety of the early and long-term use of clopidogrel plus aspirin with those of aspirin alone in patients with ACS without ST-segment elevation	Randomised trial; early and long-term clopidogrel (300-mg bolus and 75 mg OD) and aspirin vs. aspirin alone given for 3–12 months	12,562	Vascular death/MI/stroke (9.3% vs. 11.4%; RR, 0.80 95% CI, 0.72–0.90; P < 0.001)	Major bleed (3.7% vs. 2.7%; RR, 1.38; P = 0.001) For every 1000 patients treated with clopidogrel, 6 required transfusion
CURE PCI [14]	To demonstrate whether aspirin and pre-treatment with clopidogrel followed by its long-term administration is superior to no pre-treatment and short-term treatment with clopidogrel after PCI	Patients with NSTEMI undergoing PCI in the CURE study for refractory ischaemia. Randomly assigned double-blind treatment with clopidogrel (n = 1313) or placebo (n = 1345). Pre-treated with aspirin and study drug for a median of 10 d before PCI	2658	CV death, MI, or urgent TVR within 30 d of PCI (4.5% vs. 6.4%; RR, 0.70; 95% CI, 0.50–0.97; P = 0.03)	Major bleed 30 d: 1.6% vs. 1.4%, P1/4.69; end of follow-up: 2.7% vs. 2.5%, P = 0.64
CLARITY-TIMI 28 [15]	To demonstrate whether addition of clopidogrel is beneficial in patients with STEMI who have received fibrinolysis and aspirin, patients were scheduled for coronary angiography 48–192 hrs after study medication	Randomised trial of patients with STEMI, 75 y or younger, presenting within 12 hrs of symptom onset	3491	Occluded IRA at angiogram (TIMI flow 0/1) or death or recurrent MI before angiography (15% vs. 21.7%; RR, 0.36; 95% CI, 0.24–0.47, P < 0.001)	Major bleed: 1.3% vs. 1.1% on day after angiography (P = 0.64); 1.9% vs. 1.7% at 30 d
COMMIT [16]	To demonstrate benefit of DAPT vs. aspirin alone on mortality and morbidity in a large Chinese population presenting with STEMI and treated with fibrinolytic therapy	Randomised trial of clopidogrel 75 mg OD (n = 22,961) or placebo (n = 22,891) in addition to aspirin 162 mg daily; 93% had STEMI	45,852	Death/reinfarction/stroke in 9.2% vs. 10.1% (P = 0.002) All-cause mortality: 7.5% vs. 8.1% (P = 0.03)	Fatal, transfused, or cerebral bleeds: 0.58% vs. 0.55% (P = 0.59)
TRITON-TIMI-38 [18]	To test whether prasugrel with a higher level of inhibition of ADP-induced platelet aggregation and a less-variable response reduces ischaemic events compared with standard-dose clopidogrel in patients with ACS undergoing PCI	Patients with ACS scheduled for PCI. Prasugrel: 60-mg loading dose and 10-mg OD maintenance dose or Clopidogrel: 300-mg loading dose and 75-mg OD maintenance dose for 6–15 mo. Drugs started after coronary anatomy known, except for primary PCI in STEMI	13,608	CV death/nonfatal MI/stroke (9.9% vs. 12.1%; HR, 0.81; 95% CI, 0.73–0.90; P < 0.001). MI rates 7.4% vs. 9.7%; (P < 0.001) and stent thrombosis 1.1% vs. 2.4% (P < 0.001)	Major bleeding was seen in 2.4% vs. 1.8% (HR, 1.32; 95% CI, 1.03–1.68; P = 0.03) Patients treated with prasugrel had higher life-threatening (1.4% vs. 0.9%; P = 0.01), nonfatal (1.1% vs. 0.9%; HR, 1.25; P = 0.23) and fatal bleeding (0.4% vs. 0.1%; P = 0.002)
TRILOGY-ACS [23]	To investigate the effect of intensified platelet inhibition with prasugrel in patients with ACS without ST-segment elevation treated medically without revascularization	Double-blind, randomised trial. Primary analysis involving 7243 patients <75 y receiving aspirin, FU for 30 mo of treatment with prasugrel (10 mg daily) vs. clopidogrel (75 mg daily)	9326	CV death/MI/stroke (13.9% vs. 16%; HR, 0.91; 0.79–1.05; P = 0.21)	TIMI major bleed in patients <75 y: 2.1% vs. 1.5% (HR, 1.31; 95% CI 0.81–2.11; P = 0.27)
PLATO [24]	To determine whether ticagrelor is superior to clopidogrel in a broad population of patients presenting with an ACS treated with invasive and conservative approaches. Treatment started upstream	Double-blind, randomised trial, compared ticagrelor (180-mg loading dose, then 90 mg twice daily) and clopidogrel (300- to 600-mg loading dose, then 75 mg OD) for the prevention of CV events in patients with ACS with/without STEMI	18,624	1-y primary end point cardiovascular death, MI, or stroke in 9.8% vs. 11.7% with clopidogrel (HR, 0.84; 95% CI, 0.77–0.92; P < 0.001)	Major bleed: 11.6% vs. 11.2% (HR, 1.04; 95% CI, 0.95–1.13; P = 0.43) Non-CABG-related major bleed: 4.5% vs. 3.8% (P = 0.03)
CHAMPION-PHOENIX [29]	To evaluate whether cangrelor reduces ischemic complications of PCI	Double-dummy, double-blind trial to receive cangrelor before PCI or clopidogrel (600 mg or 300 mg) immediately after PCI	11,145	All-cause death/MI/ischemia-driven revascularization/stent thrombosis at 48 hrs: 4.7% vs. 5.9% (OR, 0.78; 95% CI, 0.66–0.93; P = 0.005)	GUSTO-defined severe bleed: 0.16% vs. 0.11% (OR, 1.50; 95% CI, 0.53–4.22; P = 0.44)

Source: Reprinted (adapted) from Singh M et al. *Mayo Clin Proc.* 2016 Oct;91(10):1413–1447.

were absent, there was a net positive clinical benefit with prasugrel in comparison to clopidogrel. Consequently, prasugrel is contra-indicated in patients with prior TIA or stroke and best avoided or used at a lower dose (5 mg daily) in elderly patients >75 years of age and those with weight <60 kg. In the ACCOST trial involving 4033 ACS (NSTEMI) patients undergoing PCI, pre-treatment with prasugrel before identifying the coronary anatomy on angiography did not result in any significant reduction in the rate of the primary outcome but led to an increased rate of TIMI major bleeding at 1 week [22]. Hence, prasugrel is not indicated in patients with ACS in whom coronary anatomy is not known and an indication for PCI is not established, except for STEMI patients scheduled to undergo immediate coronary catheterisation and PCI, if clinically indicated. Similarly, among medically managed patients with ACS, the use of prasugrel is not recommended, since it has not been found to provide any benefit over clopidogrel in preventing ischaemic events, but rather has been shown to increase bleeding risk in patients not undergoing PCI [23].

TICAGRELOR

It is a cyclopentyl-triazolo-pyrimidine ADP antagonist. Ticagrelor has distinct pharmacokinetic and pharmacodynamic properties and binds directly to the P2Y12 receptor, thereby altering its con-formation and resulting in reversible inhibition. It is not a prodrug and does not require metabolic activation. It, therefore, exhibits a relatively rapid onset (30 minutes) of action. The drug has a short half-life of 6 to 12 hours and needs to be administered twice daily to achieve a steady-state ADP inhibition [2,3]. A large randomised trial involving 18,624 patients with ACS (PLATO trial) showed a significant reduction in vascular death, MI, or stroke with the use of ticagrelor in comparison with clopidogrel (9.8% vs. 11.7%; P < 0.001). This benefit was consistent regardless of the presentation (STEMI or NSTEMI) and whether the patients were treated conservatively or underwent an invasive approach for ACS [24]. In addition to the reduction in MI and stent thrombosis, ticagrelor also led to a reduc-tion in the rates of vascular as well as all-cause mortality. Ticagrelor resulted in an increased incidence of major bleeding not related to coronary artery bypass grafting (CABG). However, there was no increase in non-CABG-related bleeding, fatal bleeding, and overall major bleeding, probably because of its reversibility. Notably, there were higher rates of dyspnoea and ventricular pauses leading to dis-continuation of therapy, the mechanism of which remains elusive and these side effects have not been shown to have any significant clinical impact [25]. Ticagrelor is superior to clopidogrel irrespec-tive of the absence or presence of CYP2C19 and/or ABCB1 loss-of-polymorphisms [26]. Ticagrelor is contraindicated in patients with severe hepatic dysfunction and prior haemorrhagic stroke.

INTRAVENOUS ANTI-PLATELET AGENTS IN ACS

CANGRELOR

It belongs to a new class of drugs termed as non-thienopyri-dine adenosine triphosphate analogues. It is an intravenous and competitive P2Y12 inhibitor and has a reversible mode of action. It has a short half-life of 5 minutes only. Cangrelor has a very rapid onset and offset of action, unlike the currently approved oral P2Y12 anti-platelet agents, which require hours to be effec-tive. Furthermore, cangrelor does not require *in vivo* bioacti-vation. It, therefore, reaches a steady-state in plasma within a few minutes of its administration and achieves more than 90% inhibition of platelet activation resulting from the P2Y12 path-way [2,3]. Multiple randomised controlled trials, comparing the use of cangrelor with the current standard therapy, have found no significant differences in the mortality or further MI when patients were treated with either cangrelor or clopidogrel before [27] or during PCI [28]. However, in a double-blind placebo-controlled randomised trial involving 11,145 patients, cangre-lor led to a significant reduction in the rate of ischaemic events during PCI, compared with clopidogrel, without any increase in severe bleeding [29]. Cangrelor was subsequently approved by US and European regulatory agencies in 2015 for use in patients undergoing PCI. It is particularly useful in patients with ACS who are unable to take oral agents due to repeated vomiting or those in a state of shock or on a ventilator. It is also very use-ful in patients with ACS who require urgent surgery, as its use avoids preloading with DAPT and thus permits early surgery without waiting 5–7 days for oral drug washout.

GLYCOPROTEIN IIB/IIIA RECEPTOR INHIBITORS IN ACS

GPIIb/IIIa inhibitors compete with the von Willebrand factor and fibrinogen for binding at the GPIIb/IIIa receptor. They thus inhibit the final pathway of platelet aggregation and provide rapid and potent anti-platelet effects. They are more potent anti-platelet agents than cangrelor since they inhibit platelet response to all the agonists [30]. GPIIb/IIIa inhibitors overcome the delayed and weak platelet inhibition caused by a clopidogrel loading dose by achieving rapid and nearly complete platelet aggregation inhibi-tion [30]. Early clinical trials demonstrated the benefits of pre-treatment with these intravenous agents in the high-risk patients undergoing angioplasty, resulting in a significant reduction in MI and urgent revascularisation [31,32]. However, these benefits were mainly shown in the era before the routine use of DAPT, potent oral P2Y12 inhibitors, direct thrombin inhibitors, the advent of new stent technologies, radial artery interventions, and thrombus aspiration. Currently, GPIIb/IIIa inhibitors are used in nearly one-third of patients undergoing PCI for ACS in the United States [33]. The use of GPIIb/IIIa inhibitors has been associated with a reduction in adverse cardiovascular events, including MI, albeit at the expense of increased bleeding and thrombocytopenia [33,34]. Many recent trials and systematic reviews, specifically in patients who are adequately pre-treated with thienopyridines, have shown conflicting evidence regard-ing the benefit of routine use of GPIIb/IIIa inhibitors [33–35]. Current guidelines recommend their use only in patients without adequate and timely preloading with P2Y12 antagonists, in bail-out/rescue situations, and in those with large thrombus burden during primary PCI [2,3,33].

WHAT DO THE GUIDELINES SAY? SELECTION AND TIMING OF INITIATION OF P2Y12 INHIBITOR IN ACS

Recommendations on the timing and selection of P2Y12 inhibitors are largely consistent between the European Society of Cardiology (ESC) and the American College of Cardiology (ACC) guidelines [36]. Both society guidelines recommend that in ACS patients with no contraindications, aspirin should be combined with either prasugrel or ticagrelor in preference to clopidogrel. While ticagrelor is a recommended option for all the patients with ACS regardless of whether patients are undergoing invasive or conservative approach, prasugrel should be used in only those patients in whom coronary anatomy is known and who are undergoing PCI. Clopidogrel should be used in ACS patients only if these newer agents are contraindicated or unavailable [36]. It might also be considered in the elderly and/or patients with increased bleeding risk. The recommendation for STEMI patients remains the same, especially those undergoing PCI, except that prasugrel can be administered before coronary angiography in STEMI patients once the indication to primary PCI is established. This strategy has been tested in the regulatory trial of prasugrel and was not shown to be harmful [18]. Additionally, in STEMI patients treated with thrombolysis, clopidogrel remains the drug of choice. This is because STEMI patients undergoing thrombolysis were excluded from the regulatory trials of ticagrelor and prasugrel, therefore there is not enough data regarding their use in these patients [36].

There has been extensive research on the optimal timing for the initiation of P2Y12 inhibitors in the setting of ACS [37–39]. Until conclusive data is available, it is a reasonable approach to start a P2Y12 inhibitor based on the timing with which the particular drug was investigated in its landmark approval study. Thus it would be appropriate to start clopidogrel and ticagrelor as soon as possible after the presentation and start prasugrel once the indication for PCI is established based on coronary anatomy. The early administration of P2Y12 inhibitors also depends on the planned

use of cangrelor during PCI, which ensures immediate platelet inhibition in oral P2Y12 inhibitor naive patients. Converting from cangrelor to the P2Y12 inhibitors after PCI is complicated by a pharmacodynamic competitive effect between cangrelor and the active metabolites of clopidogrel and prasugrel, which cannot bind to P2Y12 when cangrelor occupies the receptor. Ticagrelor forms an ideal combination with cangrelor since no such interaction is seen between them. Ticagrelor, therefore, can be given at any time before, during, or at the end of cangrelor infusion. On the contrary, since earlier use of clopidogrel and prasugrel during cangrelor infusion can increase and hasten platelet recovery, it is recommended that clopidogrel is given at the time of cangrelor infusion discontinuation and prasugrel to be given 30 minutes before the end of infusion of cangrelor to avoid any competitive interaction between the active metabolites and cangrelor occupied P2Y12 receptors [40]. This, however, does leave a potential time window for clot formation and stent thrombosis, a phenomenon not seen with ticagrelor and cangrelor combination [40].

There is a consensus that early administration of oral P2Y12 inhibitors outweighs any potential risks if the coronary anatomy is known or the probability of PCI is high like in STEMI patients. ESC gives class 1 recommendation for pre-treatment with a P2Y12 inhibitor in ACS patients in whom coronary anatomy is known and the decision to proceed to PCI is made as well as in patients with STEMI [41]. In patients with ACS undergoing invasive management, ticagrelor (180 mg loading dose, followed by 90 mg twice daily), or clopidogrel (600 mg loading dose, followed by 75 mg daily dose) if ticagrelor is not an option, should be considered as soon as the diagnosis is established (class IIa recommendation). In ACS patients in whom coronary anatomy is not known, it is not recommended to administer prasugrel (class III recommendation).

PRACTICAL SUGGESTIONS

The various advantages and disadvantages of the three standard oral P2Y12 receptor antagonists are listed in Table 11.3. With

Table 11.3 Pros and cons of three commonly used oral P2Y12 antagonists

Drug	Advantages	Disadvantages
Clopidogrel	1. Inexpensive 2. Greater familiarity 3. Can be used in both medically managed and PCI patients 4. Only agent with proven efficacy following thrombolysis 5. Once-daily dosing	1. Variable efficacy 2. Slow onset of action 3. Drug–drug interactions 4. Genetic response variation 5. Weaker anti-platelet effect than the newer agents
Prasugrel	1. Rapid onset of action 2. Greater efficacy in STEMI/DM 3. Less drug–drug interactions 4. More effective than clopidogrel 5. Single-daily dosing	1. Expensive (higher cost than clopidogrel) 2. Major bleeding higher 3. Can be used only in PCI patients 4. Cannot be preloaded until coronary anatomy is known 5. Longer off-drug period before CABG
Ticagrelor	1. Rapid onset and offset of action 2. Reversible platelet inhibition 3. Greater efficacy than clopidogrel 4. Bleeding risk comparable to clopidogrel 5. Mortality benefit 6. Can be used in both medically managed and PCI patients	1. Most expensive of all three 2. Twice-daily dosing 3. Side effects of dyspnoea and ventricular pauses 4. Higher withdrawal rates 5. Higher non-CABG-related bleeding

the increasing number and complexity of PCI in ACS, more prolonged and intensified anti-platelet therapy is required. All possible DAPT strategies need to be assessed objectively. The concern with clopidogrel is the variable and frequent weak response; while bleeding and cost are the major problems with prasugrel and ticagrelor, respectively. How do we decide which agent to use for a particular patient? The answer is not simple. Clopidogrel is still commonly used in those with a low ischaemic burden and high bleeding risk and especially in those patients who have received thrombolysis. Ticagrelor and prasugrel have proven superiority over clopidogrel. But the question arises: Which is better, ticagrelor or prasugrel? Ticagrelor is proposed by many as the best choice when balancing ischaemic and bleeding risk, with an additional advantage of decreased mortality and myocardial infarction. With ticagrelor, the dose of aspirin must be less than 100 mg per day. Additionally, the reversible action of ticagrelor makes it an attractive choice in situations when DAPT needs to be interrupted. Furthermore, ticagrelor provides better efficacy and safety in medically managed ACS patients, unlike prasugrel, which is recommended for use only in patients undergoing PCI. However, prasugrel is a good choice in those patients of ACS who undergo PCI with high ischaemic risk and low bleeding risk. It is an appropriate choice for relatively younger patients with ACS and diabetes and also in those who have had stent thrombosis or recurrent ACS while on clopidogrel. In the recently published randomised, controlled ISAR-REACT 5 trial [42], involving 4018 patients with acute coronary syndromes (41.1% of whom had ST-segment elevation myocardial infarction [STEMI]) for whom invasive evaluation was planned, a prasugrel-based strategy was superior to a ticagrelor-based strategy in reducing the incidence of death, myocardial infarction, or stroke at 1 year (6.9% vs. 9.3%, P = 0.006), with a number needed to treat of 42. This result was driven primarily by a significant reduction of 1.8% age points in the incidence of recurrent (spontaneous and PCI associated) myocardial infarction, with no significant between-group differences in the incidence of major bleeding. Thus the ISAR-REACT 5 trial has tilted the table towards prasugrel for use among ACS patients undergoing PCI. However, we need further data to establish this superiority. Remember that prasugrel should not be used in patients with a history of stroke or transient ischaemic attack and at reduced doses in elderly patients more than 75 years of age and in those with a low body weight of less than 60 kg.

ANTI-PLATELET THERAPY IN PATIENTS TREATED WITH CORONARY ARTERY BYPASS SURGERY FOR ACS

No dedicated study exists comparing the effect of dual anti-platelet therapy in ACS patients undergoing coronary artery bypass grafting (CABG) compared to aspirin monotherapy. In the CURE trial, the outcome in the CABG subpopulation was consistent with the overall results of the study [43]. In the CABG substudies of the TRITON-TIMI 38 and the PLATO trials where, respectively, prasugrel and ticagrelor were tested against clopidogrel in combination with ASA, both newer P2Y12 inhibitors were more effective

than clopidogrel in preventing fatal outcomes, with a higher risk for bleeding in the former but not the latter trial [44,45]. However, it is comprehensively proven that the continuation of DAPT until CABG increases the risk of excessive perioperative bleeding, transfusions, and re-exploration for bleeding [41]. Therefore, it is recommended that the P2Y12 inhibitors should be discontinued whenever possible before elective CABG [41]. Alternatively, elective operations may be postponed until the DAPT treatment period is completed. It is recommended that the heart team should estimate the individual ischaemic and bleeding risks and guide the antithrombotic management as well as the timing of CABG. In patients who are on aspirin therapy and need a non-emergent cardiac surgery, it is recommended to continue aspirin at a low dose daily throughout the perioperative period. On the other hand, for patients who are taking P2Y12 inhibitors and need to undergo a non-emergent cardiac surgery, it is recommended to postpone surgery for at least 3, 5, and 7 days after discontinuation of ticagrelor, clopidogrel, and prasugrel, respectively [41].

In urgent cases, most often patients with ACS, the risk of thrombotic episodes while waiting for the effect of the P2Y12 inhibitor to cease must be weighed against the risk of perioperative bleeding complications. In extreme high-risk patients requiring urgent CABG, e.g. those with recent DES implantation, bridging therapy with cangrelor or a glycoprotein IIb/IIIa blocker may be considered. After both non-emergent and urgent CABG in the ACS setting, resumption of P2Y12 inhibitor therapy should be as soon as it is deemed safe after the surgery and continuation of up to 12 months is recommended [41].

NEWER DEVELOPMENTS

Thrombin, the most potent platelet activator, activating platelets at an extremely low concentration, is not influenced by P2Y12 receptor antagonists or aspirin. PAR-1 antagonists antagonise the thrombin-induced platelets' activation and aggregation by blocking the binding of thrombin to PAR-1. Importantly, this blockade does not interfere with the thrombin-mediated fibrin generation that is essential for hemostasis [2]. Currently, two PAR-1 inhibitors are under clinical development for the prevention of arterial thrombosis: voraxapar and atopaxar [46]. Vorapaxar, a PAR-1 antagonist, was studied in the TRACER trial, involving 12,944 patients with ACS without ST-segment elevation who were randomised to vorapaxar versus standard treatment [47]. The primary composite end point of cardiovascular death, stroke, MI, recurrent ischaemia with rehospitalisation, or urgent coronary revascularisation after a median follow-up of 502 days was not significantly less with vorapaxar (18.5% vs. 19.9%; HR, 0.92; 95% CI, 0.85–1.01; P = 0.07). The secondary ischaemic outcomes of cardiovascular death, MI, or stroke occurred in 14.7% of patients treated with vorapaxar compared with 16.4% treated with placebo (HR, 0.89; 95% CI, 0.81–0.98; P = 0.02). The trial had to be prematurely terminated because of higher rates of severe bleeding in the vorapaxar group, including intracranial haemorrhage. Vorapaxar was also studied in a CHARISMA-like secondary prevention population. In the TRAP 2 P-TIMI 50 trial [48], 26,449 patients with MI, prior stroke, and peripheral artery disease (PAD) were randomised to vorapaxar treatment versus placebo. At 3 years, the primary end point of cardiovascular death, MI, or stroke occurred in fewer vorapaxar-treated patients (9.3% vs. 10.5%; P < 0.001), although major bleeding was increased with vorapaxar, especially in patients with prior stroke. Atopaxar, another PAR-1 inhibitor, is still in the early phase of clinical development. Two phase II studies, the LANCELOT-ACS (Lessons from Antagonising the Cellular Effects of Thrombin–Acute Coronary Syndromes) and the LANCELOT-CAD (Lessons from Antagonising the Cellular Effects of Thrombin–Coronary Artery Disease), have demonstrated a good safety profile in terms of bleeding risk of atopaxar compared with placebo in subjects with ACS and CAD, respectively [49,50]. However, there were some concerning signals about transient elevation in liver transaminases and prolongation of the QTc interval with the highest dose of atopaxar. Larger trials would be required to establish the real clinical value of this new agent.

Besides these, various agents targeting a number of platelet signalling pathways have been addressed in preclinical or early phase clinical studies [2,17], including serotonin receptor blocker (APD791), prostaglandin E receptor 3 antagonists (DG-041), nitric oxide donors (LA846, LA419), glycoprotein VI antagonists (kistomin, revacept) or glycoprotein Ib antagonist (6B4-Fab monoclonal antibody), and phosphatidylinositol 3-kinase inhibitors (TGX-221).

REFERENCES

1. Hanson, G.K. Inflammation, atherosclerosis and coronary artery disease. *N Engl J Med*. 2005;352:1685–1895.
2. Dash D. Current status of antiplatelet therapy in acute coronary syndrome. *Cardiovasc Hematol Agents Med Chem*. 2015;13(1):40–49.
3. Layne K, Ferro A. Antiplatelet therapy in acute coronary syndrome. *Eur Cardiol*. 2017 Aug;12(1):33–37.
4. Lewis HD Jr, Davis JW, Archibald DG et al. Protective effects of aspirin against acute myocardial infarction and death in men with unstable angina. Results of a Veterans Administration Cooperative Study. *N Engl J Med*. 1983;309:396–403.
5. Fuster V, Dyken ML, Vokonas PS, Hennekens C. Aspirin as a therapeutic agent in cardiovascular disease. Special Writing Group. *Circulation*. 1993;87:659–675.
6. Antithrombotic Trialists' (ATT) Collaboration, Baigent C, Blackwell L, Collins R et al. Aspirin in the primary and secondary prevention of vascular disease: Collaborative meta-analysis of individual participant data from randomised trials. *Lancet*. 2009;373:1849–1860.
7. CURRENT-OASIS 7 Investigators, Mehta SR, Bassand JP, Chrolavicius S et al. Dose comparisons of clopidogrel and aspirin in acute coronary syndromes. *N Engl J Med*. 2010;363(10):930–942.
8. Pamukcu B, Oflaz H, Oncul A, Umman B, Mercanoglu F, Ozcan M, Meric M, Nisanci Y. The role of aspirin resistance on outcome in patients with acute coronary syndrome and the effect of clopidogrel therapy in the prevention of major cardiovascular events. *J Thromb Thrombolysis*. 2006 Oct;22(2):103–110.
9. Santilli F, Rocca B, De Cristofaro R et al. Platelet cyclooxygenase inhibition by low-dose aspirin is not reflected consistently by platelet function assays: Implications for aspirin "resistance". *J Am Coll Cardiol*. 2009;53:667–677.
10. Storey, R.F., Newby, L.J., Heptinstall, S. Effects of P2Y (1) and P2Y(12) receptor antagonists on platelet aggregation induced by different agonists in human whole blood. *Platelets*. 2001;12:443–447.
11. Kovacs KMJ, Soong PY, Chin-Yee IH. Thrombotic thrombocytopenic purpura associated with ticlopidine. *Ann Pharmacother*. 1993;27:1060–1061.
12. Wijeyeratne YD, Heptinstall S. Anti-platelet therapy: ADP receptor antagonists. *Br J Clin Pharmacol*. 2011;72:647–657.
13. Yusuf S, Zhao F, Mehta SR, Chrolavicius S, Tognoni G, Fox KK. Effects of clopidogrel in addition to aspirin in patients with acute coronary syndromes without ST-segment elevation. *N Engl J Med*. 2001;345(7):494–502.
14. Mehta SR, Yusuf S, Peters RJ et al. Clopidogrel in Unstable angina to prevent Recurrent Events trial (CURE) Investigators. Effects of pretreatment with clopidogrel and aspirin followed by long-term therapy in patients undergoing percutaneous coronary intervention: The PCI-CURE study. *Lancet*. 2001;358(9281):527–533.
15. Sabatine MS, Cannon CP, Gibson CM et al.; CLARITY-TIMI 28 Investigators. Addition of clopidogrel to aspirin and fibrinolytic therapy for myocardial infarction with ST-segment elevation. *N Engl J Med*. 2005;352(12):1179–1189.
16. Chen ZM, Jiang LX, Chen YP, Xie JX, Pan HC, Peto R, Collins R, Liu LS; COMMIT (ClOpidogrel and Metoprolol in Myocardial Infarction Trial) collaborative group. Addition of clopidogrel to aspirin in 45,852 patients with acute myocardial infarction: Randomised placebo-controlled trial. *Lancet*. 2005;366(9497):1607–1621.
17. Ferreiro, J.L., Angiolillo D.J. New directions in antiplatelet therapy. *Circ Cardiovasc Interv* 2012;5:433–445.
18. Wiviott SD, Braunwald E, Mccabe CH et al., TRITON-TIMI 38 Investigators. Prasugrel versus clopidogrel in patients with acute coronary syndromes. *N Engl J Med*. 2007;357:2001–2015.
19. Wiviott S.D, Braunwald E., Angiolillo D.J. et al., TRITON-TIMI 38 Investigators Greater clinical benefit of more intensive oral antiplatelet therapy with prasugrel in patients with diabetes mellitus in the trial to assess improvement in therapeutic outcomes by optimizing platelet inhibition with prasugrel-Thrombolysis in Myocardial Infarction 38. *Circulation*. 2008;118:1626–1636.
20. Montalescot G, Wiviott S.D., Braunwald E, Murphy S.A, Gibson C.M., McCabe C.H., Antman E.M., TRITON-TIMI 38 investigators. TRITON-TIMI 38 Investigators. Prasugrel compared with clopidogrel in patients undergoing percutaneous coronary intervention for ST-elevation myocardial infarction (TRITON- TIMI 38): Double-blind, randomized controlled trial. *Lancet*. 2009;373:723–731.
21. Murphy SA, Antman EM, Wiviott SD, Weerakkody G, Morocutti G, Huber K, Lopez-Sendon J, McCabe C.H, Braunwald, E, TRITON-TIMI 38 Investigators. Reduction in recurrent cardiovascular events with prasugrel compared

with clopidogrel in patients with acute coronary syndromes from the TRITON-TIMI 38 trial. *Eur Heart J.* 2008;29:2473–2479.

22. Montalescot G, Bolognese L, Dudek D et al. Pretreatment with prasugrel in non-ST-segment elevation acute coronary syndromes. *N Engl J Med.* 2013;369:999–1010.

23. Roe MT, Armstrong P, Fox KAA et al., TRILOGY ACS Investigators. Prasugrel versus clopidogrel for acute coronary syndromes without revascularization. *N Engl J Med.* 2012;367:1297–1309.

24. Wallentin L, Becker RC, Budaj A et al., for the PLATO Investigators. Ticagrelor versus clopidogrel in patients with acute coronary syndromes. *N Engl J Med.* 2009;361:1045–1057.

25. Scirica BM, Cannon CP, Emanuelsson H et al. PLATO Investigators. The incidence of bradyarrhythmias and clinical bradyarrhythmic events in patients with acute coronary syndromes treated with ticagrelor or clopidogrel in the PLATO (Platelet Inhibition and Patient Outcomes) trial: Results of the continuous electrocardiographic assessment substudy. *J Am Coll Cardiol.* 2011;57:1908–1916.

26. Wallentein L, James S, Storey RF et al., PLATO investigators. Effect of CYP2C19 and ABCB1 single nucleotide polymorphisms on outcomes of treatment with ticagrelor versus clopidogrel for acute coronary syndromes: A genetic substudy of the PLATO trial. *Lancet.* 2010;376:1320–1328.

27. Harrington RA, Stone GW, McNulty S et al. Platelet inhibition with cangrelor in patients undergoing PCI. *N Engl J Med.* 2009;361:2318–2329.

28. Bhatt DL, Lincoff AM, Gibson CM et al., CHAMPION PLATFORM Investigators. Intravenous platelet blockade with cangrelor during PCI. *N Engl J Med.* 2009;361:2230–2341.

29. Bhatt DL, Stone GW, Mahaffey KW et al., Genereux P, Liu T, Prats J, Todd M, Skerjanec S, White H.D, Harrington R.A, CHAMPION PHOENIX Investigators. Effect of platelet inhibition with cangrelor during PCI on ischemic events. *N Engl J Med.* 2013;368:1303–1313.

30. Gurbel PA, Bliden KP, Zaman KA, Yoho JA, Hayes KM, Tantry US. Clopidogrel loading with eptifibatide to arrest the reactivity of platelets: Results of the Clopidogrel loading with eptifibatide to arrest the reactivity of platelets (CLEAR PLATELETS) study. *Circulation.* 2005;111:1153–1159.

31. ESPRIT Investigators. Enhanced suppression of the platelet IIb/IIIa receptor with integrilin therapy. Novel dosing regimen of eptifibatide in planned coronary stent implantation (ESPRIT): A randomised, placebo-controlled trial. *Lancet.* 2000;356:2037–2044.

32. Safley DM, Venkitachalam L, Kennedy KF, Cohen DJ. Impact of glycoprotein IIb/IIIa inhibition in contemporary percutaneous coronary intervention for acute coronary syndromes: Insights from the national cardiovascular data registry. *JACC Cardiovasc Interv.* 2015;8:1574–1582.

33. Muñiz-Lozano A, Rollini F, Franchi F, Angiolillo DJ. Update on platelet glycoprotein IIb/IIIa inhibitors: Recommendations for clinical practice. *Ther Adv Cardiovasc Dis.* 2013;7:197–213.

34. Sethi A, Bajaj A, Bahekar A, Bhuriya R, Singh M, Ahmed A, Khosla S. Glycoprotein IIb/IIIa inhibitors with or without thienopyridine pretreatment improve outcomes after primary percutaneous coronary intervention in high-risk patients with ST elevation myocardial infarction--a meta-regression of randomized controlled trials. *Catheter Cardiovasc Interv.* 2013;82:171–181.

35. Winchester DE, Wen X, Brearley WD, Park KE, Anderson RD, Bavry AA. Efficacy and safety of glycoprotein IIb/IIIa inhibitors during elective coronary revascularization: A meta-analysis of randomized trials performed in the era of stents and thienopyridines. *J Am Coll Cardiol.* 2011;57:1190–1199.

36. Capodanno D, Alfonso F, Levine GN, Valgimigli M, Angiolillo DJ. ACC/AHA Versus ESC guidelines on dual antiplatelet therapy: JACC guideline comparison. *J Am Coll Cardiol.* 2018 Dec 11;72(23 Pt A):2915–2931.

37. Roffi M, Patrono C, Collet JP et al. 2015 ESC Guidelines for the management of acute coronary syndromes in patients presenting without persistent ST-segment elevation: Task. Force for the management of acute coronary syndromes in patients. Presenting without persistent ST-segment elevation of the European Society of. Cardiology (ESC). *Eur Heart J.* 2016;37:267–315.

38. Valgimigli M. Pretreatment with P2Y12 inhibitors in non-ST-segment-elevation. acute coronary syndrome is clinically justified. *Circulation.* 2014;130:1891–1903; discussion 1903.

39. Collet JP, Silvain J, Bellemain-Appaix A, Montalescot G. Pretreatment with P2Y12. inhibitors in non-ST-segment-elevation acute coronary syndrome: An outdated. and harmful strategy. *Circulation.* 2014;130:1904–1914.

40. Erlinge D. Cangrelor for ST-segment-elevation myocardial infarction. *Circulation.* 2019 Apr 2;139(14):1671–1673.

41. Valgimigli M, Bueno H, Byrne RA et al.; ESC Scientific Document Group; ESC Committee for Practice Guidelines (CPG); ESC National Cardiac Societies. 2017 ESC focused update on dual antiplatelet therapy in coronary artery disease developed in collaboration with EACTS: The Task Force for dual antiplatelet therapy in coronary artery disease of the European Society of Cardiology (ESC) and of the European Association for Cardio-Thoracic Surgery (EACTS). *Eur Heart J.* 2018 Jan 14;39(3):213–260.

42. Schüpke S, Neumann FJ, Menichelli M et al.; ISAR-REACT 5 Trial Investigators. Ticagrelor or Prasugrel in patients with acute coronary syndromes. *N Engl J Med.* 2019 Oct 17;381(16):1524–1534.

43. Fox KA, Mehta SR, Peters R, Zhao F, Lakkis N, Gersh BJ, Yusuf S. Benefits and risks of the combination of clopidogrel and aspirin in patients undergoing surgical revascularization for non-ST-elevation acute coronary syndrome: The Clopidogrel in unstable angina to prevent recurrent ischemic events (CURE) Trial. *Circulation.* 2004;110:1202–1208.

44. Held C, Asenblad N, Bassand JP et al. Ticagrelor versus clopidogrel in patients with acute coronary syndromes undergoing coronary artery bypass surgery: Results from the PLATO (Platelet Inhibition and Patient Outcomes) trial. *J Am Coll Cardiol.* 2011;57:672–684.

45. Smith PK, Goodnough LT, Levy JH, Poston RS, Short MA, Weerakkody GJ, Lenarz LA. Mortality benefit with prasugrel in the TRITON-TIMI 38 coronary artery bypass grafting cohort: Risk-adjusted retrospective data analysis. *J Am Coll Cardiol.* 2012;60:388–396.

46. Angiolillo D.J, Capodanno D, Goto S. Platelet thrombin receptor antagonism and atherosclerosis. *Eur Heart J.* 2010;31:17–28.

47. Tricoci P, Huang Z, Held C et al., TRACER Investigators. Thrombin-receptor antagonist vorapaxar in acute-coronary syndromes. *N Engl J Med.* 2012;366:20–33.

48. Morrow DA, Braunwald E, Bonaca MP et al. TRA 2P-TIMI 50 Steering Committee and Investigators. Vorapaxar in the secondary prevention of atherothrombotic events. *N Engl J Med.* 2012;366:1404–1413.

49. O'Donoghue ML, Bhatt DL, Wiviott SD et al., LANCELOT-ACS Investigators. Safety and tolerability of atopaxar in the treatment of patients with acute coronary syndromes: The lessons from antagonizing the cellular effects of thrombin-acute coronary syndromes trial. *Circulation.* 2011;123:1843–1853.

50. Wiviott SD, Flather MD, O'Donoghue ML et al., LANCELOT-CAD Investigators. Randomized trial of atopaxar in the treatment of patients with coronary artery disease: The lessons learned from antagonizing the cellular effect of thrombin-coronary artery disease trial. *Circulation.* 2011;123:1854–1863.

51. Singh M, Bhatt DL, Stone GW et al., Antithrombotic approaches in acute coronary syndromes: Optimizing benefit vs bleeding Risks. *Mayo Clin Proc.* 2016 Oct;91(10): 1413–1447.

12

Current status of fibrinolytic therapy

SAUBHIK KANJILAL AND SOUMITRA KUMAR

INTRODUCTION

ST-elevated myocardial infarction remains one of the major public health problems, the incidence of which is on the rise all over the world, especially in developing countries, despite advancement in the diagnosis and management. Over the years, the primary mode of care of STEMI patients has changed from a primary pharmacologic strategy to a catheter-based one. Progressive loss of myocyte after a STEMI is linearly related to the duration of occlusion of infarct related artery. Hence, the goal of therapy of such patients is to do reperfusion of the occluded artery at the earliest. For most patients of STEMI, primary PCI is the preferred option. RCTs have shown that if time delay is similar, then primary PCI is superior to fibrinolysis in reducing mortality, reinfarction and stroke [1–5]. Fibrinolytic therapy is to be offered in a timely manner (in absence of any contraindications) to all patients who do not have the option of primary PCI, especially if they present early in their window period. As the time of presentation increases, the efficacy and clinical benefit of fibrinolytic therapy decreases [7]. It can prevent 30 deaths out of 1000 patients treated within 6 hours of onset of AMI [6]. Such pharmacologic therapy is capable of establishing antegrade flow in 75% of cases. However, there is 30% chance of re-occlusion after fibrinolysis alone.

INDICATIONS OF FIBRINOLYTIC THERAPY

Patients having chest pain suggestive of ischaemia, who present up to 12 hours of onset of symptoms, are candidates of reperfusion therapy if ECG criteria for diagnosis of AMI match. The 'golden hour' for such reperfusion therapy is within 3 hours of onset of chest pain. Any further delay beyond such period yields lesser benefit to the patients, although the final outcome of any reperfusion therapy after occlusion of an artery also depends on factors other than duration of occlusion preconditioning, presence of collaterals, comorbidities like diabetes, spontaneous recanalization, etc. All patients who cannot receive PCI in the proper time period should be considered for fibrinolysis as the reduction of death with this mode of therapy is generally between 15% and 30% in different trials compared with placebo.

PRE-HOSPITAL FIBRINOLYSIS

STEMI is a dynamic process that evolves over hours. Hence, pre-hospital fibrinolysis seems to be a good option to save time if logistics for achieving proper care is anticipated to be delayed by more than expected. However, a proper setup is mandatory for carrying out such a process. Well-organised EMS systems, full time trained paramedics and physicians capable of detecting and treating complications of fibrinolytic therapy are essential parts of it. Multiple observational studies and RCTs have shown no significant mortality reduction, but a meta-analysis suggested a 17% mortality reduction with this strategy, particularly when administered within 2 hours of symptom onset [8]. The CAPTIM trial reported a trend toward lower mortality when pre-hospital thrombolysis was compared with PPCI, especially when they were treated within 2 hours of onset of chest pain. Similarly, in the STREAM trial, pre-hospital thrombolysis was shown to be of similar benefit to PPCI within 3 hours of chest pain in patients who could not undergo PPCI within 1 hour of FMC [9].

LATE THERAPY

The best outcome of fibrinolytic therapy is achieved when used within 2–3 hours of chest pain in patients with less bleeding risks. But the window of this treatment option may be extended up to 12 hours according to two trials (LATE and EMERAS), which demonstrated some mortality benefit during 6–12 hours use of fibrinolysis. However, no benefit was shown beyond a 12-hour period in these studies. Though in selected cases of young patients (<65 yrs) with ongoing chest pain and unavailable PPCI facilities, late thrombolysis may provide some benefit. Because of the risk of cardiac rupture with late thrombolysis in elderly patients, such patients, when seen for the first time beyond 12 hours of the window period, should better be managed with PCI.

CHOICE OF FIBRINOLYTIC AGENT

All fibrinolytic agents act by converting plasminogen to plasmin, which is an active enzyme catalysing the conversion of fibrinogen to fibrin. These days only fibrin specific agents are preferred [10]. Presence of fibrin makes their catalytic efficiency many times better. Non-fibrin specific agents can act in the absence of fibrin also. Due to cost issues, non-fibrin specific agents are still being used in developing countries.

Comparative features of all available fibrinolytic agents are given in the following sections (Table 12.1).

Both tenecteplase and reteplase are of comparable efficacy with a patency rate that is almost the same as alteplase. But their administration is more convenient, especially by paramedics, as they can be given in bolus doses. Both these new agents have mortality benefits like that of the standard fibrin specific agent alteplase. However, in one large trial, TNK had a lower rate of major bleeding than alteplase [11].

The choice of fibrinolytics in hospital should be based on cost, efficacy, ease of administration and other institutional preferences.

Patients presenting early after AMI with less chance of bleeding benefit more with fibrin specific agents. For those patients who have low risk of MI (IWMI without RV involvement) and those with higher risk of intracranial haemorrhage (uncontrolled hypertension), administration of non-fibrin specific streptokinase is reasonable.

Bolus fibrinolytics have the advantage of less error of dosing, less chance of non-cerebral haemorrhage and the potential for pre-hospital fibrinolysis.

INTRACORONARY FIBRINOLYSIS

In current clinical practice, most of the patients with STEMI are treated with either a primary PCI or IV fibrinolysis. There has been rekindled interest using those agents, especially alteplase or tenecteplase in cases where there is a high thrombus burden. Doses used are one fifth of the systemic dose over 5–10 minutes time. However, use of such intracoronary thrombolysis draws controversies as some studies show no benefit when compared with intracoronary abciximab. Even stent thrombosis incidences are higher. On the contrary, cases of complicated PCI have been reported where use of IC fibrinolysis yielded better outcome.

Therefore, the use of IC fibrinolysis is restricted to adjunctive use in selected cases of complicated PCI.

ADJUNCTIVE USE OF ANTI-PLATELETS

Addition of aspirin to fibrinolytic agents is beneficial [12]. Initial non-enteric coated 150–300 mg aspirin is to be crushed and chewed followed by 75–100 mg tablets to be continued for an indefinite period. Clopidogrel is used along with aspirin, with an initial bolus dose of 300 mg followed by 75 mg daily [13]. Patients older than 75 years are given only 75 mg as an initial dose followed by the usual dose of clopidogrel. No other anti-platelets are used adjunct to fibrinolysis (Table 12.2).

ADJUNCTIVE USE OF ANTITHROMBOTICS

Parenteral anti-coagulation should be used along with fibrinolysis until revascularisation (if PCI is performed). In other cases it is continued for at least 48 hours and preferably until hospitalisation, i.e., for 8 days.

Low molecular weight heparin (LMWH) has been compared with unfractionated heparin (UFH) in different trials as an adjunct to fibrinolysis.

The ASSENT-3 trial showed improved net clinical benefit of LMWH [14]. Despite the increased risk of major bleeding, LMWH is preferred to UFH.

Table 12.1 Doses of fibrinolytic agents

Fibrinolytic agents	Fibrin specificity	Dose	Patency rate
Streptokinase	Nil	1.5 MU IV over 30–60 minutes	60%–70%
Alteplase (t-PA)	2+	15 mg bolus, infusion of 0.75 mg/kg for 30 min and then 0.5 mg/kg over next 60 min (total dose <100 mg)	73%–84%
Tenecteplase (TNK)	4+	Single IV weight-based bolus Half the dose for patients >75 yrs	85%
Reteplase (r-PA)	2+	Two bolus doses 10 U each 30 min apart	84%

Table 12.2 Anti-platelets used with thrombolysis

Anti-platelet agents	Dose
Aspirin	Initial dose of 150–300 mg orally followed by 75–100 mg daily. IV aspirin can be used in the dose of 75–250 mg, if oral ingestion is not possible.
Clopidogrel	Loading dose of 300 mg followed by 75 mg daily. For patients ≥ 75 yrs, only 75 mg bolus is used.

In the EXTRACT-TIMI 25 trial, enoxaparin was found to reduce death and reinfarction at 30 days when compared with weight adjusted UFH [15]. A reduced dose of enoxaparin was used for patients >75 years and those with impaired renal function. However, major non-cerebral bleeding occurred more with enoxaparin, shown in the ASSENT-3 trial. Still, the net clinical benefit suggested the use of LMWH over UFH.

Fondaparinux was studied in the OASIS-6 trial [16]. The reduction of mortality and reinfarction was better compared to placebo or UFH, especially when such patients were treated with streptokinase.

Bivalirudin is a direct thrombin inhibitor. This agent showed a reduction of reinfarction when 48 hours infusion of bivalirudin was compared with UFH after thrombolysis with streptokinase. A non-significant increase in non-cerebral haemorrhage was seen. Interestingly, bivalirudin was never tried with a fibrin specific fibrinolytic. Hence, its use after fibrinolysis in the current era is limited (Table 12.3).

HAZARDS OF FIBRINOLYTIC THERAPY

1. Intracranial bleeding, 0.9%–1.0% incidence [11], occurring mainly on the first day of therapy. More common in uncontrolled hypertension, female sex, previous history of stroke and low body weight [18].

Table 12.3 Anti-coagulants with their doses used with thrombolysis

Anti-coagulant	Dose
Enoxaparin	In patients <75 yrs, 30 mg IV followed 15 min later by s/c injection of 1 mg/kg every 12 hrs till revascularisation is performed
	In patients >75 yrs, No IV bolus dose, s/c dose of 0.75 mg/kg twice
	For patients with eGFR<30, Single-daily s/c dose
UFH	60 U/kg IV bolus (max 4000 U) followed by 12 U/kg/hr (max 1000 U) for 24–48 hrs, target aPTT 50–70 secs (to be monitored at 3, 6,12 and 24 hrs)
Fondaparinux	2.5 mg IV bolus followed by s/c dose of 2.5 mg daily

2. Major non-cerebral bleeding occurring in 4%–13% of patients [10].
3. Hypotension and allergic reaction with streptokinase.

CONTRAINDICATIONS OF FIBRINOLYSIS

See Table 12.4.

TRANSFER OF PATIENTS AFTER FIBRINOLYSIS

Indications

1. Patient developing severe heart failure or cardiogenic shock.
2. Non-invasive pre-hospital discharge study showing intermediate/high-risk features.
3. Evidence of spontaneous/easily provable myocardial ischaemia.
4. Evidence of failed reperfusion.
5. As a part of routine PCI in a stable patient 3–24 hours after fibrinolysis.

Transfer of a stable patient for performing non-emergency PCI after a fibrinolysis, known as pharmaco-invasive therapy, has been shown to reduce the rate of reinfarction in different studies. TRANSFER-AMI is the largest of those studies and has shown that early transfer after fibrinolysis resulted in composite end points of death, recurrent ischaemia, new onset heart failure or shock at 30 days. In a meta-analysis involving seven such RCTs, the strategy of routine PCI after 3 hours of fibrinolysis was associated with 35% reduction of recurrent MI and death [17,19].

Early (<2–3 hours) PCI after fibrinolysis is associated with increased bleeding. Hence an early procedure is reserved only for evidence of failed thrombolysis (rescue PCI) or development of shock, where bleeding risk is negated by the benefits of early PCI.

Table 12.4 Contraindications of fibrinolysis

Absolute	1. Previous ICH anytime
	2. Ischaemic stroke within 6 months
	3. Major trauma, surgery, head injury <1 month
	4. CNS neoplasm or AVM
	5. Active GI bleeding
	6. Bleeding diathesis
	7. Non-compressible puncture <24 hrs
	8. Aortic dissection
Relative	1. On oral anti-coagulation
	2. Pregnancy or within 1 week post-partum
	3. TIA within 6 months
	4. Uncontrolled hypertension
	5. Prolonged resuscitation
	6. Active peptic ulcer
	7. Advanced liver disease
	8. Infective endocarditis

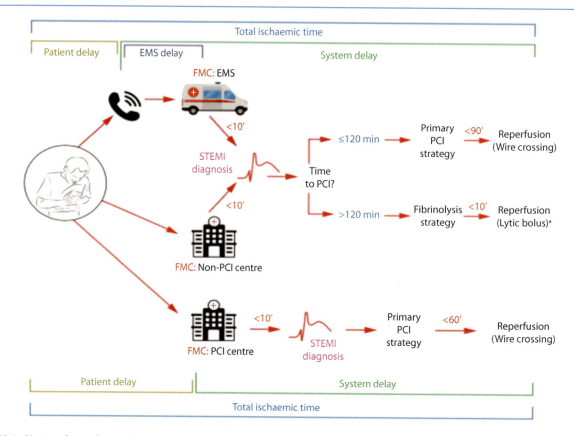

Figure 12.1 Choice of reperfusion therapy with time. EMS, emergency medical system; FMC, first medical contact; PCI, percutaneous coronary intervention; STEMI, ST-segment elevation myocardial infarction.

CHOICE OF REPERFUSION THERAPY

The choice of reperfusion therapy will depend on the anticipated time delay from STEMI diagnosis and proper reperfusion of the culprit vessel. Such delay in time will incalculate the fact if the centre is PCI capable or not. See Figure 12.1.

REFERENCES

1. Lassen JF, Botker HE, Terkelsen CJ. Timely and optimal treatment of patients with STEMI. *Nat Rev Cardiol.* 2013;10(1):41–48.
2. Zijlstra F, Hoorntje JC, de Boer MJ et al. Long-term benefit of primary angioplasty as compared with thrombolytic therapy for acute myocardial infarction. *N Engl J Med.* 1999;341(19):1413–1419.
3. Keeley EC, Boura JA, Grines CL. Primary angioplasty versus intravenous thrombolytic therapy for acute myocardial infarction: A quantitative review of 23 randomised trials. *Lancet.* 2003;361(9351):13–20.
4. Widimsky P, Budesinsky T, Vorac D et al., 'PRAGUE' Study Group Investigators. Long distance transport for primary angioplasty vs immediate thrombolysis in acute myocardial infarction. Final results of the randomized national multicentre trial—PRAGUE-2. *Eur Heart J.* 2003;24(1):94–104.
5. Andersen HR, Nielsen TT, Rasmussen K et al., DANAMI-2 Investigators. A comparison of coronary angioplasty with fibrinolytic therapy in acute myocardial infarction. *N Engl J Med.* 2003;349(8):733–742.
6. Fibrinolytic Therapy Trialists' (FTT) Collaborative Group. Indications for fibrinolytic therapy in suspected acute myocardial infarction: Collaborative overview of early mortality and major morbidity results from all randomised trials of more than 1000 patients. *Lancet.* 1994;343(8893):311–322.
7. Pinto DS, Frederick PD, Chakrabarti AK et al. National Registry of Myocardial Infarction Investigators. Benefit of transferring ST-segment-elevation myocardial infarction patients for percutaneous coronary intervention compared with administration of onsite fibrinolytic declines as delays increase. *Circulation.* 2011;124(23):2512–2521.
8. Morrison LJ, Verbeck PR, McDonald AC, Sawadsky BV, Cook DJ. Mortality and prehospital thrombolysis for acute myocardial infarction: A meta-analysis. *JAMA.* 2000;283(20):2686–2692.
9. Sinnaeve PR, Armstrong PW, Gershlick AH et al., STREAM Investigators. ST-segment-elevation myocardial infarction patients randomized to a pharmaco-invasive strategy or primary percutaneous coronary intervention: Strategic Reperfusion Early After. Myocardial Infarction (STREAM) 1-year mortality follow-up. *Circulation.* 2014;130(14):1139–1145.

10. The GUSTO Investigators. An international randomized trial comparing four thrombolytic strategies for acute myocardial infarction. *N Engl J Med.* 1993;329(10):673–682.

11. Assessment of the Safety and Efficacy of a New Thrombolytic (ASSENT-2) Investigators, Van de Werf F, Adgey J, Ardissino D et al. Single-bolus tenecteplase compared with front-loaded alteplase in acute myocardial infarction: The ASSENT-2 double-blind randomised trial. *Lancet.* 1999;354(9180):716–722.

12. ISIS-2 (Second International Study of Infarct Survival) Collaborative Group. Randomised trial of intravenous streptokinase, oral aspirin, both, or neither among 17,187 cases of suspected acute myocardial infarction: ISIS-2. *Lancet.* 1988;2(8607):349–360.

13. Sabatine MS, Cannon CP, Gibson CM et al., CLARITY-TIMI 28 Investigators. Addition of clopidogrel to aspirin and fibrinolytic therapy for myocardial infarction with ST-segment elevation. *N Engl J Med.* 2005;352(12):1179–1189.

14. Assessment of the Safety and Efficacy of a New Thrombolytic Regimen (ASSENT)-3Investigators. Efficacy and safety of tenecteplase in combination with enoxaparin, abciximab, or unfractionated heparin: The ASSENT-3 randomised trial in acute myocardial infarction. *Lancet.* 2001;358(9282):605–613.

15. Giraldez RR, Nicolau JC, Corbalan R et al. Enoxaparin is superior to unfractionated heparin in patients with ST elevation myocardial infarction undergoing fibrinolysis regardless of the choice of lytic: An ExTRACT-TIMI 25 analysis. *Eur Heart J.* 2007;28(13):1566–1573.

16. Peters RJ, Joyner C, Bassand JP et al., OASIS-6 Investigators. The role of fondaparinux as an adjunct to thrombolytic therapy in acute myocardial infarction: A subgroup analysis of the OASIS-6 trial. *Eur Heart J.* 2008;29(3):324–331.

17. Scheller B, Hennen B, Hammer B, Walle J, Hofer C, Hilpert V, Winter H, Nickenig G, Bohm M, SIAM III Study Group. Beneficial effects of immediate. stenting after thrombolysis in acute myocardial infarction. *J Am Coll Cardiol.* 2003;42(4):634–641.

18. Van de Werf F, Barron HV, Armstrong PW et al., ASSENT-2 Investigators, Assessment of the Safety and Efficacy of a New Thrombolytic. Incidence and predictors of bleeding events after fibrinolytic therapy with fibrin-specific agents: A comparison of TNK-tPA and rt-PA. *Eur Heart J.* 2001 Dec;22(24):2253–2261.

19. Le May MR, Wells GA, Labinaz M et al. Combined angioplasty and pharmacological intervention. versus thrombolysis alone in acute myocardial infarction (CAPITAL AMI study). *J Am Coll Cardiol.* 2005;46(3):417–424.

13

Anti-coagulation in acute coronary syndrome

NITIN PARASHAR, DEEPTI SIDDHARTHAN AND SIVASUBRAMANIAN RAMAKRISHNAN

INTRODUCTION

Early intravenous anti-coagulation along with anti-platelets is the cornerstone for the management of acute coronary syndrome patients. The primary aim of early anti-coagulation is to reduce the ischaemic burden in the myocardium without increasing the haemorrhagic events. Acute coronary syndrome (ACS) occurs due to complete or incomplete coronary thrombosis following atherosclerotic plaque rupture. ACS includes the patients having unstable angina (UA), non-ST-elevation myocardial infarction (NSTEMI) and ST-elevation myocardial infarction (STEMI). The umbrella term NSTE-ACS is used for UA and NSTEMI patients.

PATHOPHYSIOLOGY OF ACS AND ROLE OF ANTI-COAGULATION

The primary pathogenesis of ACS starts from the development of coronary atherosclerotic plaques and subsequent consequences due to rupture/erosion of unstable coronary plaques. Rupture of the plaques leads to activation of platelets and coagulation cascade as a result of injury to blood vessels. Pathophysiology of ACS includes platelet activation and thrombin production, among others [1]. Thrombin production and generation of a prothrombotic state in ACS have paved the role for treatment with anti-coagulation during an acute stage.

Initial management of ACS includes oxygen therapy, anti-platelets, nitrates, analgesics, beta-blockers and statins. Due to the generation of platelet-rich thrombus and prothrombotic state, the anti-coagulants such as unfractionated heparin (UFH), low

molecular weight heparin (LMWH) and other antithrombotic agents are indicated in these patients. Following this initial acute coronary event, thrombin remains elevated for a long time, and these patients are at risk of recurrence of ACS. Research is ongoing to determine the role of long-term anti-coagulants to prevent subsequent coronary events once the acute stage is over.

ANTI-COAGULANTS USED IN ACS

The commonly used anti-coagulants in ACS include UFH, LMWH, bivalirudin and fondaparinux. The characteristics of various anti-coagulants used in ACS are discussed in Table 13.1. Doses of anti-coagulants for ACS and duration of anti-coagulation are discussed in Tables 13.2 and 13.3, respectively.

UFH is the most affordable, oldest and remains the most frequently used anti-coagulant in ACS. It binds with anti-thrombin III and inhibits factors IIa (thrombin) and Xa indirectly by activation of antithrombin. Heparin requires parenteral administration and is usually given via a continuous intravenous route. Clearance of heparin is extra-renal; hence, it is safe in renal dysfunction. Levels of heparin-binding proteins vary from person to person inside the blood circulation, which results in unpredictable and variable anti-coagulant responses of heparin. Because of intra- and inter-individual variability, monitoring of the anti-coagulation effect either by aPTT, activated clotting time (ACT) or anti-factor Xa level is essential to ensure a therapeutic response [2,3]. Activity of heparin may be reduced in the vicinity of platelet-rich thrombus by neutralisation of heparin by high concentration of PF4 released from activated platelets. Another important limitation is risk of

Table 13.1 Characteristics of various anti-coagulants used in acute coronary syndrome

Anti-coagulant	Structure	Molecular weight	Onset of action	Half-life	Mechanism of action	Monitoring
Heparin	Sulfated muco-polysaccharide	15000 daltons (4000–30000 daltons)	Immediate	1 hr	Antithrombin mediated inhibition of factors II and X	aPTT, Anti-factor Xa activity, or ACT (200–250 s during PCI with GPI or 250–300 s without GPI)
Enoxaparin	Fractionation and depolymerisation of heparin	5000 daltons (3000–5000 daltons)	IV: Immediate SC: 2 hrs	4 hrs	Antithrombin mediated inhibition of X≫II	No need of monitoring
Bivalirudin	Synthetic 20-amino acid analogue of hirudin	2000 daltons	Immediate	25 min	Direct thrombin (II) inhibitor	ACT
Fondaparinux	Synthetic pentasaccharide, derived from cleavage of heparin sulfate	1700 daltons	IV: Immediate SC: 2 hrs	17 hrs	Antithrombin mediated inhibitor of factor X	No need of monitioring

Abbreviations: ACT, activated clotting time; aPTT, activated partial thromboplastin time; GPI, Glycoprotein IIb/IIIa inhibitor; HIT, heparin induced thrombocytopenia; hr, hour; IV, intravenous; PCI, percutaneous coronary intervention; SC, subcutaneous.

Table 13.2 Dosing of anti-coagulants used in acute coronary syndrome

Anti-coagulant	NSTE ACS/Ischemia-guided therapy	Thrombolysis	Primary PCI
UFH	60 units/kg bolus (max 4000 units) + 12 units/kg/hr (max 1000 units) IV infusion titrated to therapeutic aPTT Obtain aPTT of 1.5–2.0 times control (approx. 50–70 s)	60 units/kg bolus (max 4000 units) + 12 units/kg/hr (max 1000 units) IV infusion titrated to therapeutic aPTT Obtain aPTT of 1.5–2.0 times control (approx. 50–70 s)	PCI with planned GPI: 50–70 units/kg IV bolus to achieve therapeutic ACT of 200–250 s PCI without planned GPI: 70–100 units/kg IV bolus to achieve therapeutic ACT of 250–300 s
Enoxaparin	1 mg/kg IV SC q12 hr (Reduce dose to 1 mg/kg/d SC if CrCl < 30 mL/min)	≤75 yr: 30 mg IV bolus, then 15 minute later 1 mg/kg SC q12 hr ≥75 yr: No bolus, 0.75 mg/kg SC q12 hr (Reduce dose to 1 mg/kg/d SC if CrCl < 30 mL/min)	0.5–0.75 mg IV bolus if no anti-coagulation previously or if more than 12 hrs of enoxaparin 0.3 mg/kg IV if last SC dose was between 8–12 hrs before PCI Without new dose if last dose < 8 hrs
Fondaparinux	2.5 mg SC daily	2.5 mg IV × 1, then 2.5 mg SC daily starting next day	Not recommended without additional anti-coagulant with anti-II activity
Bivalirudin	0.10 mg/kg IV loading followed by 0.25 mg/kg/hr infusion	–	0.75 mg/kg IV bolus + 1.75 mg/kg/hr infusion

Abbreviations: ACT, activated clotting time; IV, intravenous; SC, subcutaneous; GPI, glycoprotein IIb/IIIa inhibitor; PCI, percutaneous coronary intervention; UFH, unfractionated heparin.

Table 13.3 Duration of anti-coagulation after acute coronary syndrome

Anti-coagulant	Duration in conservative treatment (NSTE-ACS, thrombolysis)	Primary PCI
Unfractionated heparin (UFH)	Maintain for 48 hrs or until revascularisation	Discontinue anti-coagulation
Enoxaparin	Maintain for 8 days or till hospitalisation or revascularisation	Discontinue anti-coagulation
Bivalirudin	Until diagnostic angiography or PCI is performed, in patients with early invasive strategy only	Maintain for 4 hrs after the procedure
Fondaparinux	For index hospitalisation up to 8 days or until revascularisation	Discontinue anti-coagulation
Warfarin	If patient has LV thrombus or LV aneurysm, 3 months to life-long therapy	

heparin-induced thrombocytopenia (HIT), which can paradoxically increase thromboembolic risk (arterial or venous thrombosis) in the patient. It is a serious and potentially life-threatening complication in the setting of ACS. It has also been postulated that heparin discontinuation causes biological rebound generation of thrombin and increases prothrombotic state [4]. The most common side effect is bleeding, and the antidote protamine can be used in patients with serious bleeding. Typically, 1 mg of intravenous protamine can neutralise 100 units of heparin.

Low molecular weight heparin (LMWH) is prepared from heparin by chemical depolymerisation. It causes inhibition of factor Xa more than factor IIa because of a short pentasaccharide chain. It has better bioavailability, predictable anti-coagulant response and longer half-life than heparin. Because of the predictable anti-coagulant response, monitoring of anti-coagulation is not necessary in most patients. Other advantages include a lower risk of HIT and osteoporosis. LMWH via a subcutaneous route can be administered at home which increases patient satisfaction. Doses have to be reduced in renal dysfunction and monitoring of anti-coagulant effects is indicated in special groups of patients such as those who are pregnant and in presence of mechanical prosthetic valves.

Fondaparinux is a synthetic analogue of antithrombin-binding sequence. It requires the presence of antithrombin for its action and causes inhibition of factor Xa only without affecting factor IIa. The drug is administered once daily by subcutaneous route. Because of its renal clearance, it should be given cautiously to patients with renal dysfunction and should be avoided when creatinine clearance is less than 20 mL/min.

Direct thrombin inhibitors (e.g. bivalirudin) potentially have an advantage over UFH or LMWH as they inhibit clot bound thrombin. Additionally, direct thrombin inhibitors don't interact with plasma proteins, provide a stable anti-coagulation effect and do not cause thrombocytopenia. Bivalirudin is a synthetic analogue of hirudin which directly binds and inhibits thrombin (factor IIa) without activation of antithrombin. Its action can be monitored by ACT and aPTT when used in high doses and low doses, respectively. It causes less bleeding than heparin and can be safely used in patients with heparin-induced thrombocytopenia who require PCI.

Warfarin, a oral vitamin K antagonist, interferes with synthesis of clotting factors II, VII, IX, and X. It is not indicated in acute coronary events. The only indication of warfarin is in patients requiring triple therapy (anti-coagulant and dual anti-platelet therapy), such as patients with atrial fibrillation, mechanical valves or deep venous thromboembolism. Frequent monitoring, increased drug interactions, food drug interactions and increased risk of bleeding when combined with dual anti-platelet therapy are the major limitations of warfarin for use in ACS. The development of novel anti-coagulants has addressed some of these limitations and these novel anti-coagulants might have a potential role in the management of ACS.

ANTI-COAGULATION IN STEMI

STEMI is associated with a heavy thrombus burden due to activation of platelet aggregation and coagulation cascade, and immediate primary PCI or thrombolysis is required within the window period. Anti-coagulation has shown to reduce mortality and recurrent ischaemic events with both thrombolysis and primary PCI. Primary PCI is usually done in high thrombotic settings and this thrombotic risk is increased by damage of the endothelium during coronary intervention [5]. Therefore, there is an increased risk of early ischaemic complications during PCI such as acute stent thrombosis. There is need of early and efficient anti-coagulation therapy to block the coagulation cascade and prevent ischaemic injury to the myocardium.

UFH

Randomised trials conducted in the pre-fibrinolytic era showed lower risk of mortality and reinfarction in patients of STEMI treated with heparin. A meta-analysis in the fibrinolytic era suggested that for every 1000 patients of STEMI treated with heparin in addition to aspirin, five fewer deaths ($p = 0.03$) and three fewer recurrent infarctions ($p = 0.04$) occurred, but at the cost of three major bleeding events ($p = 0.001$) [6]. Guidelines support the use of heparin for at least 48 hours after fibrinolysis or until PCI is done [7,8].

ENOXAPARIN

LMWH reduces the rates of re-occlusion of the infarct-related artery, reinfarction or recurrent ischaemic events [9]. Several trials compared LMWH with UFH as part of a pharmacologic reperfusion strategy, and found LMWH to be superior [10]. The ASSENT trial showed that enoxaparin reduced 30-day mortality and in-hospital reinfarction as compared to heparin with similar rates of intracranial haemorrhage [11]. ExTRACT-TIMI 25 was a double-blind trial which showed that enoxaparin reduced the primary end point of mortality and recurrent MI by 17% with enoxaparin but increased major bleeding significantly (1.4% vs. 2.1%) as compared to heparin [12]. Montalescot et al. (ATOLL trial) found that bleeding rates and bleeding events were reduced with enoxaparin when compared with heparin in STEMI patients undergoing primary PCI [13]. Enoxaparin was also associated with significant reduction in recurrence or complications of MI.

FONDAPARINUX

The OASIS-6 trial included 12,000 subjects with STEMI and randomised them to receive UFH or fondaparinux. Overall it was associated with a reduced rate of death and bleeding, and it showed a high rate of periprocedural catheter thrombosis and coronary complications in the subgroup treated by primary PCI [14]. Consequently, it has been given class III recommendation in STEMI when used as sole anti-coagulant [7,8].

BIVALIRUDIN

In patients undergoing fibrinolysis, bivalirudin reduced recurrent MI by 25%–30% compared with heparin without affecting mortality at the expense of higher rates of major bleeding [15].

In contrast, the HORIZONS-AMI trial compared bivalirudin with UFH plus GPI in STEMI patients undergoing primary

PCI [16]. Bivalirudin reduced net adverse clinical events (rate of major bleeding or major CV events including reinfarction and target vessel revascularisation) primarily driven by a significant 40% reduction in major bleeding events. However, patients in the bivalirudin group were found to have a four-fold increase in acute stent thrombosis.

The EUROMAX trial in the era of radial artery PCI access also presented similar findings with reduced primary outcome of death or major bleeding events but at the expense of five-fold increase of acute stent thrombosis events in the bivalirudin group [17]. These events led to a downgrade of recommendations in recent updates from the previous class I to class IIa [8].

ANTI-COAGULATION IN NSTEMI

As soon as diagnosis of NSTE-ACS is made, anti-coagulation is indicated in addition to dual anti-platelet therapy.

UFH

A meta-analysis by Oler et al. in 1996 showed that the addition of heparin to aspirin resulted in a 33% reduction of death and ischaemic outcomes [18]. These findings were confirmed in other meta-analyses also. Presently, UFH is a class IB recommendation in both the American College of Cardiology (ACC) and the European Society of Cardiology (ESC) NSTE-ACS guidelines [19,20].

ENOXAPARIN

NSTE-ACS patients were studied in the ESSENCE trial, in which the patients were randomised to receive UFH or enoxaparin. Enoxaparin was found to reduce the composite of death, recurrent MI and invasive procedures at 30 days with sustained benefit at 1 year [21]. However, there was no difference in ischaemic outcomes in the SYNERGY trial with enoxaparin when compared with UFH [22]. Petersen et al., in a systematic review of 20000 patients, described a reduction of combined death and myocardial infarction in patients treated with enoxaparin compared with UFH, with similar major bleeding events [23]. Silvain et al., in their meta-analysis of 23 trials, demonstrated superiority of enoxaparin in terms of ischaemic outcomes and bleeding complications [24]. Enoxaparin is given class IA recommendation in the ACC and IB recommendation in the ESC guidelines for the management of patients with NSTE-ACS [19,20].

FONDAPARINUX

Fondaparinux (2.5 mg, subcutaneous) was compared with enoxaparin in the OASIS-5 trial and was associated with decreased bleeding complications and mortality in patients with high risk NSTE-ACS [25]. No difference was found in primary ischaemic composite outcomes. However, it was associated with significant three-fold increase in catheter and periprocedural thrombosis. It has been given class IB recommendation in the ACC and ESC guidelines for NSTEMI in patients being managed non-invasively [19,20].

BIVALIRUDIN

The ACUITY trial compared three anti-coagulation strategies in NSTEMI patients: (1) bivalirudin monotherapy, (2) bivalirudin plus GPI and (3) UFH plus GPI [26]. Three groups had similar ischaemic outcomes but major bleedings were reduced in the bivalirudin group. ISAR REACT 4 showed similar results when comparing bivalirudin to UFH plus abciximab [27]. The MATRIX study randomised ACS patients (44% patients with high risk ACS) in whom PCI was planned to receive either bivalirudin or UFH and found that rates of MACE or mortality did not differ between the treatment groups. However, in NSTE-ACS patients, major bleeding was reduced in the bivalirudin group by almost 50% [28]. Presently, bivalirudin is given class IB recommendation in the ACC and IA in the ESC guidelines for management of NSTEMI [19,20].

NEWER ANTI-COAGULANTS IN ACS

Novel anti-coagulants such as anti-Xa therapies (apixaban, rivaroxaban, otamixaban) and direct thrombin inhibitors (dabigatran) have been tried in patients with ACS.

Anti-Xa drugs (apixaban and rivaroxaban) were found to increase the rate of bleeding in a dose-related manner when added with anti-platelet therapy in the phase III trials. The APPRAISE-2 study had to be stopped prematurely due to excessive bleeding with apixaban regimen in addition to DAPT [29].

The Anti-Xa Therapy to Lower Cardiovascular Events in Addition to Aspirin with or without Thienopyridine Therapy in Subjects with ACS Thrombolysis In MI 46 (ATLAS ACS-TIMI 46) study was done to assess the effect of rivaroxaban after ACS. It was a randomised, double-blind, placebo-controlled, phase II, dose-escalation trial in which 3491 participants were randomly assigned to rivaroxaban 5, 10, 15 or 20 mg once daily or placebo [30]. Rivaroxaban reduced major ischaemic outcomes including death, myocardial infarction or stroke but at the cost of increased bleeding in dose dependent manner.

In the ATLAS ACS 2- TIMI 51 study, low-dose (5 mg twice daily) and very low-dose rivaroxaban (2.5 mg twice daily) was added to double anti-platelet therapy in patients with established ACS, and rivaroxaban significantly decreased the primary composite outcomes (death, MI or stroke) by 16% in those patients [31]. As very low dose rivaroxaban had a more favourable safety profile, 2.5 mg twice daily rivaroxaban has been recommended by ESC in combination with aspirin and clopidogrel in patients with ACS [20].

Further safety of low-dose rivaroxaban was assessed in the GEMINI-ACS-1 trial, in which 3037 patients with ACS were randomised to receive aspirin or rivaroxaban in addition to a thienopyridine (clopidogrel or ticagrelor). This trial was different as rivaroxaban was used in place of aspirin, not simultaneously. The primary end point was TIMI clinically significant bleeding; low dose rivaroxaban was found to have similar risk of clinically significant bleeding as aspirin when added to a thienopyridine (p = 0.580). They did not assess the efficacy of rivaroxaban in this trial [32].

Table 13.4 Guidelines by the American College of Cardiology (2013) and the European Society of Cardiology (2017) regarding anti-coagulation in ST-elevation myocardial infarction

	ACC guidelines Class (level)	ESC guidelines Class (level)
Primary PCI		
Routine use of UFH with or without GPI to achieve therapeutic ACT	I (C)	I (C)
Routine use of enoxaparin	NA	IIa (A)
Routine use of bivalirudin	I (B)	IIa (A)
Fondaparinux is not recommended for primary PCI as a sole anti-coagulant	III (B)	III (B)
Fibrinolysis		
Routine use of UFH	I (C)	I (B)
Routine use of enoxaparin	I (A)	I (A)
Routine use of fondaparinux	I (B)	IIa (B)

Abbreviations: GPI, glycoprotein IIb/IIIa inhibitor; IV, intravenous; NA, not available; NSTEMI, non-ST elevation myocardial infarction; PCI, percutaneous coronary intervention; SC, subcutaneous; UFH, unfractionated heparin.

Table 13.5 Guidelines by the American College of Cardiology (2014) and the European Society of Cardiology (2015) regarding anti-coagulation in non-ST-elevation acute coronary syndrome

Recommendation	ACC guidelines Class (level)	ESC guidelines Class (level)
SC enoxaparin for duration of hospitalisation or until PCI is performed	I (A)	I (B)
Bivalirudin until diagnostic angiography or PCI is performed in patients with early invasive strategy only	I (B)	I (A)
SC fondaparinux for the duration of hospitalisation or until PCI is performed	I (B)	I (B)
Administer additional anti-coagulant with anti-IIa activity if PCI is performed while patient is on fondaparinux	I (B)	
IV UFH for 48 hrs or until PCI is performed	I (B)	I (B)
Discontinuation of anti-coagulation after PCI	NA	IIa (C)
Cross over between UFH and enoxaparin is not recommended	NA	III (B)
In NSTEMI patients with no prior stroke/TIA and at high ischaemic risk as well as low bleeding risk receiving aspirin and clopidogrel, low-dose rivaroxaban (2.5 mg twice daily for approximately 1 year) may be considered after discontinuation of parenteral anti-coagulation	NA	IIb (B)

Abbreviations: IV, intravenous; NA, not available; NSTEMI, non-ST elevation myocardial infarction; PCI, percutaneous coronary intervention; SC, subcutaneous; TIA, transient ischaemic attack; UFH, unfractionated heparin.

Dabigatran was added to DAPT in ACS patients in the RE-DEEM study and was associated with dose-dependent increase in bleeding events [33]. A phase III trial of intravenous anti-Xa otamixaban was not found to be useful in patients with NSTE-ACS undergoing early PCI. Otamixaban did not reduce ischaemic event rates, but significantly increased bleeding rates when compared with UFH plus eptifibatide [34].

The use of newer anti-coagulants in ACS is limited by increased risk of bleeding as they are given in addition to dual anti-platelet drugs. Only rivaroxaban, out of the novel anti-coagulants, has been approved in Europe at present for the use in ACS patients. Further studies are ongoing for other novel anti-coagulants.

GUIDELINES

The use of various anti-coagulants has been advised in guidelines for the management of patients with STEMI and NSTE-ACS but different classes of recommendations are given based on available evidence which are summarised in Tables 13.4 and 13.5, respectively.

FUTURE VISION

Large randomised trials of newer anti-coagulants are required in the current setting of modern techniques and stronger P2Y12 inhibitors. Trials evaluating ticagrelor and prasugrel in STEMI used UFH and enoxaparin mostly during periprocedural time, while bivalirudin was used in less than 5% of patients [35,36]. Optimum anti-coagulation in the presence of newer anti-platelets is not known. Further trials will clarify these issues.

CONCLUSION

Anti-coagulation along with anti-platelets has been the standard of care and first line therapy in patients admitted with acute coronary syndrome. It is limited to treatment during initial hospitalisation and revascularisation at present. Anti-coagulants have improved mortality and decreased recurrent ischaemic events in both STEMI as well as NSTEMI patients. There is not a single anti-coagulant that is suitable for all patients in all conditions.

The anti-coagulant should be chosen on the basis of availability in hospital and type of procedure being planned for the patient. A patient-centric approach should be followed to balance ischaemic and bleeding risks.

REFERENCES

1. Undas A, Szułdrzyński K, Brummel-Ziedins KE et al. Systemic blood coagulation activation in acute coronary syndromes. *Blood*. 26 Feb 2009;113(9):2070–2078.

2. Montalescot G, Cohen M, Salette G et al. Impact of anticoagulation levels on outcomes in patients undergoing elective percutaneous coronary intervention: Insights from the STEEPLE trial. *Eur Heart J*. Feb 2008;29(4):462–471.

3. Brener SJ, Moliterno DJ, Lincoff AM et al. Relationship between activated clotting time and ischemic or hemorrhagic complications: Analysis of 4 recent randomized clinical trials of percutaneous coronary intervention. *Circulation*. 2004;110:994–998.

4. Montalescot G, Bal-dit-Sollier C, Chibedi D et al. Comparison of effects on markers of blood cell activation of enoxaparin, dalteparin, and unfractionated heparin in patients with unstable angina pectoris or non-ST-segment elevation acute myocardial infarction (the ARMADA study). *Am J Cardiol*. 2003;91:925.

5. Zeitouni M, Kerneis M, Nafee T et al. Anticoagulation in acute coronary syndrome—State of the art. *Prog Cardiovasc Dis*. Feb 2018;60(4–5):508–513.

6. Collins R, MacMahon S, Flather M et al. Clinical effects of anticoagulant therapy in suspected acute myocardial infarction: Systematic overview of randomised trials. *BMJ*. 14 Sep 1996;313(7058):652–659.

7. O'Gara PT, Kushner FG, Ascheim DD et al. 2013 ACCF/AHA guideline for the management of ST-elevation myocardial infarction: A report of the American College of Cardiology Foundation/American Heart Association Task Force on Practice Guidelines. *Circulation*. 29 Jan 2013;127(4):e362–e425.

8. Ibanez B, James S, Agewall S et al. 2017 ESC Guidelines for the management of acute myocardial infarction in patients presenting with ST-segment elevation The Task Force for the Management of Acute Myocardial Infarction in patients presenting with ST-segment elevation of the European Society of Cardiology (ESC). *Eur Heart J*. 7 Jan 2018;39(2):119–177.

9. Singh S, Bahekar A, Molnar J, Khosla S, Arora R. Adjunctive low molecular weight heparin during fibrinolytic therapy in acute ST-segment elevation myocardial infarction: A meta-analysis of randomized control trials. *Clin Cardiol*. Jul 2009;32(7):358–364.

10. O'Connor RE, Bossaert L, Arntz H-R et al. Part 9: Acute coronary syndromes: 2010 International Consensus on Cardiopulmonary Resuscitation and Emergency Cardiovascular Care Science With Treatment Recommendations. *Circulation*. 19 Oct 2010;122(16 Suppl 2):S422–S465.

11. Armstrong PW, Westerhout CM, Van de Werf F et al. Refining clinical trial composite outcomes: An application to the Assessment of the Safety and Efficacy of a New Thrombolytic-3 (ASSENT-3) trial. *Am Heart J*. May 2011;161(5):848–854.

12. Welsh RC, Armstrong PW. Contemporary pharmacological reperfusion in ST elevation myocardial infarction. *Curr Opin Cardiol* 2012;27(4):340–346.

13. Montalescot G, Zeymer U, Silvain J et al. Intravenous enoxaparin or unfractionated heparin in primary percutaneous coronary intervention for ST-elevation myocardial infarction: The international randomised open-label ATOLL trial. *Lancet*. 20 Aug 2011;378(9792):693–703.

14. Yusuf S, Mehta SR, Chrolavicius S et al. Effects of fondaparinux on mortality and reinfarction in patients with acute ST-segment elevation myocardial infarction: The OASIS-6 randomized trial. *JAMA*. 5 Apr 2006;295(13):1519–1530.

15. Coppens M, Eikelboom JW, Gustafsson D, Weitz JI, Hirsh J. Translational success stories: Development of direct thrombin inhibitors. *Circ Res*. 14 Sep 2012;111(7):920–929.

16. Stone GW, Witzenbichler B, Guagliumi G et al. Heparin plus a glycoprotein IIb/IIIa inhibitor versus bivalirudin monotherapy and paclitaxel-eluting stents versus bare-metal stents in acute myocardial infarction (HORIZONS-AMI): Final 3-year results from a multicentre, randomised controlled trial. *Lancet*. 25 Jun 2011;377(9784):2193–2204.

17. Steg PG, van 't Hof A, Hamm CW et al. Bivalirudin started during emergency transport for primary PCI. *N Engl J Med*. 5 Dec 2013;369(23):2207–2217.

18. Oler A, Whooley MA, Oler J, Grady D. Adding heparin to aspirin reduces the incidence of myocardial infarction and death in patients with unstable angina. A meta-analysis. *JAMA* 1996;276:811–815.

19. Amsterdam EA, Wenger NK, Brindis RG et al. 2014 AHA/ACC Guideline for the Management of Patients with Non-ST-Elevation Acute Coronary Syndromes: A report of the American College of Cardiology/American Heart Association Task Force on Practice Guidelines. *J Am Coll Cardiol*. 23 Dec 2014;64(24):e139–e228.

20. Roffi M, Patrono C, Collet J-P et al. 2015 ESC Guidelines for the management of acute coronary syndromes in patients presenting without persistent ST-segment elevation: Task Force for the Management of Acute Coronary Syndromes in Patients Presenting without Persistent ST-Segment Elevation of the European Society of Cardiology (ESC). *Eur Heart J*. 14 Jan 2016;37(3):267–315.

21. Goodman SG, Cohen M, Bigonzi F et al. Randomized trial of low molecular weight heparin (enoxaparin) versus unfractionated heparin for unstable coronary artery disease: One-year results of the ESSENCE Study. Efficacy and Safety of Subcutaneous Enoxaparin in Non-Q Wave Coronary Events. *J Am Coll Cardiol*. Sep 2000;36(3):693–698.

22. White HD, Kleiman NS, Mahaffey KW et al. Efficacy and safety of enoxaparin compared with unfractionated heparin in high-risk patients with non-ST-segment elevation acute coronary syndrome undergoing percutaneous coronary intervention in the Superior Yield of the New Strategy of Enoxaparin, Revascularization and Glycoprotein

IIb/IIIa Inhibitors (SYNERGY) trial. *Am Heart J*. Dec 2006;152(6):1042–1050.

23. Petersen JL, Mahaffey KW, Hasselblad V et al. Efficacy and bleeding complications among patients randomized to enoxaparin or unfractionated heparin for antithrombin therapy in non-ST-Segment elevation acute coronary syndromes: A systematic overview. *JAMA*. 7 Jul 2004;292(1): 89–96.

24. Silvain J, Beygui F, Barthélémy O et al. Efficacy and safety of enoxaparin versus unfractionated heparin during percutaneous coronary intervention: Systematic review and meta-analysis. *BMJ*. 3 Feb 2012;344:e553.

25. Fifth Organization to Assess Strategies in Acute Ischemic Syndromes Investigators, Yusuf S, Mehta SR, Chrolavicius S et al. Comparison of fondaparinux and enoxaparin in acute coronary syndromes. *N Engl J Med*. 6 Apr 2006;354(14):1464–1476.

26. Stone GW, White HD, Ohman EM et al. Bivalirudin in patients with acute coronary syndromes undergoing percutaneous coronary intervention: A subgroup analysis from the Acute Catheterization and Urgent Intervention Triage Strategy (ACUITY) trial. *Lancet Lond Engl*. 17 Mar 2007;369(9565):907–919.

27. Kastrati A, Neumann F-J, Schulz S et al. Abciximab and heparin versus bivalirudin for non–ST-elevation myocardial infarction. *N Engl J Med*. 24 Nov 2011;365(21): 1980–1989.

28. Valgimigli M, Frigoli E, Leonardi S et al. Bivalirudin or unfractionated heparin in acute coronary syndromes. *N Engl J Med*. 10 Sep 2015;373(11):997–1009.

29. Alexander JH, Lopes RD, James S et al. Apixaban with antiplatelet therapy after acute coronary syndrome. *N Engl J Med*. 25 Aug 2011;365(8):699–708.

30. Mega JL, Braunwald E, Mohanavelu S et al. Rivaroxaban versus placebo in patients with acute coronary syndromes (ATLAS ACS-TIMI 46): A randomised, double-blind, phase II trial. *Lancet Lond Engl*. 4 Jul 2009;374(9683): 29–338.

31. Mega JL, Braunwald E, Wiviott SD et al. Rivaroxaban in patients with a recent acute coronary syndrome. *N Engl J Med*. 5 Jan 2012;366(1):9–19.

32. Ohman EM, Roe MT, Steg PG et al. Clinically significant bleeding with low-dose rivaroxaban versus aspirin, in addition to P2Y12 inhibition, in acute coronary syndromes (GEMINI-ACS-1): A double-blind, multicentre, randomised trial. *Lancet*. 6 May 2017;389(10081):1799–1808.

33. Oldgren J, Budaj A, Granger CB et al. Dabigatran vs. placebo in patients with acute coronary syndromes on dual antiplatelet therapy: A randomized, double-blind, phase II trial. *Eur Heart J*. Nov 2011;32(22):2781–2789.

34. Steg PG, Mehta SR, Pollack CV et al. Anticoagulation with otamixaban and ischemic events in non-ST-segment elevation acute coronary syndromes: The TAO randomized clinical trial. *JAMA*. 18 Sep 2013;310(11):1145–1155.

35. Wallentin L, Becker RC, Budaj A et al. Ticagrelor versus clopidogrel in patients with acute coronary syndromes. *N Engl J Med*. 2009;361(11):1045–1057.

36. Wiviott SD, Braunwald E, McCabe CH et al. Prasugrel versus clopidogrel in patients with acute coronary syndromes. *N Engl J Med*. 2007;357(20):2001–2015.

14

Contentious issues in primary angioplasty
Deferred stenting, manual thrombectomy, culprit versus complete revascularisation, microvasculature in ACS

AJ SWAMY AND K SARAT CHANDRA

MANUAL THROMBECTOMY

Manual thrombectomy during treatment of primary angioplasty has been widely used since its introduction more than a decade ago. Beyond restoring epicardial flow, limiting distal embolisation and restoring microvascular integrity have been the targets of primary angioplasty. Manual thrombectomy offers an attractive and intuitive reduction of the thrombus burden in a patient with complete occlusion of the infarct-related vessel. This should lead to theoretical benefits in terms of lesser slow-flow, better microvascular perfusion, smaller infarct sizes and thus better clinical outcomes in the short and long term [1,2].

Primary percutaneous intervention is a high risk due to the attendant risks of thrombosis and no-reflow that can complicate the procedure. Initial studies showed a benefit of the use of manual thrombectomy devices [1,2]. However, inconsistent results led to many further studies that were designed more rigorously. These produced equivocal results, and large randomised trials demonstrated that routine use of aspiration thrombectomy had no benefit on mortality.

A meta-analysis by Jolly et al. evaluated the use of thrombus aspiration during primary PCI [3]. This meta-analysis included randomised controlled trials that studied at least 1000 patients comparing routine manual thrombectomy with PCI and PCI alone in patients with STEMI. There were three eligible randomised trials (TAPAS [Thrombus Aspiration during Percutaneous Coronary Intervention in Acute Myocardial Infarction], TASTE [Thrombus Aspiration in ST-Elevation Myocardial Infarction in Scandinavia], and TOTAL [Trial of Routine Aspiration Thrombectomy with PCI Versus PCI Alone in Patients with STEMI]). These together enrolled 19,047 patients, of whom 18,306 underwent PCI and were included in the primary analysis [4–6].

Cardiovascular death at 30 days occurred in 2.4% of patients randomised to thrombus aspiration versus 2.9% randomised to PCI alone (hazard ratio, 0.84; 95% confidence interval, 0.70–1.01; $P = 0.06$). Stroke/transient ischaemic attack (TIA) occurred in 66 (0.8%) randomised to thrombus aspiration and 46 (0.5%) randomised to PCI alone (odds ratio, 1.43; 95% confidence interval, 0.98–2.10; $P = 0.06$). There were no significant differences in recurrent myocardial infarction, stent thrombosis, heart failure or target vessel revascularisation [3]. However, in the subgroup with high thrombus burden (TIMI [Thrombolysis in Myocardial Infarction] thrombus grade $\geq$3), thrombus aspiration was associated with significantly fewer cardiovascular deaths (170 versus 205; $P = 0.03$) but with more stroke (0.9% versus 0.5%; $P = 0.04$).

The conclusions drawn were that routine thrombus aspiration did not help in patients undergoing primary angioplasty and that it might help cardiovascular outcomes in patients with large thrombus burdens but at the cost of an increased stroke risk. Further studies on improving the modality of thrombus removal might reduce the risk of stroke associated with manual thrombectomy in patients with large thrombus burdens.

Current ACC-AHA guidelines give a IIb recommendation for manual thrombectomy in patients with large thrombus burdens and class III recommendation for routine manual thrombectomy in patients undergoing primary angioplasty [7].

Authors' comment

It is notable that although there were fewer deaths in the thrombectomy group overall, this only just failed to reach significance.

Additionally, it is possible that if the thrombectomy technique was refined or improved, the stroke risk may also be reduced. Intuitively, patients with larger thrombus burdens have a prothrombotic state and the occurrence of stroke in them is due to the embolisation of clot fragments from the thrombosuction catheter into the systemic circulation, and if negative pressure on the catheter was not released until the catheter is exteriorised, this may be significantly reduced. Although routine use of the thrombosuction catheter may not be recommended in patients with high thrombus burdens, there appears to be significant benefit, especially with respect to cardiovascular outcomes at the cost of a slightly higher stroke risk.

DEFERRED STENTING

The reopening of an infarct-related (usually thrombotic) occlusion of an epicardial coronary vessel is the goal of the primary angioplasty. However, there is a large element of microvascular obstruction that negatively impacts the results in the short and long term. Even after wire passage and balloon dilatation, there is a significant residual thrombus that, after deployment of a stent, might result in distal embolisation and coronary slow flow with associated complications and impaired prognosis. Systematic manual thrombectomy has not been shown to consistently prevent or abolish this problem [3].

The concept of deferred stenting, proposed for the first time by Isaaz et al. [8], refers to the practice of restoring flow by mechanical means (wire passage, balloon dilatation) and performing the stenting procedure at a second sitting. Observational studies suggested that deferred stenting was associated with higher rates of procedural success, higher 6-month left ventricular ejection fraction (LVEF), and lower rates of adverse events compared with immediate stenting [9–11]. A meta-analysis was performed that suggested better angiographic outcomes although cardiovascular outcomes were not improved [12]. However, randomised multi-centre trials with reproducible and consistent results are not easily designed and completed.

A large meta-analysis that included all the randomised studies that evaluated deferred stenting was reported recently [13]. Multiple end points were evaluated and reported, including slow-flow/no-reflow, incidence of MACE, major bleeding, all-cause mortality, myocardial infarction, target vessel revascularisation and long-term LV ejection fraction. Improved long-term LV function was found in the deferred-stenting group, although there was no significant difference in hard clinical outcomes such as MACE [13]. In another substudy with cardiac magnetic resonance (CMR) after deferred stenting, there was no difference in the final infarct size on CMR between the group who underwent deferred stenting and those that underwent routine primary PCI with stenting [14].

Certain caveats are important in the concepts of deferred stenting. It is mandatory to obtain TIMI III flow in the epicardial vessel before the consideration of deferred stenting is made. Less robust flow is not the subset being discussed, as the reason for the same has to be established prior to a decision. This interesting concept has been advocated by some dedicated interventionists but needs more detailed study before it is either adopted or rejected universally. As of now, it is not routinely recommended, as firm evidence is scant.

CULPRIT-ONLY REVASCULARISATION VERSUS COMPLETE REVASCULARISATION

A significant proportion of patients who undergo primary angioplasty have significant lesions in other parts of the coronary vasculature [15]. This group is at higher risk of adverse events including repeat ACS in non-culprit territories. The assessment and management of these has received constant and rigorous assessment over the last quarter century with significant advancement in knowledge but an incomplete picture as of now.

Traditionally, in patients without cardiogenic shock, only infarct-related artery revascularisation was recommended based on initial experience with primary percutaneous intervention (PCI). In fact, at one point, non-infarct vessel-related PCI was considered inappropriate [16]. However, in patients with cardiogenic shock, non-infarct vessel revascularisation was recommended. Both these concepts have been challenged by studies in the last decade [17–20].

The PRAMI (PReventive Angioplasty in Myocardial Infarction) trial assessed complete revascularisation or infarct-related PCI only in 465 patients with acute myocardial infarction. The primary end point of CV death, MI or refractory angina occurred twice as frequently in the infarct-artery only group over 23 months as compared to the complete revascularisation group achieving significance of a very high order (p < 0.001) [17]. Similar results were also found in the CvLPRIT trial [18]. It was noted that there was a small increase in the CMR detected non-IRA MI in the multi-vessel PCI group but there was no significant difference in the overall total infarct size between the two groups on CMR [21].

The DANAMI-3-PRIMULTI (Third DANish Study of Optimal Acute Treatment of Patients with ST-segment Elevation Myocardial Infarction: PRImary PCI in MULTI-vessel Disease) and the Compare-Acute (Fractional Flow Reserve-Guided Multivessel Angioplasty in Myocardial Infarction) studies evaluated the role of physiology in the assessment of the non-infarct-related vessel and the timing of revascularisation [19,20].

In Compare-Acute, patients with MI were randomised to either FFR-guided complete revascularisation or infarct-only revascularisation. Eighty per cent of patients in the FFR group had a planned revascularisation within 3 days of the index procedure at the operator's discretion. FFR was performed in the second group also but the primary care physician was not informed of the results. In the infarct-only group, 10% had a planned revascularisation within 45 days that was not included in the primary end point (PEP). The two groups were compared for end points that included repeat revascularisation (death, non-fatal myocardial infarction, revascularisation and cerebrovascular events). The results favoured the FFR-guided revascularisation group but this was mostly driven by repeat revascularisation and not hard end points. Additionally, two patients in the infarct-only group suffered a complication related to the pressure wire, both resulting in dissection in the non-infarct-related vessel and one in death [20].

The DANAMI-3-PRIMULTI trial was similar in design, however, a magnetic resonance imaging substudy revealed additional findings. A significant number of patients had fresh subendocardial scars in the non-infarct-related artery segments (probably fresh Type 4a myocardial infarction) and many had remote scars that were picked up at this time [22].

The issue is by no means completely resolved and ongoing trials like COMPLETE (Complete vs. Culprit-only Revascularisation to Treat Multi-vessel Disease After Early PCI for STEMI) (NCT01740479), and FULL-REVASC (Ffr-gUidance for compLete Non-cuLprit REVASCularization) (NCT02862119) compare FFR-guided revascularisation versus conservative management. The FLOWER-AMI (FLOW Evaluation to Guide Revascularization in Multi-vessel ST-elevation Myocardial Infarction) (NCT02943954) trial compares angiography-guided PCI versus FFR-guided PCI. These trials have superiority designs. The BioVasc (NCT03621501) and iMODERN (iFR Guided Multi-vessel Revascularization During Percutaneous Coronary Intervention for Acute Myocardial Infarction) (NCT03298659) trials have non-inferiority designs; however, the comparator group in the iMODERN trial evaluates management guided by stress perfusion CMR at 6 weeks.

Thus, revascularisation of the non-infarct vessel definitely reduces ischaemia-driven revascularisation although the spontaneous event rate may be unclear. A physiology-driven strategy seems to be the current gold standard, but this strategy has its limitations as the vast majority of clinical events occur in non-obstructive lesions. The optimal timing currently seems to be during the index hospitalisation although clinical judgement is paramount. A wealth of information is likely to be available in the near future on this issue that will definitely impact decisions.

REVASCULARISATION IN PATIENTS WITH CARDIOGENIC SHOCK

Among patients with acute MI, nearly 5%–10% present with cardiogenic shock and they have higher mortality [23]. Guidelines recommend complete revascularisation in this subset; however, the evidence base for this is not very large and most studies were small with multiple confounding factors as cardiogenic shock was an exclusion criteria for most trials for primary PCI. In fact, the CULPRIT SHOCK trial suggested a better prognosis for the patients who underwent staged revascularisation [24].

In the CULPRIT SHOCK trial, 706 patients were randomly assigned to culprit-lesion only or multi-vessel PCI and clinical outcomes at 30 days and 1 year were evaluated. End points included all-cause death, repeat revascularisation and rehospitalisation for recurrent heart failure. At 30 days, death or renal replacement occurred in 45.9% of patients in the culprit-only group versus 55.4% in the multi-vessel group. At 1 year, death occurred in 50.9% in the culprit-only versus 56.9% in the multi-vessel group. Recurrent infarction was 1.7% in the culprit-only patients versus 2.1% in the multi-vessel group. Repeat revascularisation and rehospitalisation for heart failure were higher in the culprit-only group (32.3% and 5.2% vs. 9.4% and 1.2%, respectively).

In contrast, a large registry-based study that looked at infarct-related only or multi-vessel PCI in patients with cardiogenic shock from Korea revealed that all-cause mortality and cardiac death at 1 year were lesser in the group that underwent multi-vessel PCI

[25]. A multivariate Cox proportional hazard model showed that multi-vessel PCI strategy was associated with a decreased risk of all-cause mortality at 1 year. A lower risk of all-cause death at 1 year was consistently observed in all subgroups (age>65, diabetes, history of cardiac arrest, LV dysfunction, left main disease) in patients who underwent multi-vessel PCI.

However, there are important differences between the two studies. The second study (KAMIR) is registry-based and not an intention to treat analysis. The mortality in the CULPRIT SHOCK trial was much higher (47.4% vs. 21.9%), and in the CULPRIT SHOCK trial all patients with CTO underwent attempts to open the CTO at the index revascularisation procedure, which is not the standard in the real world.

Acute MI with cardiogenic shock and multi-vessel disease remains a high-risk group with high mortality and multiple issues that may not be apparent at the time of the intervention, as this is an emergency. A rapid and skilled analysis of the clinical situation and anatomy should prompt the treatment strategy. The interventionist has the daunting task of walking the tight rope between doing too little, leaving significant ischaemic myocardium, or too much, and with excessive procedure time and contrast burden negatively impacting outcomes. Definitely, in a given situation, the best strategy as outlined by the patient's risk group, anatomy and available expertise is recommended.

REFERENCES

1. Fernandez-Rodriguez D, Regueiro A, Brugaletta S et al. EXAMINATION Investigators Optimization in stent implantation by manual thrombus aspiration in ST-segment-elevation myocardial infarction: Findings from the EXAMINATION trial. *Circ Cardiovasc Interv.* 2014;7:294–300.
2. Liistro F, Grotti S, Angioli P, Falsini G, Ducci K, Baldassarre S, Sabini A, Brandini R, Capati E, Bolognese L. Impact of thrombus aspiration on myocardial tissue reperfusion and left ventricular functional recovery and remodeling after primary angioplasty. *Circ Cardiovasc Interv.* 2009;2:376–383.
3. Jolly SS, James S, Džavík V et al. Thrombus aspiration in ST-segment-elevation myocardial infarction: An individual patient meta-analysis: Thrombectomytrialists collaboration. *Circulation.* 2017;135:14352.
4. Vlaar PJ, Svilaas T, van der Horst IC et al. Cardiac death and reinfarction after 1 year in the Thrombus Aspiration during Percutaneous coronary intervention in Acute myocardial infarction Study (TAPAS): A 1-year follow-up study. *Lancet.* 2008;371:1915–1920.
5. Fröbert O, Lagerqvist B, Gudnason T, Thuesen L, Svensson R, Olivecrona GK, James SK. Thrombus Aspiration in ST-Elevation myocardial infarction in Scandinavia (TASTE trial): A multicenter, prospective, randomized, controlled clinical registry trial based on the Swedish angiography and angioplasty registry (SCAAR) plat- form: Study design and rationale. *Am Heart J.* 2010;160:1042–1048.
6. Lagerqvist B, Fröbert O, Olivecrona GK et al. Outcomes 1 year after thrombus aspiration for myocardial infarction. *N Engl J Med.* 2014;371:1111–1120.

7. Levine GN, Bates ER, Blankenship JC et al. 2015 ACC/AHA/SCAI Focused Update on Primary Percutaneous Coronary Intervention for Patients with ST-Elevation Myocardial Infarction: An Update of the 2011 ACCF/AHA/SCAI Guideline for Percutaneous Coronary Intervention and the 2013 ACCF/AHA Guideline for the Management of ST-Elevation Myocardial Infarction. *J Am Coll Cardiol.* 2016;67:1235–1250.

8. Isaaz K, Robin C, Cerisier A, Lamaud M, Richard L, Da Costa A, Sabry MH, Gerenton C, Blanc JL. A new approach of primary angioplasty for ST-elevation acute myocardial infarction based on minimalist immediate mechanical intervention. *Coron Artery Dis.* 2006;17:261–269.

9. Meneveau N, Seronde MF, Descotes-Genon V, Dutheil J, Chopard R, Ecarnot F, Briand F, Bernard Y, Schiele F, Bassand JP. Immediate versus delayed angioplasty in infarct-related arteries with TIMI III flow and ST segment recovery: A matched comparison in acute myocardial infarction patients. *Clin Res Cardiol.* 2009;98:257–264.

10. Ke D, Zhong W, Fan L, Chen L. Delayed versus immediate stenting for the treatment of ST-elevation acute myocardial infarction with a high thrombus burden. *Coron Artery Dis.* 2012;23:497–506.

11. Pascal J, Veugeois A, Slama M, Rahal S, Belle L, Caussin C, Amabile N. Delayed stenting for ST-elevation acute myocardial infarction in daily practice: A single- centre experience. *Can J Cardiol.* 2016;32:988–995.

12. Freixa X, Belle L, Joseph L et al. Immediate vs. delayed stenting in acute myocardial infarction: A systematic review and meta-analysis. *Euro-Intervention.* 2013;8:1207–1216.

13. Qiao J, Pan L, Zhang B et al. Deferred Versus immediate stenting in patients with ST-segment Elevation Myocardial Infarction: A systematic Review and Meta-Analysis. *J Am Heart Assoc.* 2017;6:e0048383.

14. Lønborg J, Engstrøm T, Ahtarovski KA et al. for the DANAMI-3 Investigators Myocardial damage in patients with deferred stenting after STEMIA DANAMI-3–DEFER substudy. *J Am Coll Cardiol.* 2017;69:2794–2804.

15. Park DW, Clare RM, Schulte PJ et al. Extent, location, and clinical significance of non-infarct- related coronary artery disease among patients with ST-elevation myocardial infarction. *JAMA.* 2014;312:2019–2027.

16. O'Gara PT, Kushner FG, Ascheim DD et al. 2013 ACCF/AHA guideline for the management of ST- elevation myocardial infarction: A report of the American College of Cardiology Foundation/American Heart Association Task Force on Practice Guidelines. *J Am Coll Cardiol.* 2013;61:e78–140.

17. Wald DS, Morris JK, Wald NJ et al. Randomized trial of preventive angioplasty in myocardial infarction. *N Engl J Med.* 2013;369:1115–1123.

18. Gershlick AH, Khan JN, Kelly DJ et al. Randomized trial of complete versus lesion-only revascularization in patients undergoing primary percutaneous coronary intervention for STEMI and multivessel disease: The CvLPRIT trial. *J Am Coll Cardiol.* 2015;65:963–972.

19. Engstrom T, Kelbaek H, Helqvist S et al. Complete revascularisation versus treatment of the culprit lesion only in patients with ST-segment elevation myocardial infarction and multivessel disease (DANAMI-3-PRIMULTI): An open-label, randomised controlled trial. *Lancet.* 2015;386:665–671.

20. Smits PC, Abdel-Wahab M, Neumann FJ et al. Fractional flow reserve-guided multivessel angioplasty in myocardial infarction. *N Engl J Med.* 2017;376:1234–1244.

21. McCann GP, Khan J.N. Greenwood JP et al. Complete Versus Lesion-Only Primary PCI: The Randomized Cardiovascular MR CvLPRIT Substudy. *J Am Coll Cardiol.* 2015;66:2713–2724.

22. Kyhl K, Ahtarovski KA, Nepper-Christensen L et al. Complete revascularization versus culprit lesion only in patients with ST-segment elevation myocardial infarction and multivessel disease: A DANAMI-3-PRIMULTI cardiac magnetic resonance substudy. *J Am Coll Cardiol. Intv.* 2019;12:721–730.

23. Abdel-Wahab M, Saad M, Kynast J et al. Comparison of hospital mortality with intra-aortic balloon counterpulsation insertion before versus after primary percutaneous coronary intervention for cardiogenic shock complicating acute myocardial infarction. *Am J Cardiol.* 2010;105:967–971.

24. Thiele H, Akin I, Sandri M et al. for the CULPRIT-SHOCK Investigators One year outcomes after PCI strategies in cardiogenic shock. *N Engl J Med.* 2018;379:1699–1710.

25. Lee JM, Rhee T-M, Hahn J-Y et al. for the KAMIR Investigators Multivessel percutaneous coronary intervention in patients with ST-Segment elevation myocardial infarction with cardiogenic shock. *J Am Coll Cardiol.* 2018;71:844–856.

15

PCI post-thrombolysis
When and for whom?

SUSHANT WATTAL AND RAJIV AGARWAL

ST-elevation myocardial infarction (STEMI) is a medical emergency and timely revascularisation is essential for reducing the infarct size and improving short-term and long-term outcomes. Thrombolysis and primary percutaneous coronary intervention (PCI) are the two most commonly used strategies to achieve timely reperfusion. Evidence from many trials underlines the superiority of primary PCI over thrombolysis in the management of ST-elevation myocardial infarction (STEMI) [1]. Primary PCI is superior to thrombolysis strategy in reducing myocardial ischaemia, reinfarction, death, intracranial bleeding and re-occlusion of the infarct-related artery in STEMI patients irrespective of the patient's risk or whether inter-hospital transfer for PCI is required [1]. As compared to thrombolysis, PCI is able to preserve the myocardium and improve clinical outcomes over a wider window period following symptom onset and is the treatment of choice for patients who present early or late after symptom onset.

However, logistic issues of transport delays and non-availability of experienced centres providing primary PCI reduce the benefits of this early invasive strategy. Delay in reperfusion has a major impact on 1-year mortality as shown by de Luca et al. [2]. The relative risk rises by 7.5% at 1-year follow-up for every 30 minutes of delay. Current guidelines recommend that primary PCI should be performed by experienced operators within 90 minutes of first medical contact in a primary PCI capable hospital (Class 1A). Due to the unavailability of primary PCI-equipped hospitals nearby and due to prolonged expected transfer time >120 minutes to a PCI equipped facility, many patients who present within 12 hours of symptom onset get treated with thrombolysis and thereafter are either treated medically or get referred for coronary angiography followed by angioplasty in various time modes. So, the questions are: Who should be referred for PCI and what should be the ideal time for performing PCI post-thrombolysis? This assumes added importance given that the national primary PCI rate remains <1% due to logistic and cost constraints. Hence, thrombolysis remains the dominant reperfusion strategy in India and it is important to have clarity of approach after thrombolysis in order to optimise the results [3].

The efficacy of thrombolysis is variable and varies with the type of lytic agent used. However, thrombolysis with even the most advanced fibrin specific lytic drug restores coronary blood flow to TIMI flow grade 3 in just over 50% of STEMI patients. Also, 5% to 10% of patients will suffer coronary artery re-occlusions after an initial successful thrombolysis. This is because the plaque/thrombosis ratio at the site of the coronary occlusion is on average 80% plaque to 20% thrombotic material [4] and it is often plaque expansion that contributes more than acute thrombosis to the acute coronary occlusion. Failure of reperfusion by thrombolysis is predicted by less than 50% resolution in ST-segment elevation, persistence of chest pain and/or hemodynamic instability or heart failure. Such patients in the past have been treated with conservative therapy and watchful waiting, repeat thrombolysis or rescue PCI.

Rescue PCI is defined as PCI done within 12 hours of a failed thrombolysis in patients with persistent or recurrent myocardial ischaemia. Patients undergoing rescue PCI have a lower mortality rate and significantly lower rates of recurrent MI and heart failure compared with patients who continue medical therapy, including repeat thrombolysis. Evidence from the REACT [5] and MERLIN [6] trials established rescue PCI as the strategy of choice in improving outcomes in STEMI patients failing thrombolysis (Class IIA). However, the drawback of this strategy is that identifying such patients takes at least 60 minutes after thrombolysis and that causes delay in transferring for PCI. Also, this strategy identifies only those patients in whom thrombolysis fails and excludes others in whom PCI may prove beneficial despite successful thrombolysis. Thus, rescue PCI may not be the most effective strategy to treat STEMI patients who have undergone thrombolysis.

The main reason for the need for PCI following thrombolysis is the suboptimal reperfusion and clinical outcomes achieved post-thrombolysis. This led to the idea of facilitated and thereafter pharmaco-invasive PCI.

Facilitated PCI refers to restoring anterograde flow in the infarct-related artery using pharmacological therapy prior to proceeding to PCI in patients with STEMI. Evidence from various trials showed that facilitated PCI is detrimental rather than beneficial for post-thrombolysis patients of STEMI. These included the ASSENT-4 PCI trial [7] showing that facilitated PCI consisting of full-dose thrombolysis (tenecteplase) plus antithrombotic co-therapy and preceding PCI by 1 to 3 hours had a worse clinical outcome versus primary PCI alone.

The FINESSE trial [8] found that facilitated PCI strategy with half-dose reteplase plus abciximab resulted in a graded rise in the rates of bleeding, intracranial haemorrhage and transfusions, with no significant difference in the clinical outcomes of composite of all-cause mortality, secondary ventricular fibrillation, cardiogenic shock and heart failure during the first 90 days when compared to the conventional PCI.

This resulted in the concept of *pharmaco-invasive PCI*, which appears to be the most promising strategy for STEMI patients post-thrombolysis. In this strategy, coronary angiogram and PCI are performed routinely 3 to 24 hours after thrombolysis. It is applicable in patients who undergo transfer from a PCI-non-capable facility to a PCI-equipped hospital. The Which Early ST-Elevation Myocardial Infarction Therapy (WEST) trial [9] and the *Grupo de Análisis de la Cardiopatía Isquémica Aguda* (GRACIA-2) trial [10] were randomised trials showing similar efficacy and safety of pharmaco-invasive and primary PCI strategies. Both studies, though, included small numbers of patients and thus were underpowered for clinical end points.

The Combined Abciximab Reteplase Stent Study in Acute Myocardial Infarction (CARESS-in-AMI) trial evaluated 600 patients treated in non–PCI-equipped hospitals with half-dose reteplase, abciximab, heparin and aspirin [11]. Patients were randomised to immediate transfer for PCI (299 patients) or standard care with transfer for rescue PCI as needed (301 patients). In the immediate PCI group, the time interval from reteplase to PCI was 2.25 hours. The primary outcome, a composite of 30-day death, reinfarction or refractory ischaemia, was found to be significantly less – 4.4% for the immediate PCI group versus 10.7% for the standard care group with rescue PCI as required ($P = 0.004$) with no significant differences in major bleeding (3.4% vs. 2.3%, $P = 0.47$) or stroke (0.7% vs. 1.3%, $P = 0.50$).

The largest such trial was the Trial of Routine Angioplasty and Stenting After Thrombolysis to Enhance Reperfusion in Acute Myocardial Infarction (TRANSFER-AMI) [12]. It studied 1059 high-risk patients with STEMI admitted in non-PCI hospitals within 12 hours from symptom onset. Patients were randomised to standard treatment group that also included rescue PCI (522 patients) or a strategy of pharmaco-invasive PCI within 6 hours (average 3.2 hours) after thrombolysis with tenecteplase (537 patients). At 30 days, the primary end point occurred significantly less in the pharmaco-invasive PCI group (11%) compared to the standard treatment group (17.2%) ($P = 0.004$), with similar bleeding rates for the two groups. The primary end-point outcomes were driven mainly by reduction in reinfarction or recurrent ischaemia.

Evidence for pharmaco-invasive PCI in STEMI is also provided by a number of meta-analyses. One of these included seven trials evaluating a total of 2961 patients comparing pharmaco-invasive PCI with standard therapy. The meta-analysis found that pharmaco-invasive PCI decreased the 30-day rate of reinfarction (2.6% vs. 4.7%, $P = 0.003$), the combined end point of death or reinfarction (5.6% vs. 8.3%, $P = 0.004$) and recurrent ischaemia (1.9% vs. 7.1%; $P < 0.001$) with similar rates of major bleeding (4.9% vs. 5.0%, $P = 0.70$) or stroke (0.7% vs. 1.3%, $P = 0.21$) [13]. The benefits of pharmaco-invasive PCI were maintained at 6 to 12 months of follow-up.

Another meta-analysis of nine trials totalling 3325 patients showed a 24% decrease in total mortality ($P = 0.06$), a decrease in recurrent MI by 45% ($P < 0.001$) and a 65% decrease in repeated episodes of ischaemia ($P < 0.001$) with similar incidences of major bleeding or stroke in patients managed with pharmaco-invasive PCI as opposed to standard care [14].

One more meta-analysis of eight trials including 3195 patients showed that the composite end point of death at 30-days, myocardial ischaemia and reinfarction were lower in the pharmaco-invasive PCI group versus the ischaemia-guided PCI group after thrombolysis (7.3% vs. 13.5%; OR, 0.47; 95% CI, 0.32 to 0.68; $P < 0.001$) with no significant difference in the major bleeding rates. This study supported the use of pharmaco-invasive PCI within 24 hours of thrombolysis when PCI was not feasible [15].

The reasons for the beneficial effects of pharmaco-invasive PCI strategy contrasting with the failure of older studies of facilitated PCI can only be speculated upon and may include better contemporary PCI techniques and stents, smaller sheaths, radial approach and elimination of routine post-procedure heparin administration as a means of reducing haemorrhage [16]. It may also relate to the intense stimulation of platelets that occurs after administration of even half-doses of lytics [17]. Delaying the subsequent PCI by 3–24 hours in the pharmaco-invasive strategy allows platelet activation to subside and thus makes a virtue out of a logistical necessity given that the patient needs to be transported to the invasive facility.

The related questions that arise are whether we may offer a pharmaco-invasive strategy involving immediate lysis and delayed PCI even if primary PCI is feasible with a small time delay. The STREAM trial suggests that patients presenting within 3 hours of STEMI may do as well with pharmaco-invasive approach with half-dose lytic therapy as with primary PCI performed at average delay of 117 minutes [18]. This probably applies to only stable patients and needs to be replicated in other settings but expands our options.

The second question relates to the fact that the 3–24-hour time window for PCI in pharmaco-invasive strategy has been worked out for third-generation lytics like tenecteplase and alteplase. The dominant thrombolytic in India remains streptokinase by virtue of cost. Streptokinase is known to have a longer half-life and more prolonged platelet activation and therefore the safe time window for PCI after administering streptokinase may be delayed. Limited evidence of safety of PCI after streptokinase including time intervals is available from the TN-STEMI project in which PCI was performed at an average of 18.2 hours after thrombolysis with streptokinase [19].

Despite the strong evidence favouring pharmaco-invasive PCI, many patients in developing countries like India find it difficult to afford thrombolysis with the best fibrinolytic agent like tenecteplase followed by a costly procedure like PCI within 24 hours. Even medical insurance may refuse to pay for two such procedures in back-to-back fashion. Thus, in such patients, translating evidence into clinical practice can prove to be a major challenge.

As a result, a more common reason for undergoing PCI post-thrombolysis in such patients seems to be recurrent onset of chest pain or asymptomatic residual ischaemia detected by exercise testing or nuclear perfusion imaging like SPECT. The benefit of revascularisation in post-thrombolysis patients having residual or recurrent ischaemia was shown in the DANAMI trial [20]. This trial showed that those patients of acute STEMI, who, post-fibrinolysis, had spontaneous symptoms of angina or positive exercise stress test and underwent PCI, had less frequency of death, re-infarction or rehospitalisations for unstable angina at 1, 2 and 4 years versus those who were treated conservatively.

More than 30% of patients of STEMI present late in India [21]. The clinical benefit of PCI in late presenters (>24 hours after thrombolysis) with no or mild symptoms is controversial. According to ACC/AHA, PCI is a class IIb indication for stable late-presenting patients (presenting after 24 hours) with hemodynamically significant stenosis in a patent infarct-related artery and not indicated (class III indication) in case of a totally occluded infarct-related artery without evidence of ischaemia.

The infarcted myocardium is a highly dynamic tissue, which is not entirely dead. According to the 'open artery hypothesis,' reperfusion beyond the window for myocardial salvage (>24 hours after STEMI) may improve survival rates by prevention of adverse ventricular remodelling, providing electrical stability and restoring blood flow to collateral coronary arteries supplying the remaining viable myocardium [22].

The BRAVE-2 trial [23] (Beyond 12 Hours Reperfusion Alternative Evaluation) evaluated 365 patients of STEMI presenting late (12–48 hours after symptoms), without persistent symptoms randomised to PCI versus medical management. The trial showed that infarct size was significantly lower in the PCI arm versus the conservative arm (8% vs. 13%, respectively; $P = 0.0002$), while there were no significant differences for mortality rates and/or MI at 30 days between the two arms. However, reperfusion with PCI in very late presenters (3–28 days) did not improve rates of death or ejection fraction of the left ventricle versus medical therapy in the OAT (Occluded Artery Trial) during 4-year follow-up [24].

However, angina and repeat revascularisation after 7 years was significantly less in the PCI arm in the OAT trial. However, the OAT trial was not representative of real-world STEMI patients with a long exclusion list (LMCA disease/triple vessel disease/severe angina/heart failure/unstable arrythmias/renal dysfunction) and had a median time to revascularisation of 8 days after STEMI, which was probably too late for benefit. Evidence from the OAT trial had too small an impact on clinical practice even in the United States [25].

A study evaluated final infarct size and myocardium salvaged in patients presenting <12 hours versus those presenting from 12–72 hours before undergoing primary angioplasty. It found the final size of infarct larger in those presenting late as expected but also concluded that significant myocardial salvage can be achieved when presenting after the 12-hour limit, even when the infarct-related artery is totally occluded [26].

A meta-analysis of 10 randomised trials tried to evaluate the benefit of late PCI in stable patients with acute STEMI by comparing percutaneous coronary intervention of the infarct-related artery with medical therapy in 3560 stable patients randomised >12 hours and up to 60 days after acute myocardial infarction. The study concluded that late PCI resulted in significant improvements in left ventricular ejection fraction and survival when compared to medical therapy [27]. So, there is no simple and specific guideline for patients of STEMI post-thrombolysis who present late. Substantial myocardial salvage is possible even when the infarct-related artery is occluded.

APPROACH TO THE PATIENT

Primary PCI should be the treatment of choice for all patients of acute ST-elevation MI and all attempts should be made to make it easily available in a timely manner. If the expected delay in transferring the patient to a primary PCI capable centre is more than 120 minutes, fibrinolysis is reasonable especially if the patient presents early, but it definitely should not be the final step in the reperfusion management for such patients. All patients post-fibrinolysis should be transferred to a primary PCI-capable facility for coronary angiography, which can be safely performed after 3 hours of thrombolysis followed by PCI if needed. The safe period for PCI after streptokinase may be delayed as compared to newer lytic drugs. Those who present late or >24 hours after fibrinolysis should be assessed clinically. Those who are unstable clinically, hemodynamically or electrically need revascularisation. Those who are stable and present after 24 hours but before 72 hours should have coronary angiogram with an intent to do PCI if suitable, even if the infarct-related artery is occluded. Those who present after 72 hours need to be screened for viability by non-invasive stress testing, and if the stress test is positive then a coronary angiogram should be done with an intent to do PCI if the anatomy is suitable.

REFERENCES

1. Keeley EC, Boura JA, Grines CL. Primary angioplasty versus intravenous thrombolytic therapy for acute myocardial infarction: A quantitative review of 23 randomised trials. *Lancet* 2003;361(9351):13–20.

2. de Luca G, Suryapranata H, Ottervanger JP, Antman EM. Time delay to treatment and mortality in primary angioplasty for acute myocardial infarction: Every minute of delay counts. *Circulation* 2004;109:1223–1225.

3. Guha S, Sethi R, Ray S et al. Cardiological Society of India: Position statement for the management of ST elevation myocardial infarction in India. *Indian Heart J.* 2017;69(Suppl 1):S63–S97.

4. Brosius FC, 3rd, Roberts WC. Significance of coronary arterial thrombus in transmural acute myocardial infarction. A study of 54 necropsy patients. *Circulation* 1981;63:810–816.

5. Carver A, Rafelt S, Gershlick AH et al. Longer-term follow-up of patients recruited to the REACT (Rescue Angioplasty Versus Conservative Treatment or Repeat Thrombolysis) trial. *J Am Coll Cardiol.* 2009;54:118–126.

6. Sutton AG, Campbell PG, Graham R et al. A randomized trial of rescue angioplasty versus a conservative approach for failed fibrinolysis in ST-segment elevation myocardial infarction: The Middlesbrough Early Revascularization to Limit Infarction (MERLIN) trial. *J Am Coll Cardiol.* 2004;44:287–296.

7. Assessment of the Safety and Efficacy of a New Treatment Strategy with Percutaneous Coronary Intervention (ASSENT-4 PCI) Investigators: Primary versus tenecteplase-facilitated percutaneous coronary intervention in patients with ST-segment elevation acute myocardial infarction (ASSENT-4 PCI): Randomised trial. *Lancet* 2006;367(9510):569–578.

8. Ellis SG, Tendera M, de Belder MA et al. Facilitated PCI in patients with ST-elevation myocardial infarction. *N Engl J Med.* 2008;358:2205–2217.

9. Armstrong PW. WEST Steering Committee: A comparison of pharmacologic therapy with/without timely coronary intervention vs. primary percutaneous intervention early after ST-elevation myocardial infarction: The WEST (Which Early ST-elevation myocardial infarction Therapy) study. *Eur Heart J.* 2006;27:1530–1538.

10. Fernandez-Aviles F, Alonso JJ, Pena G et al. Primary angioplasty vs. early routine post-fibrinolysis angioplasty for acute myocardial infarction with ST-segment elevation: The GRACIA-2 noninferiority, randomized, controlled trial. *Eur Heart J.* 2007;28:949–960.

11. Di Mario C, Dudek D, Piscione F et al. Immediate angioplasty versus standard therapy with rescue angioplasty after thrombolysis in the Combined Abciximab REteplase Stent Study in Acute Myocardial Infarction (CARESS-in-AMI): An open, prospective, randomised, multicentre trial. *Lancet* 2008;371(9612):559–568.

12. Cantor WJ, Fitchett D, Borgundvaag B et al. Routine early angioplasty after fibrinolysis for acute myocardial infarction. *N Engl J Med.* 2009;360:2705–2718.

13. Borgia F, Goodman SG, Halvorsen S et al. Early routine percutaneous coronary intervention after fibrinolysis vs. standard therapy in ST-segment elevation myocardial infarction: A metaanalysis. *Eur Heart J.* 2010;31:2156–2169.

14. Desch S, Eitel I, Rahimi K et al. Timing of invasive treatment after fibrinolysis in ST elevation myocardial infarction–a metaanalysis of immediate or early routine versus deferred or ischemia-guided randomised controlled trials. *Heart* 2010;96:1695–1702.

15. D'Souza SP, Mamas MA, Fraser DG, Fath-Ordoubadi F. Routine early coronary angioplasty versus ischaemia-guided angioplasty after thrombolysis in acute ST-elevation myocardial infarction: A meta-analysis. *Eur Heart J.* 2011;32:972–982.

16. Ibanez B, James S, Agewall S et al. 2017 ESC Guidelines for the management of acute myocardial infarction in patients presenting with ST-segment elevation. *Eur Heart J.* 2018;39:119–177.

17. Moser M, Nordt T, Peter K et al. Platelet function during and after thrombolytic therapy for acute myocardial infarction with reteplase, alteplase, or STK. *Circulation* 1999;100:1858–1864.

18. Armstrong PW, Gershlick AH, Goldstein P et al. Fibrinolysis or primary PCI in ST-segment elevation myocardial infarction. *N Engl J Med.* 2013;368:1379–1387.

19. Mishra S. What is the ideal fibrinolysis to PCI time: Pharmaco-invasive strategy with streptokinase? *Indian Heart J.* 2017;69:569–570.

20. Madsen JK, Grande P, Saunamaki K et al. Danish multicentre randomized study of invasive versus conservative treatment in patients with inducible ischemia after thrombolysis in acute myocardial infarction (DANAMI). DANish trial in Acute Myocardial Infarction. *Circulation* 1997;96:748.

21. Xavier D, Pais P, Devereaux PJ et al.; CREATE Registry investigators. Treatment and outcomes of acute coronary syndromes in India (CREATE): A prospective analysis of registry data. *Lancet* 2008;371(9622):1435–1442.

22. Braunwald E. Myocardial reperfusion, limitation of infarct size, reduction of left ventricular dysfunction, and improved survival. Should the paradigm be expanded? *Circulation* 1989;79:441–444.

23. Ndrepepa G, Kastrati A, Mehilli J, Antoniucci D, Schömig A. Mechanical reperfusion and long-term mortality in patients with acute myocardial infarction presenting 12 to 48 hours from onset of symptoms. *JAMA* 2009;301:487–488.

24. Hochman JS, Lamas GA, Buller CE et al. Occluded Artery Trial Investigators. Coronary intervention for persistent occlusion after myocardial infarction. *N Engl J Med.* 2006;355:2395–2407.

25. Deyell MW, Buller CE, Miller LH et al. Impact of national clinical guideline recommendations for revascularization of persistently occluded infarct-related arteries on clinical practice in the United States. *Arch Intern Med.* 2011;171:1636–1643.

26. Busk M, Kaltoft A, Nielsen SS et al. Infarct size and myocardial salvage after primary angioplasty in patients presenting with symptoms for <12 h vs. 12–72 h. *Eur Heart J.* 2009;30:1322–1330.

27. Abbate A, Biondi-Zoccai GG, Appleton DL et al. Survival and cardiac remodeling benefits in patients undergoing late percutaneous coronary intervention of the infarct-related artery: Evidence from a meta-analysis of randomized controlled trials. *J Am Coll Cardiol.* 2008;51:956–964.

16

PCI in unstable angina and NSTEMI

SMIT SHRIVASTAVA AND ABHIKRISHNA SINGH

INTRODUCTION

The treatment of non-ST elevation myocardial infarction (NSTEMI) can be pharmacological or interventional or a combination of both. The NSTEMI, unlike ST-elevation myocardial infarction (STEMI), is deprived of the vantage of treating with thrombolytics, thus necessitating an invasive treatment for most of the NSTEMI. NSTEMI remains the leading cause of mortality and morbidity, despite the aggressive treatment.

The range of presentation of coronary syndromes varies, including silent ischaemia, anginal equivalents, chronic stable angina, unstable angina, NSTEMI, STEMI, heart failure and sudden death. Unstable angina (UA) and NSTEMI are clinically indistinguishable except for the elevation of cardiac enzymes. These two presentations are regarded as interchangeable entities in this chapter.

EPIDEMIOLOGY AND NATURAL HISTORY

The higher incidence of NSTEMI is consistently evident from registry data. The incidence, though it varies between regions, is about 3 NSTEMI per 1000 people per year [1]. For in-hospital mortality, though it is higher for STEMI (7% vs. 3%–5%), the rates equate at 6 months and mortality for NSTEMI increases two-fold beyond 4 years. As the NSTEMI patients tend to be more elderly, with more comorbidities, the mortality rates tend to be higher. The incidences of NSTEMI, STEMI and bundle branch block myocardial infarction (BBBMI) were 54%, 39% and 6%, and the 1-year mortalities for the same were 31%, 21% and 55%, respectively, in a study of 654 patients [2].

PATHOPHYSIOLOGY

The mismatch of myocardial oxygen supply and demand is the principal underlying mechanism for NSTEMI. The most common precipitating factor is coronary artery stenosis resulting from a partially occlusive thrombus over an eroded atherosclerotic lesion with or without superimposed coronary vasospasm or stenosis. The pathological hallmark of NSTEMI is erosion of vulnerable plaque; culminating platelet activation and adhesion within the lipid core, the protruding thrombus then showers clumps of platelets into the downstream myocardium, causing its necrosis [3]. Very rarely, non-atherosclerotic causes like arteritis, trauma, dissection, thromboembolism, catheterisation or pharmacogenetic mechanism may be responsible. It is vital to understand that the vulnerable plaque concept underlies the aetiological mechanism for NSTEMI and hence, the thin capped large atheromatous plaque is the target for treatment strategies [4].

Plaque rupture is the most common cause of acute coronary syndrome in males while pre-menopausal females more frequently have erosion, and again plaque rupture shows progressive occurrence in post-menopausal females. Culprit lesions responsible for acute coronary syndrome are less calcified than those for stable angina, stressing the stability of calcified lesions [5].

DIAGNOSIS

The chief presentation of NSTEMI is with typical angina. The working diagnosis of NSTEMI is based on exclusion of persisting ST-elevation in electrocardiogram (ECG) and the positive cardiac biomarkers. NSTEMI, like other acute coronary syndromes, presents with atypical symptoms especially in the elderly, women, diabetics and chronic kidney disease patients. The established ECG-specific criteria for NSTEMI by the joint ESC/ACCF/AHA/WHF committee for the fourth universal definition is: Horizontal or down-sloping ST-segment depression greater than or equal to 0.5 mm in 2 contiguous leads and/or T inversion greater than 1 mm in 2 contiguous leads with prominent R wave or R/S ratio greater than 1 [6].

Physical examination needs to be directed to uncover precipitating comorbidities, to assess warning signs for complications of acute coronary syndrome and to rule out non-ischaemic and non-cardiac causes for the presentation.

The electrocardiogram should be obtained within 10 minutes of medical contact. NSTEMI patients present with acute onset chest pain without persistent ST-segment elevation. The ECG changes can include no manifested changes, pseudo-normalisation, flattening, inversion of T waves or persistent or transient ST-segment depression. The specificity for ECG diagnosis of NSTEMI is high (97%), while the sensitivity is poor (28%) [7]. However, the unavailability of biomarkers' diagnosis in the initial 4 hours makes ECG more important for the diagnosis.

The biomarkers, especially troponin elevation, separate NSTEMI from unstable angina. The troponin elevation is more sensitive and specific than other cardiac biomarkers. Recent ultrasensitive troponin assays have 100 times more analytical sensitivity. The serial changes in the level of biomarkers are more confirmatory especially in patients of chronic stable angina. The clinical importance of false positive rise of troponin (Table 16.1) as in aortic dissection or pulmonary embolism mandates emphasis.

The imaging by coronary arteriography is recommended to be performed prior to and post-intracoronary vasodilator injection. The TIMI IIIB [8] and FRISC studies [9] determined in acute coronary settings the incidences of single vessel disease, double vessel disease and left main as 30%–38%, 44%–59% and 4%–8%, respectively. The subset of left main with multi-vessel disease was obviously at the highest risk. Biomarkers like BNP, CRP and NT Pro BNP may portend the prognosis, while chemokine ligand 5 and ligand 18, [10] interleukin 6, [11] heart type fatty acid binding protein, [12] pentraxin, [13] mid-regional proadrenomedullin and copeptin [14] are promising newer markers for diagnosis and prognosis. A prospective observational study of 478 patients suggests superiority of hs-cTn with supplementary copeptin over a repeat hs-cTn [15].

Table 16.1 Important causes of false troponin rise

Common	Less common
1. Chronic or acute renal derangement	1. Aortic dissection and valvular diseases
2. Advanced heart failure	2. Cardiomyopathy
3. Hypertensive crisis	3. Cardiac trauma
4. Cardiac arrhythmias	4. Hypothyroidism
5. Pulmonary embolism/hypertension	5. Drug myotoxicity
6. Myocarditis	6. Moderate to severe burns
7. Neurological stroke or haemorrhage	7. Rhabdomyolysis
	8. Severe sepsis

Table 16.2 The differential diagnosis of NSTEMI

Cardiac	Myocarditis	Pericarditis
	Cardiomyopathy	Valvular disease
	Trauma	
Pulmonary	Pulmonary embolism/infarction	Pneumonitis/pleuritis
	Pneumothorax	
Haematological	Severe anaemia	Sickle cell crisis
Vascular	Aortic aneurysm/dissection	Cerebrovascular disease
Gastrointestinal	Oesophagitis/SAPM	Acid peptic disease
Thoracic	Cervical radiculopathy	Rib fractures
	Thoracic myositis/herpes zoster	Costochondritis

DIFFERENTIAL DIAGNOSIS

The differential diagnosis for NSTEMI revolves around acute chest pain presentation and rise in cardiac biomarkers (see Table 16.2).

RISK ASSESSMENT

NSTEMI due to high association with comorbidities has a higher short-term and long-term mortality than other coronary syndromes. This necessitates timely risk stratification to devise appropriate treatment strategies (Table 16.3). The Global Registry of Acute Coronary Events (GRACE) score provides most accurate quantification for both risk at admission and at discharge compared to the TIMI risk score [16].

MANAGEMENT

The principles of management of NSTEMI (1) general measures, (2) anti-ischaemic measures, (3) antithrombotic measures, (4) invasive treatment and (5) rehabilitation are outlined in Table 16.4.

1. *General measures*: The importance of good directed history underlies the fact that NSTEMI can initially have negative cardiac biomarkers and a normal-appearing ECG. A repeated measure of rising cardiac biomarkers and serial ECG recording and the recent hs-cTn prevent missing early patients with NSTEMI.

2. *Anti-ischaemic measures*: The risk prediction algorithms and scores help in determining the patients who need to be subjected to pharmacological or invasive anti-ischaemic measures. The principal mechanism of anti-ischaemic drugs is to lower myocardial oxygen demand by reducing heart rate, afterload, preload and myocardial contractility, and by facilitating myocardial oxygen supply by coronary vasodilatation.

3. *Antithrombotic measures*: Platelet aggregations that follow platelet activation in NSTEMI are the key therapeutic targets in treating acute coronary syndromes.
   a. *Aspirin*: Aspirin reduces myocardial infarction or death in unstable angina (odds ratio 0.47; CI 0.37–0.61;

Table 16.3 Risk scores in NSTEMI

	Factors	Predicts	Score	Trials
TIMI Risk Score (1 score for each factor present)	1. Age 2. Three or more traditional CAD risk factors - hypertension, diabetes, hyperlipidaemia, smoking 3. Aspirin in prior 7 days 4. Known coronary artery disease 5. Anginal episode in past 24 hrs 6. ST-segment deviation $\geq$0.5 mm 7. Elevated cardiac biomarkers	Risk of death, death or myocardial infarction at 14 days	0–2 low 3–4 intermediate 5–7 high	Validated in TIMI-IIB and ESSENCE
GRACE Risk Score	1. Age 2. Systolic blood pressure 3. Pulse rate 4. Serum creatinine 5. Killip Class 6. Cardiac arrest at admission 7. Elevated biomarkers 8. ST deviation	Mortality in hospital and at 6 months	In-hospital mortality: $\leq$108 low 109–140 intermediate >140 high At 6 months: <88 low 89–117 intermediate >118 high	

Note: Other risk scores like PREDICT, AMIS, EMMACE and SRI (simple risk score) have not found wide acceptability. The CRUSADE Registry Bleeding Risk Score is utilised to assess in-hospital major bleeding risk.

Table 16.4 Principles for management of NSTEMI

General measures	1. Directed history 3. ECG within 10 min 5. Bed rest 7. Continuous ECG monitoring with telemetry	2. Relevant physical examination 4. Cardiac markers Quantitative assay repeated after 3–6 hrs 6. Inhaled oxygen if SpO_2 < 90% or heart failure	
Anti-ischaemic measures	1. Beta-blockers 2. Nitrates 3. Calcium channel blocker 4. Nicorandil 5. Trimetazidine 6. Ranolazine 7. Cyclosporine	Decreases mortality No benefit in mortality No benefit in mortality Decreases arrhythmias and transient ischaemia Decreased short time mortality Decreases arrhythmias and transient ischaemia Reduces infarct size in small studies	
Antithrombotic measures	1. Aspirin 2. P2Y12 inhibitor 3. Anti-coagulant	Recommendation IA Recommendation IB Recommendation IB	
Invasive treatment			
Rehabilitation			

p < 0.001) [17]. Dose of chewed plain aspirin of 150–300 mg is recommended for loading. Intravenous aspirin is not available widely. There is a recommended daily maintenance dose of 75–100 mg of anti-platelet activity similar to higher doses at reduced gastrointestinal bleeding potential as suggested by the PCI-CURE [18] and CURRENT OASIS-7 [19] trial outcomes.

   b. *Thienopyridines*: Ticlopidine, clopidogrel and prasugrel irreversibly block the P2Y12 receptors through their metabolites, independent of aspirin action.

      i. *Clopidogrel*: Showed 20% reduction in cardiovascular death, MI and stroke in 12,562 to patients in CURE (Clopidogrel in Unstable Angina to Prevent Recurrent Events) trial [18]. The PCI-CURE subset was associated with a 31% reduction in cardiovascular death or MI [20]. The conversion of prodrug to active metabolites varies with polymorphism of hepatic CYP pathways. However, the Gauging Responsiveness with a Verify-now Assay Impact on Thrombosis and Safety (GRAVITAS) trial—did not suggest any improvement with genetic testing for platelet functions [21]. The Clopidogrel and the Optimisation of Gastrointestinal Events Trial (CONGENT) showed no clinical difference in cardiovascular outcomes with omeprazole and placebo [22]. The US Food and Drug Administration warns against the concomitant use of clopidogrel with esomeprazole and omeprazole. The anti-platelet action of clopidogrel is irreversible and takes several days for optimal effect without a loading dose.

ii. *Prasugrel*: Scores over other thienopyridines with better biotransformation to active metabolite. Prasugrel in loading as well as in maintenance doses has more rapid onset, more P2Y12 inhibition and less variability than others. The TRINITON-TIMI 38 [23] study showed the benefits of prasugrel were similar in patients with NSTEMI (HR 0.82; 95% CI 0.73 to 0.93; p = 0.02). The pre-specified landmark analysis in this trial to detect outcomes attributable to loading dose of study drugs showed that prasugrel is superior to clopidogrel in early and maintenance phases. A significant bleeding hazard, especially in prior stroke patients, patients beyond 75 years of age and of weight less than 60 kg, contraindicates prasugrel use in these cohorts. The ACCOAST [24] trial with 4033 patients of NSTEMI compared pre-treatment with prasugrel and placebo; TIMI major bleeding was significantly higher in the pre-treatment cohort with no significant difference in primary outcomes.

iii. *Ticagrelor*: Is a directly active drug that binds reversibly to P2Y12 receptors at a different site from ATP or thienopyridine binding. It is primarily metabolised by CYP3A hepatic mechanism. A loading dose of ticagrelor 180 mg provides an IPA with ADP 20 mmol/L of 41% at 30 minutes and 88% at 2 hours compared with 8% and 41% after clopidogrel 600 mg loading dose, respectively [25]. The PLATO trial randomised 18,624 patients with both STEMI and NSTEMI to show a significant reduction in the primary composite end points compared with clopidogrel at 1 year (9.8% vs. 11.7%; HR 0.84; 95% CI 0.77 to 0.92; p < 0.001). Instances of fatal intracerebral haemorrhage were higher with ticagrelor; however, that was balanced by more non-intracranial major bleeding with clopidogrel. A subgroup analysis showed that significant reduction of primary end points was seen with NSTEMI patients only and not with unstable angina patients [26]. Ticagrelor is associated with dyspnoea, hyperuricaemia and ventricular pauses secondary to lesser adenosine degradation and erythrocyte uptake. In the dose confirmation study assessing anti-platelet effects of AZD-6140 versus clopidogrel in non-ST-segment elevation myocardial infarction (DISPERSE-2), dyspnoea was seen in 10.5% of those who received ticagrelor 90 mg twice a day compared to 6.4% with clopidogrel (p = 0.07) [27]. CYP3a inhibitors such as itraconazole and diltiazem increase plasma concentration of ticagrelor, while ticagrelor increases simvastatin levels [28].

iv. *Cangrelor*: The intravenous rapid and direct-acting inhibitor of P2Y12 receptor with short half-life of 3 minutes, which achieves greater than 95% IPA within 15 minutes of 4 microgram per kg per minute dose [29].

c. *Cilostazol*: Is a selective phosphodiesterase inhibitor that does not have studies for an NSTEMI subset. The pharmacodynamic studies suggest greater inhibition of ATP (adenosine triphosphate)-induced platelet inhibition compared with aspirin and clopidogrel alone, resulting in reduced risk of stent thrombosis, restenosis and major adverse cardiac event without increased breathing risk. It should be noted that any amount of left ventricular dysfunction contraindicates use of cilostazol due to increased mortality.

d. *Glycoprotein IIIa/IIb inhibitors*: The glycoprotein IIa/IIb inhibitors target the final common pathway of platelet activation and aggregation. The latest ACC/AHA guidelines recommend use of these agents in very high-risk cases especially when newer anti-platelets cannot be used.

i. *Abciximab*: The ISAR-REACT trial assessed incremental benefits of glycoprotein IIa/IIb inhibitors in 2022 patients with acute coronary syndrome with clopidogrel 600 mg for at least 2 hours compared to placebo. The abciximab significantly reduced the primary end points of death, MI and target vessel revascularisation at 30 days only in patients with elevated troponin.

ii. *Eptifibatide*: The Platelet Glycoprotein IIb/IIIa in Unstable Angina: Receptor Suppression Using Integrilin Therapy (PURSUIT) Trial showed 10% reduction in the relative risk of death and MI at 30 days [30]. The EARLY-ACS study randomised 9492 patients treated invasively to either upstream or early eptifibatide. The study showed increased bleeding and transfusion need in the prior eptifibatide group. The benefits of glycoprotein IIb/IIIa are limited to moderate- to high-risk patients only, according to a meta-analysis [31].

iii. *Tirofiban*: The Platelet Receptor Inhibition in Ischaemic Syndrome Management (PRISM) trial randomised 3232 patients with unstable angina between unfractionated heparin and tirofiban for 48 hours; no significant difference was noted at the end of 30 days [32]. The Platelet Receptor Inhibition in Ischaemic Syndrome Management in Patient Limited by Unstable Signs and Symptoms (PRISM-PLUS) compared patients receiving tirofiban alone, heparin alone and both. The patients receiving both heparin and tirofiban showed benefits at the end of 7 days, 30 days and 6 months [33].

e. *Direct thrombin inhibitors*: Bivalirudin is administered at 0.1 mg/kg bolus and 0.25 mg/kg/hr infusion in

NSTEMI interventions. The ACUITY trial demonstrated that bivalirudin alone was non-inferior to UFH (unfractionated heparin) and GP IIb/IIIa inhibitor and it had significantly lower major bleeding [34].

f. *Newer oral anti-coagulants*: The apixaban in APPRAISE-2 trial was stopped early owing to high bleeding. The rivaroxaban in ALTAS-ACS-TIMI51 trial showed reduction in composite of cardiovascular death, myocardial infarction and stroke by 16% as compared to clopidogrel and aspirin alone [35].

4. *Invasive measures*: The high-risk subset of NSTEMI with hemodynamic instability, heart failure, persisting ischaemia, mechanical complications and arrhythmias needs to undergo coronary angiography urgently [3]. The rest of patients can be triaged under three strategies: (1) the ischaemia-guided strategy (48–72 hours or later); (2) the early invasive strategy (less than 48–72 hours); and (3) the very early (within 12 hours) (see Table 16.5).

a. *The ischaemia-guided strategy*: Or, the initial conservative strategy, utilises intensive medical therapy with anti-platelets, anti-coagulants, beta-blockers, statins

Table 16.5 Optimal timing for invasive treatment

Study	Randomisation	Results	Limitations
TIMACS [46] 3031 NSTEMI pts	Early (<24 hrs) vs. delayed (>36 hrs)	No difference in the rates of death, MI or stroke	'Early' intervention was not actually early
ICTUS trial [47] 1200 NSTEMI	Early (within 24–48 hrs) vs. selectively invasive groups (beyond 48 hrs)	No difference in mortality or spontaneous MI, at 1 year and 10 years follow-up there was a 5% absolute increase (15% vs. 10%) in myocardial infarction in the early invasive group	Excluded reperfusion therapy, hemodynamic instability or overt congestive heart failure
ELISA [48] 220 patients	Early (median 6 hrs) vs. late (median 50 hrs)	No difference in clinical outcomes at 30 days	Detailed ECG and angiographic analysis not performed, refractory chest pain was excluded
ISAR-COOL Study [49] 410 patients	Early (median 2.4 hrs) vs. late (86 hrs)	Significantly higher rate of death or 'large' MI in the delayed strategy group compared to the early invasive group (11.6% vs. 5.9%, p = 0.04)	Detailed ECG and angiographic analysis not performed
LIPSIA-NSTEMI Trial [50] 401 patients	Early (median 1.1 hrs) vs. late (18.6 hrs)	No difference in death or MI within 6 months	Detailed ECG and angiographic analysis not performed, refractory chest pain was excluded
Montalescot [51] 352 patients	Immediate (70 min) vs. next day (21 hrs)	Median peak troponin I values did not differ between the two groups (2.1 vs. 1.7 ng/mL) No difference in the secondary end point at 1-month follow-up (13.7% vs. 10.2%)	Detailed ECG and angiographic analysis not performed, refractory chest pain was excluded
Sisca [52] 170 patients	Early (median 2.8 hrs) vs. late (20.9 hrs)	The primary end point at 30 days was significantly lower for early invasive strategy group (2% vs. 24%, p < 0.01)	14 patients in the delayed strategy group who received urgent revascularisation; very small sample size
RIDDLE-NSTEMI [53] 323 patient	Immediate intervention (<2 hrs) Delayed intervention groups (2–72 hrs)	The primary end point (occurrence of death or new MI at 30-day follow-up) was less frequent in the immediate group (4.3% vs. 13%, p = 0.008)	Detailed ECG and angiographic analysis not performed
VERDICT [36] 2147 patients	Very early invasive group (4.7 hrs after *randomisation*) standard invasive care group, (cath at a median of 61.6 hrs)	With GRACE risk score, a very early invasive treatment strategy improved the primary outcome (HR, 0.81; 95% CI, 0.67–1.01; p = 0.023), overall no benefits	Time to cath is after randomisation, not symptoms Refractory ischaemia, hemodynamic or electric instability, acute heart failure, mechanical complication or cardiac arrest patients were excluded

and nitrates for the initial 48–72 hours. If the patient becomes asymptomatic, this is typically followed by stress imaging. However, for symptomatic patients, invasive treatment is then proposed.

b. *The early invasive strategy:* The patients are treated with intensive medical therapy followed by early coronary angiography within 48–72 hours and necessary revascularisation.

c. *The very early (within 12 hours):* The Very EaRly vs. Deferred Invasive evaluation using Computerised Tomography (VERDICT) study randomised 2147 patients into 1075 in the 'very early invasive' group (cath at a median of 4.7 hours) and another 1072 in the 'standard invasive care' group (cath at a median of 61.6 hours). After a median follow-up time of 4.3 years, the primary end point occurred in 296 (27.5%) of participants in the very early group and 316 (29.5%) in the standard care group (hazard ratio, 0.92; 95% CI, 0.78–1.08). This study excluded the patients who had emergent needs for invasive coronary arteriography as very high-risk NSTE-ACS, including ongoing ischaemia despite intravenous nitroglycerin infusion, hemodynamic or electric instability, acute heart failure, mechanical complications or cardiac arrest [36].

The initial studies done in the pre-stent era like TIMI IIIB [8], Veterans Affairs Non-Q-Wave Infarction Strategies in Hospital (VANQUISH) [37] and Medicine versus Angiography in Thrombolytic Exclusion (MATE) [38] did not reveal superiority of early invasive strategy or ischaemia-guided strategy. The trials done in the contemporary PCI era like Fast Revascularisation during Instability of Coronary Artery (FRISC-II), [9] Treat Angina with Aggrastat and Determine Cost of Therapy with an Invasive or Conservative Strategy-Thrombolysis in Myocardial Infarction (TACTICS-TIMI 18) [39], Value of First Day Angiography/Angioplasty in Evolving Non-ST-Segment Elevation Myocardial Infarction (VINO), Randomised Intervention Trial of unstable Angina–3 (RITA-3) and Invasive versus Conservative Treatment in Unstable Coronary Syndrome (ICTUS) found statistically significant advantage with early invasive strategy except in the RITA-3 and ICTUS trials. In the RITA-3 trial, significant mortality benefit was seen late after 5 years, particularly in the high-risk group that underwent early investing strategy. The mortality benefit, however, did not persist to 10 years.

In the early invasive strategy, the optimal timing of intervention has not been determined. The Can Rapid Risk Stratification of Unstable Angine Patients Suppress Adverse Outcomes With Early Implementation of the ACC/AHA Guidelines (CRUSADE) registers between the early (23.4 hours) and later (46.3 hours) catheterisation group. The Intracoronary Stenting with Antithrombotic Regimen-Cooling Off (ISAR-COOL) found a significant reduction in combined death MI rate for very early invasive strategy. The early or late intervention in unstable angina (ELISA) showed no difference in clinical outcomes at 30 days; however, the enzymatic infarct size (LDHQ48) was less in patients with delayed angiography after pre-treatment with tirofiban. The optimal timing of

coronary angiography and potential intervention in non-ST-elevation acute coronary syndrome (OPTIMA), though, which was terminated early for poor enrollment, demonstrated that the early invasive group had higher rates of MI.

5. *Rehabilitation*: The frequent and high association of multiple comorbidities in patients of NSTEMI mandates emphasis on patient education for lifestyle changes, blood pressure and glycemic and lipid control and management of comorbidities with reduction of risk factors.

SPECIAL CONSIDERATIONS

AGE

The elderly present more frequently with NSTEMI than STEMI and also with more atypical symptoms like dyspnoea. The mortality with NSTEMI doubles in patients beyond 75 years of age, and so does the risk of bleeding, especially with enoxaparin owning to renal impairment. The OASIS-5 [40] trial showed a lower risk of bleeding with fondaparinux. The TACTICS-TIMI 18 trial showed the largest benefit of early invasive treatment in patients with an age more than 75 years at a cost of increased risk of major bleeding [39].

DIABETICS

The mortality rate in NSTEMI at 30 days is double in diabetics as compared to non-diabetics (2.1% vs. 1.1%, p < 0.001) and at 1 year (HR 1.65 vs. 1.22) [41]. The 2012 ACCF/AHA focussed update recommends early invasive strategy for patients with NSTEMI. The diabetic subgroup in the FRISC-II and TACTICS-TIMI 18 trials showed improved outcomes with invasive strategy [9,39].

WOMEN

Women more often present with NSTEMI than STEMI. The long-term outcomes with very early invasive strategy are better in women compared to men (OR 0.65; 95% CI, 0.28–0.92) [42].

CHRONIC KIDNEY DISEASE (CKD)

The Swedish Web-system for Enhancement and Development of Evidence-based care in heart disease evaluated according to recommended therapeutics (SWEDEHEART) observed 36% lower mortality rate with early revascularisation in NSTEMI patients with mild to moderate CKD but not with severe CKD. The 2012 ACCF/AHA focussed update comments and early invasive strategy in patients with mild to moderate CKD based on physician's discretion [43].

RADIAL ROUTE APPROACH

The Trans-radial versus Trans-femoral Percutaneous Coronary Intervention (PCI) Access Site Approach in Patients With Unstable Angine or Myocardial Infarction Managed With an Invasive Strategy (RIVAL) [44] did not show a significant reduction in mortality or primary end point in the NSTEMI subgroup. The observational study radial versus femoral access in mortality reduction in non-ST-elevation myocardial infarction (REALITY-NSTEMI) showed that the transradial as compared to transfemoral access was associated with significantly low rates of bleeding

(0.23% vs. 0.97%, p = 0.001) and access site complications (0.35% vs. 1.00%, p = 0.003) [45].

CONCLUSION

The NSTEMI has high incidence, limited pharmacological treatment and a high long-term mortality. The recent hs-cTn has increased sensitivity to pick up these patients early. The ticagrelor and prasugrel have benefits over clopidogrel. The use of GP IIb/IIIa inhibitors is recommended only in high-risk cases where newer anti-platelets cannot be used. The optimal timing for early invasive strategy remains to be determined. The elderly, women, moderate chronic kidney disease patients and diabetics are better treated with early invasive strategy.

REFERENCES

1. Fox KAA, Eagle KA, Gore JM, Steg PG, Anderson FA. The global registry of acute coronary events, 1999 to 2009-GRACE. *Heart [Internet]*. 1 Jan 2010 [cited 4 Nov 2019];96(14):1095–1101.

2. Terkelsen CJ, Lassen JF, Nørgaard BL et al. Mortality rates in patients with ST-elevation vs. non-ST-elevation acute myocardial infarction: Observations from an unselected cohort. *Eur Heart J*. 2005;26(1):18–26.

3. Jneid H, Anderson JL, Wright RS et al. 2012 ACCF/AHA focused update of the guideline for the management of patients with unstable angina/non–ST-elevation myocardial infarction (updating the 2007 guideline and replacing the 2011 focused update). *J Am College Cardiol [Internet]*. 1 Jan 2012 [cited 4 Nov 2019];60(7):645–681.

4. Stone GW, Maehara A, Lansky AJ et al. A prospective natural-history study of coronary atherosclerosis. *N Engl J Med [Internet]*. 1 Jan 2011 [cited 4 Nov 2019];364(3):226–235.

5. Falk E, Nakano M, Bentzon JF, Finn AV, Virmani R. Update on acute coronary syndromes: The pathologists' *view*. 1 Jan 2013 [cited 4 Nov 2019];34(10):719–728.

6. Thygesen K, Alpert JS, Jaffe AS et al. Fourth universal definition of myocardial infarction. *J Am College Cardiol. [Internet]*. 1 Jan 2018 [cited 4 Nov 2019];72(18):2231–2264.

7. Fesmire FM, Percy RF, Bardoner JB, Wharton DR, Calhoun FB. Usefulness of automated serial 12-lead ECG monitoring during the initial emergency department evaluation of patients with chest pain. *Ann Emerg Med [Internet]*. 1 Jan 1998 [cited 4 Nov 2019];31(1):3–11.

8. Effects of tissue plasminogen activator and a comparison of early invasive and conservative strategies in unstable angina and non-Q-wave myocardial infarction. Results of the TIMI IIIB Trial. Thrombolysis in myocardial ischemia. *Circulation [Internet]*. 1 Jan 1994 [cited 4 Nov 2019];89(4):1545–1556. Available from: 10.1161/01.CIR.89.4.1545

9. FRagmin Fast Revascularisation during In Stability in Coronary artery disease (FRISC II) Investigators. Long-term low-molecular-mass heparin in unstable coronary-artery disease: FRISC II prospective randomised multicentre study. *Lancet [Internet]*. 1 Jan 1999 [cited 4 Nov 2019];354(9180):701–707. Available from: 10.1016/S0140-6736(99)07350-X

10. Kraaijeveld AO, de Jager SCA, de Jager WJ et al. CC Chemokine Ligand-5 (CCL5/RANTES) and CC Chemokine Ligand-18 (CCL18/PARC) are specific markers of refractory unstable angina pectoris and are transiently raised during severe ischemic symptoms. *Circulation [Internet]*. 1 Jan 2007 [cited 4 Nov 2019];116(17):1931–1941.

11. Beygui F, Silvain J, Pena A et al. Usefulness of biomarker strategy to improve GRACE score's prediction performance in patients with non-ST-segment elevation acute coronary syndrome and low event rates. *Am J Cardiol [Internet]*. 1 Jan 2010 [cited 4 Nov 2019];106(5):650–658.

12. Viswanathan K, Kilcullen N, Morrell C et al. Heart-type fatty acid-binding protein predicts long-term mortality and re-infarction in consecutive patients with suspected acute coronary syndrome who are troponin-negative. *J Am Coll Cardiol [Internet]*. 1 Jan 2010 [cited 4 Nov 2019];55(23):2590–2598.

13. Koga S, Ikeda S, Yoshida T et al. Elevated levels of systemic pentraxin 3 are associated with thin-cap fibroatheroma in coronary culprit lesions. *JACC: Cardiovasc Interv [Internet]*. 1 Jan 2013 [cited 4 Nov 2019];6(9):945–954.

14. O'Malley RG, Bonaca MP, Scirica BM et al. Prognostic performance of multiple biomarkers in patients with non-ST-segment elevation acute coronary syndrome. *J Am Coll Cardiol [Internet]*. 1 Jan 2014 [cited 4 Nov 2019];63(16):1644–1653.

15. Thelin J, Melander O. Dynamic high-sensitivity troponin elevations in atrial fibrillation patients might not be associated with significant coronary artery disease. *BMC Cardiovasc Disord [Internet]*. 1 Jan 2017 [cited 4 Nov 2019];17(1). Available from: 10.1186/s12872-017-0601-7

16. Antman EM, Cohen M, Bernink PJLM et al. The TIMI risk score for unstable angina/non-ST Elevation MI. *JAMA [Internet]*. 1 Jan 2000 [cited 4 Nov 2019];284(7):835.

17. Théroux P, Ouimet H, McCans J et al. Aspirin, heparin, or both to treat acute unstable angina. *N Engl J Med [Internet]*. 1 Jan 1988 [cited 4 Nov 2019];319(17):1105–1111.

18. Yusuf S, Zhao F, Mehta SR, Chrolavicius S, Tognoni G, Fox KK; Clopidogrel in Unstable Angina to Prevent Recurrent Events Trial Investigators. Effects of clopidogrel in addition to aspirin in patients with acute coronary syndromes without ST-segment elevation. *N Engl J Med [Internet]*. 2001 Jan 1 [cited 4 Nov 2019];345(7):494–502. Available from: 10.1056/NEJMoa010746

19. Mehta SR, Tanguay J-F, Eikelboom JW et al. Double-dose versus standard-dose clopidogrel and high-dose versus low-dose aspirin in individuals undergoing percutaneous coronary intervention for acute coronary syndromes (CURRENT-OASIS 7): A randomised factorial trial. *Lancet [Internet]*. 1 Jan 2010 [cited 4 Nov 2019];376(9748):1233–1243.

20. Mehta SR, Yusuf S, Peters RJ et al. Effects of pretreatment with clopidogrel and aspirin followed by long-term therapy in patients undergoing percutaneous coronary intervention: The PCI-CURE study. *Lancet [Internet]*. 1 Jan 2001 [cited 4 Nov 2019];358(9281):527–533.

21. Price MJ. Standard- vs high-dose clopidogrel based on platelet function testing after percutaneous coronary intervention. *JAMA [Internet]*. 1 Jan 2011 [cited 4 Nov 2019];305(11):1097.

22. Farkouh ME. A COGENT argument for gastrointestinal protection with low-dose aspirin. *J Am Coll Cardiol [Internet]*. 1 Jan 2016 [cited 4 Nov 2019];67(14):1672–1673.

23. Wiviott SD, Braunwald E, McCabe CH et al. Prasugrel versus clopidogrel in patients with acute coronary syndromes. *N Engl J Med [Internet]*. 1 Jan 2007 [cited 4 Nov 2019];357(20):2001–2015.

24. Silvain J, Rakowski T, Lattuca B et al. Interval from initiation of prasugrel to coronary angiography in patients with non-ST-segment elevation myocardial infarction. *J Am Coll Cardiol [Internet]*. 1 Jan 2019 [cited 4 Nov 2019];73(8):906–914.

25. Best PJM, Lennon R, Ting HH et al. The impact of renal insufficiency on clinical outcomes in patients undergoing percutaneous coronary interventions. *J Am Coll Cardiol [Internet]*. 1 Jan 2002 [cited 4 Nov 2019];39(7):1113–1119.

26. Wallentin L, Becker RC, Budaj A et al. Ticagrelor versus clopidogrel in patients with acute coronary syndromes. *N Engl J Med [Internet]*. 1 Jan 2009 [cited 4 Nov 2019];361(11):1045–1057.

27. Cannon CP, Husted S, Harrington RA et al. Safety, tolerability, and initial efficacy of AZD6140, the first reversible oral adenosine diphosphate receptor antagonist, compared with clopidogrel, in patients with non-ST-segment elevation acute coronary syndrome. *J Am Coll Cardiol [Internet]*. 1 Jan 2007 [cited 4 Nov 2019];50(19):1844–1851.

28. Anavekar NS, McMurray JJV, Velazquez EJ et al. Relation between renal dysfunction and cardiovascular outcomes after myocardial infarction. *N Engl J Med [Internet]*. 1 Jan 2004 [cited 4 Nov 2019];351(13):1285–1295.

29. Greenbaum AB, Grines CL, Bittl JA et al. Initial experience with an intravenous P2Y12 platelet receptor antagonist in patients undergoing percutaneous coronary intervention: Results from a 2-part, phase II, multicenter, randomized, placebo- and active-controlled trial. *Am Heart J [Internet]*. 1 Jan 2006 [cited 4 Nov 2019];151(3):689.e1–689.e10.

30. Lauer MA, Houghtaling PL, Peterson JG et al; Platelet IIb/IIIa in Unstable Angina; Receptor Suppression Using Integrilin Therapy (PURSUIT) Trial Investigators. Inhibition of platelet glycoprotein IIb/IIIa with eptifibatide in patients with acute coronary syndromes. *N Engl J Med [Internet]*. 1 Jan 1998 [cited 4 Nov 2019];339(7):436–443. Available from: 10.1056/NEJM199808133390704

31. Boersma E, Harrington RA, Moliterno DJ et al. Platelet glycoprotein IIb/IIIa inhibitors in acute coronary syndromes: A meta-analysis of all major randomised clinical trials. *Lancet [Internet]*. 1 Jan 2002 [cited 4 Nov 2019];359(9302):189–198.

32. Platelet Receptor Inhibition in Ischemic Syndrome Management (PRISM) Study Investigators. A comparison of aspirin plus tirofiban with aspirin plus heparin for unstable angina. *N Engl J Med [Internet]*. 1 Jan 1998 [cited 4 Nov 2019];338(21):1498–1505. Available from: 10.1056/NEJM199805213382103

33. Platelet Receptor Inhibition in Ischemic Syndrome Management in Patients Limited by Unstable Signs and Symptoms (PRISM-PLUS) Study Investigators. Inhibition of the platelet glycoprotein IIb/IIIa receptor with tirofiban in unstable angina and non-Q-wave myocardial infarction. *N Engl J Med [Internet]*. 1 Jan 1998 [cited 4 Nov 2019];338(21):1488–1497. Available from: 10.1056/NEJM199805213382102

34. Stone GW, McLaurin BT, Cox DA et al. Bivalirudin for patients with acute coronary syndromes. *N Engl J Med [Internet]*. 1 Jan 2006 [cited 4 Nov 2019];355(21):2203–2216.

35. Mega JL, Braunwald E, Wiviott SD et al. Rivaroxaban in patients with a recent acute coronary syndrome. *N Engl J Med [Internet]*. 1 Jan 2012 [cited 4 Nov 2019];366(1):9–19.

36. Kofoed KF, Kelbæk H, Hansen PR et al. Early versus standard care invasive examination and treatment of patients with non-ST-segment elevation acute coronary syndrome. *Circulation [Internet]*. 1 Jan 2018 [cited 4 Nov 2019];138(24):2741–2750.

37. Boden WE, O'Rourke RA, Crawford MH et al. Outcomes in patients with acute non-Q-wave myocardial infarction randomly assigned to an invasive as compared with a conservative management strategy. *N Engl J Med [Internet]*. 1 Jan 1998 [cited 4 Nov 2019]; 338(25):1785–1792.

38. McCullough PA, O'Neill WW, Graham M et al. A prospective randomized trial of triage angiography in acute coronary syndromes ineligible for thrombolytic therapy. *J Am Coll Cardiol [Internet]*. 1 Jan 1998 [cited 4 Nov 2019];32(3):596–605.

39. Cannon CP, Weintraub WS, Demopoulos LA et al. Comparison of early invasive and conservative strategies in patients with unstable coronary syndromes treated with the glycoprotein IIb/IIIa inhibitor tirofiban. *N Engl J Med [Internet]*. 1 Jan 2001 [cited 4 Nov 2019];344(25):1879–1887.

40. The Fifth Organization to Assess Strategies in Acute Ischemic Syndromes Investigators; Yusuf S, Mehta SR, Chrolavicius S et al. Comparison of fondaparinux and enoxaparin in acute coronary syndromes. *N Engl J Med [Internet]*. 1 Jan 2006 [cited 4 Nov 2019];354(14):1464–1476. Available from: 10.1056/NEJMoa055443

41. Donahoe SM, Stewart GC, McCabe CH et al. Diabetes and mortality following acute coronary syndromes. *JAMA [Internet]*. 1 Jan 2007 [cited 4 Nov 2019];298(7):765.

42. Mueller C, Neumann F-J, Roskamm H et al. Women do have an improved long-term outcome after non-ST-elevation acute coronary syndromes treated very early and predominantly with percutaneous coronary intervention. *J Am Coll Cardiol [Internet]*. 1 Jan 2002 [cited 4 Nov 2019];40(2):245–250.

43. Lindholm D, Alfredsson J, Angerås O et al. Timing of percutaneous coronary intervention in patients with non-ST-elevation myocardial infarction: A SWEDEHEART study. *Eur Heart J Qual Care Clin Outcomes [Internet].* 1 Jan 2017 [cited 4 Nov 2019];3(1):53–60.

44. Mehta SR, Jolly SS, Cairns J et al. Effects of radial versus femoral artery access in patients with acute coronary syndromes with or without ST-segment elevation. *J Am Coll Cardiol [Internet].* 1 Jan 2012 [cited 4 Nov 2019]; 60(24):2490–2499.

45. Iqbal MB, Arujuna A, Archbold A et al. TCT-42 superior outcomes associated with radial versus femoral access in non-ST elevation myocardial infarction: An observational cohort study of 10,095 patients. Results of the radial versus femoral access in mortality reduction in non-ST elevation myocardial infarction (REALITY-NSTEMI) study. *J Am Coll Cardiol [Internet].* 1 Jan 2013 [cited 4 Nov 2019];62(18):B14.

46. Mehta SR, Granger CB, Boden WE et al. Early versus delayed invasive intervention in acute coronary syndromes. *N Engl J Med [Internet].* 1 Jan 2009 [cited 4 Nov 2019];360(21):2165–2175.

47. Hoedemaker NPG, Damman P, Woudstra P et al. Early invasive versus selective strategy for non-ST-segment elevation acute coronary syndrome. *J Am Coll Cardiol [Internet].* 1 Jan 2017 [cited 4 Nov 2019];69(15):1883–1893.

48. van 't Hof A. A comparison of two invasive strategies in patients with non-ST elevation acute coronary syndromes: Results of the Early or Late Intervention in unstable Angina (ELISA) pilot study 2b/3a upstream therapy and acute coronary syndromes. *Eur Heart J [Internet].* 1 Jan 2003 [cited 4 Nov 2019];24(15):1401–1405.

49. Neumann F-J, Kastrati A, Pogatsa-Murray G et al. Evaluation of prolonged antithrombotic pretreatment. *JAMA [Internet].* 1 Jan 2003 [cited 4 Nov 2019];290(12). Available from: 10.1001/jama.290.12.1593

50. Thiele H, Rach J, Klein N et al. Optimal timing of invasive angiography in stable non-ST-elevation myocardial infarction: The Leipzig immediate versus early and late PercutaneouS coronary Intervention triAl in NSTEMI (LIPSIA-NSTEMI Trial). *Eur Heart J.* 2012;33(16):2035–2043.

51. Montalescot G, Cayla G, Collet J-P et al. Immediate vs delayed intervention for acute coronary syndromes. *JAMA [Internet].* 1 Jan 2009 [cited 4 Nov 2019];302(9):947.

52. Reuter P-G, Rouchy C, Cattan S et al. Early invasive strategy in high-risk acute coronary syndrome without ST-segment elevation. The Sisca randomized trial. *Int J Cardiol [Internet].* 1 Jan 2015 [cited 4 Nov 2019];182:414–418.

53. Milosevic A, Vasiljevic-Pokrajcic Z, Milasinovic D et al. Immediate versus delayed invasive intervention for non-STEMI patients. *JACC: Cardiovasc Interv [Internet].* 1 Jan 2016 [cited 4 Nov 2019];9(6):541–549.

17

Bleeding in acute coronary syndrome

VARSHA KOUL AND UPENDRA KAUL

INTRODUCTION

Acute coronary syndrome (ACS) is a potentially life-threatening condition. A multi-modality approach involving the combined use of early invasive coronary procedures as well as adjunctive potent anti-platelet therapy and antithrombotic drugs has completely revolutionised the management of acute coronary syndrome. These include oral anti-platelet drugs (aspirin and thienopyridines), parenteral antithrombin (unfractionated heparin, low molecular weight heparins, fondaparinux or bivalirudin) and glycoprotein IIb/IIIa receptor blocker. Anti-platelet and antithrombotic agents, in addition to their role in interventional cardiology, also play an important role in the treatment of those patients with ACS who have been medically managed. However, the enormous strides achieved in the reduction of ischaemic events in these patients have been at the cost of an increased incidence of bleeding complications. Bleeding is known to have an adverse impact on clinical outcomes. Therefore, all patients with ACS should ideally be evaluated for the risk of developing bleeding complications and their treatment should be individualised in order to minimise the number of these complications.

INCIDENCE AND SITE OF BLEEDING IN ACS

Rates of bleeding in ACS and PCI trials vary widely, and bleeding complications have been reported to occur in about 1 in 10 patients [1–4] and major bleeding is at present one of the most common non-cardiac complications in patients with ACS [5,6]. Major bleeding is defined as life-threatening bleeding requiring transfusion of more than two units of blood, a haematocrit decrease of 10% or more or bleeding resulting in death, subdural haematoma or intra-cerebral bleed in about 4% of patients with ACS [7].

In patients with STEMI, intra-cranial bleeding occurs in about 1% of the patients treated with fibrinolysis whereas major non-cerebral bleeds occur in about 4%–13% of these patients [8]. On the other hand, primary percutaneous coronary intervention (PCI) results in less than 2% of major bleeds [9]. In patients who undergo PCI, more than half of the bleeding events occur at the arterial access site, ranging from subcutaneous access site haematoma to fatal retroperitoneal bleeding [10].

The most common bleeding event during the index admission is procedure related, which is about 50%, followed by gastrointestinal bleeding (16%), whereas in subsequent admissions gastrointestinal bleeding makes up about 50% of the bleeding events. The occurrence of other types of bleeding (like respiratory, intra-cranial, intra-ocular, urogenital, etc.) is similar for both index and subsequent admissions [11].

BLEEDING DEFINITIONS

There is heterogeneity in the definition of bleeding. The overall aim of classifications is to systematically report and categorise bleeding events in order to allow comparisons across various data sets. These classification systems have improved over time to become more objective and also account for blood transfusions. These bleeding definitions were originally used to study thrombolytic regimens in acute myocardial infarction but have subsequently been used in many PCI studies.

The TIMI (thrombolysis in myocardial infarction) score was the first to be developed and is widely used, but the disadvantage is that it has low sensitivity as the haemoglobin needs to be reduced by 5 g/dL for bleeding to be considered severe [12].

The CRUSADE bleeding score [13] includes eight factors: female sex, history of diabetes, prior vascular disease, heart rate, systolic blood pressure, signs of congestive heart failure (CHF), baseline haematocrit <36% and creatinine clearance, providing a quantitative method to assess bleeding risk for in-hospital major bleeding, across all modes of treatments for ACS. The bleeding risk in the CRUSADE score is classified as very low risk (3.1% risk of major bleeding), low risk (5.5%), moderate risk (8.5%), high risk (11.9%) and very high risk (19.5%).

The DAPT score [14] has been developed as a risk prediction tool to identify patients who may benefit from prolonged (>12 months) DAPT after PCI. It ranges from −2 to 10, with a higher score conferring greater ischaemic risk and increased benefit of long-term DAPT therapy. The factors included are age, smoking, diabetes, MI at presentation, prior PCI or prior MI, paclitaxel-eluting stent, stent diameter <3 mm, CHF or left ventricular ejection fraction <30% and vein graft stent. Patients with a DAPT score of ≥2 have reduced rates of ischaemic MACE and stent thrombosis with prolonged DAPT, with only a small increase in bleeding. However, patients with a DAPT score of <2 have a lesser reduction in ischaemic events, a marked increase in bleeding and higher all-cause mortality with prolonged DAPT.

North American institutions have recently created the Bleeding Academic Research Consortium (BARC) to standardise the definitions of bleeding [5]. This score stratifies bleeding on a scale from 0 (no bleeding) to 5 (fatal bleeding) and provides the ability to assess patients subjected to myocardial revascularisation procedures and anti-platelet therapy.

RISK FACTORS FOR BLEEDING IN ACS

Several clinical trials have tried to identify significant baseline predictors which increase the risk of bleeding in patients with ACS in order to provide tailored dual anti-platelet therapy according to the bleeding risk of the patient. These include advanced age, female sex, low body weight, obesity, hypertension, heart failure or shock, diabetes mellitus, chronic kidney disease, anaemia, sepsis, prior history of GI bleeding or stroke, NSTEMI (vs unstable angina), use of invasive procedures and use of anti-platelet and/or antithrombotic drugs [8,15–19].

Advanced age, lower weight, female sex, previous cerebrovascular disease and systolic and diastolic hypertension on admission are significant predictors of intra-cranial haemorrhage (ICH) with an incremental risk beginning at systolic pressures more than160–170 mmHg [19,20].

The risk factors identified which increase the chances of haemorrhagic complications during primary PCI include inappropriate dosing of antithrombotic drugs, femoral access, number of punctures, sheath size, late removal of sheath post-procedure, prolonged duration of the procedure, intra-aortic balloon pump, use of GP IIa/IIIb inhibitors and low molecular weight heparin within 48 hours of PCI [9,18].

EFFECT OF DRUGS ON BLEEDING IN ACS

Patients with ACS require potent anti-platelet agents and anti-coagulants to reduce ischaemic and thromboembolic risk, all of which increase bleeding to some degree according to their mechanism of action, potency and duration of treatment, a risk which is further modified by specific patient characteristics. Overall, there is no evidence of decreased efficacy but clear evidence of increased safety with lower doses of aspirin [21].

Compared with clopidogrel, prasugrel significantly reduces the rates of MI, urgent target-vessel revascularisation and stent thrombosis but at the cost of excess major bleeding including life-threatening and fatal bleeding [22].

Similarly, ticagrelor [23] results in a higher rate of major bleeding not related to CABG as compared with clopidogrel. Also, there are more instances of fatal intra-cranial bleeding but fewer instances of fatal bleeding from other sources. In ACS patients treated with PCI and ticagrelor or prasugrel, BARC 3–5 bleedings negatively impact the prognosis [1].

Higher doses of unfractionated heparin (UFH) are independently associated with higher rates of bleeding. The incidence of major or minor bleeding within 48 hours of the procedure increased with increasing ACT [24]. Bleeding is significantly more frequent with enoxaparin than with fondaparinux (a factor Xa inhibitor) in patients with ACS managed conservatively [3].

Although the GP IIb/IIIa inhibitors including abciximab, eptifibatide and tirofiban have demonstrated considerable efficacy in reducing the risk of adverse ischaemic events in patients undergoing PCI for NSTE-ACS or STEMI compared to UFH, these agents can be associated with substantial bleeding risk [25,26]. The use of these agents is now reserved only for bailout indications.

The direct thrombin inhibitor bivalirudin is associated with considerably less risk of bleeding complications than UFH or a GP IIb/IIIa inhibitor plus UFH, while maintaining similar protection from ischaemic events in patients undergoing PCI or patients with ACS [27]. There were also reports of higher stent thrombosis. In the unfractionated Heparin versus Bivalirudin in Primary Percutaneous Coronary Intervention (HEAT-PPCI) study [28], bleeding was not decreased with bivalirudin as compared to UFH and the overall efficacy outcome favoured UFH.

Another issue in 10%–20% of patients undergoing PCI is that they require chronic OAC in addition to DAPT. In low-risk patients treated with warfarin undergoing a non-complex PCI, discontinuation of aspirin is associated with a marked reduction in bleeding complications, without any increase in ischaemic complications as compared to continued triple therapy [29]. Among patients with atrial fibrillation who undergo PCI, the risk of bleeding is lower among those who receive dual therapy with dabigatran and a P2Y12 inhibitor than among those who receive triple therapy with warfarin, a P2Y12 inhibitor and aspirin without any increase in the risk of thromboembolic events [30]. In patients with atrial fibrillation undergoing PCI, the administration of either low-dose rivaroxaban plus a P2Y12 inhibitor or very low-dose rivaroxaban plus DAPT is associated with a lower rate of clinically significant bleeding than standard therapy with a vitamin K antagonist plus DAPT [31].

ADVERSE OUTCOMES WITH BLEEDING IN ACS

Bleeding is often merely regarded as an unpleasant event, which increases the length of hospital stay and costs without adversely affecting survival. Consequences of bleeding include hypotension, anaemia and reduction in oxygen delivery. Furthermore, severe bleeding increases the risk of acute myocardial infarction, stroke and the need for urgent myocardial revascularisation [17,20]. In post-PCI patients it also requires stoppage of DAPT leading to a high risk of stent thrombosis.

Major bleeding is associated with a subsequent increase in late mortality, potentially negating the long-term benefits of ACS treatment [3,7]. Major bleeding events increase in-hospital mortality as well as mortality after discharge at 30 days and 1 year [32].

Gastrointestinal and intra-cranial bleedings carry a worse prognosis [20]. Despite major bleeding, blood transfusion in this setting is associated with increased mortality. Potential mechanisms for the detrimental effects of transfusions include platelet activation and aggregation, impaired oxygen and nitric oxide delivery capabilities [33].

MANAGEMENT OF BLEEDING IN ACS

Sudden interruption of DAPT related to bleeding episodes may result in adverse ischaemic events like acute stent thrombosis which have been independently associated with increased mortality, so cessation of DAPT should only be undertaken after consideration of the potential repercussions. Minor bleeding can be managed without the interruption of anti-platelet drugs. For severe GI bleed, consideration should be given to continuing DAPT along with endoscopic management of a visibly bleeding vessel [13].

Patients experiencing major bleeding during an ACS should be closely monitored, preferably in an intensive care unit. Proton pump inhibitors should be the preferred agents for the therapy and prophylaxis of aspirin-associated gastrointestinal bleed [34]. Major bleeding may require interruption and/or neutralisation of both anti-coagulant and anti-platelet therapy, unless bleeding can be adequately controlled by specific haemostatic interventions. As often as possible, oral anti-platelet therapy must be restarted after the bleeding event is resolved. Blood transfusions should be considered in haemodynamically unstable patients, but they may have deleterious effects on outcome and should therefore be judiciously used [17].

PREVENTION OF BLEEDING IN ACS

Fondaparinux, low molecular weight heparins (LMWHs), bivalirudin and GP IIb/IIIa blocker are largely cleared by the kidneys and should therefore not be used or the dose should be modified in patients with severe renal failure [35]. Unfractionated heparin is the anti-coagulant of choice in this particular situation. Unfractionated heparin, LMWH, direct thrombin inhibitors, TNK-tPA and GP IIb/IIIa blockers all require careful weight-adjusted dosing [2].

The risk of aspirin-related ulcer gastrointestinal bleed is significantly increased in elderly patients, those with serious comorbidities and those with concomitant use of non-steroidal anti-inflammatory drugs (NSAIDs), systemic corticosteroids, anti-coagulants or other anti-platelet agents. Adding a proton-pump inhibitor to reduce gastrointestinal bleeding events in patients at high risk of gastrointestinal toxicity who receive long-term treatment with aspirin is recommended [34]. Reduced arterial sheath size, timely sheath removal and the use of radial instead of femoral artery access [18] for PCI are associated with a significant decrease in peri-procedural bleeding rates accompanied by a reduction in all-cause mortality.

CONCLUSION

The use of potent contemporary antithrombotic and anti-platelet agents in conjunction with an early invasive strategy has improved ischaemic outcomes in patients presenting with acute coronary syndromes. However, these have an inherent tendency to increase the risk of bleeding complications. Bleeding events and the need for blood transfusions have a significant impact on early and long-term morbidity and mortality in ACS. Each patient should undergo an individualised assessment of the baseline haemorrhagic risk as well as the ischaemic risk. Minimisation of bleeding events while maintaining anti-ischaemic effectiveness should be the therapeutic target in the management of ACS in order to reduce morbidity, mortality and health care costs.

REFERENCES

1. D'Ascenzo F, Grosso A, Abu-Assi E et al. Incidence and predictors of bleeding in ACS patients treated with PCI and prasugrel or ticagrelor: An analysis from the RENAMI registry. *Int J Cardiol*. 2018;273:29–33.
2. Stone GW, White HD, Ohman EM et al. Bivalirudin in patients with acute coronary syndromes undergoing percutaneous coronary intervention: A subgroup analysis from the Acute Catheterization and Urgent Intervention Triage strategY (ACUITY) trial. *Lancet*. 2007;369(9565):907–919.
3. Yusuf S, Mehta SR, Chrolavicius S, Afzal R, Pogue J, Granger CB. Fifth Organization to Assess Strategies in Acute Ischemic Syndromes Investigators. Comparison of fondaparinux and enoxaparin in acute coronary syndromes. *N Engl J Med*. 2006;354(14):1464–1476.
4. Ferguson JJ, Califf RM, Antman EM et al. Enoxaparin vs unfractionated heparin in high-risk patients with non-ST-segment elevation acute coronary syndromes managed with an intended early invasive strategy: Primary results of the SYNERGY randomized trial. *JAMA*. 2004;292(1):45–54.
5. Mehran R, Rao SV, Bhatt DL et al. Standardized bleeding definitions for cardiovascular clinical trials: A consensus report from the Bleeding Academic Research Consortium. *Circulation*. 2011;123(23):2736–2747.

6. Abu-Assi E, Raposeiras-Roubín S, García-Acuña JM, González-Juanatey JR. Bleeding risk stratification in an era of aggressive management of acute coronary syndromes. *World J Cardiol.* 2014;6(11):1140.

7. Moscucci M, Fox KAA, Cannon CP, Klein W, López-Sendón J, Montalescot G, White K, Goldberg RJ. Predictors of major bleeding in acute coronary syndromes: The Global Registry of Acute Coronary Events (GRACE). *Eur Heart J.* 2003;24(20):1815–1823.

8. Ibanez B, James S, Agewall S et al. 2017 ESC Guidelines for the management of acute myocardial infarction in patients presenting with ST-segment elevation: The Task Force for the Management of Acute Myocardial Infarction in patients presenting with ST-segment elevation of the European Society of Cardiology (ESC). *Eur Heart J.* 2017;39(2):119–177.

9. Hermanides RS, Ottervanger J-P, Dambrink JH, Hoorntje JC, Gosselink AT, Suryapranata H. Incidence, predictors and prognostic importance of bleeding after primary PCI for ST-elevation myocardial infarction. *EuroIntervention.* 2010;6(1):106–111.

10. Kinnaird TD, Stabile E, Mintz GS, Lee CW. Incidence, predictors, and prognostic implications of bleeding and blood transfusion following percutaneous coronary interventions. *Am J Cardiol.* 2003;92(8):930–935.

11. Voss WB, Lee M, Devlin G, Kerr AJ. Incidence and type of bleeding complications early and late after acute coronary syndrome admission in a New Zealand cohort (ANZACS-QI-7). *N Z Med J.* 2016;129(1437):27.

12. Mehran R, Pocock SJ, Nikolsky E et al. A risk score to predict bleeding in patients with acute coronary syndromes. *J Am Coll Cardiol.* 2010;23(55):2556–2566.

13. Subherwal S, Bach RG, Chen AY et al. Baseline risk of major bleeding in non-ST-segment-elevation myocardial infarction: The CRUSADE (Can Rapid risk stratification of Unstable angina patients Suppress ADverse outcomes with Early implementation of the ACC/AHA Guidelines) Bleeding Score. *Circulation.* 2009;119(14):1873–1882.

14. Yeh RW, Secemsky EA, Kereiakes DJ et al. Development and validation of a prediction rule for benefit and harm of dual antiplatelet therapy beyond 1 year after percutaneous coronary intervention. *JAMA.* 2016;315(16):1735–1749.

15. Eikelboom JW, Mehta SR, Anand SS, Xie C, Fox KAA, Yusuf S. Adverse impact of bleeding on prognosis in patients with acute coronary syndromes. *Circulation.* 2006;114(8):774–782.

16. Manoukian SV, Voeltz MD, Eikelboom J. Bleeding complications in acute coronary syndromes and percutaneous coronary intervention: Predictors, prognostic significance, and paradigms for reducing risk. *Clin Cardiol.* 2007;30(S2):II-24.

17. Steg PG, Huber K, Andreotti F et al. Bleeding in acute coronary syndromes and percutaneous coronary interventions: Position paper by the Working Group on Thrombosis of the European Society of Cardiology. *Eur Heart J.* 2011;32(15):1854–1864.

18. Valgimigli M, Gagnor A, Calabró P et al. Radial versus femoral access in patients with acute coronary syndromes undergoing invasive management: A randomised multicentre trial. *Lancet.* 2015;385(9986):2465–2476.

19. Alfredsson J, Neely B, Neely ML et al. Predicting the risk of bleeding during dual antiplatelet therapy after acute coronary syndromes. *Heart.* 2017;103(15):1168–1176.

20. O'gara, PT, Kushner FG, Ascheim DD et al. 2013 ACCF/AHA guideline for the management of ST-elevation myocardial infarction: Executive summary: A report of the American College of Cardiology Foundation/American Heart Association Task Force on Practice Guidelines. *J Am Coll Cardiol.* 2013;61(4):485–510.

21. Current–Oasis 7 Investigators. Dose comparisons of clopidogrel and aspirin in acute coronary syndromes. *N Eng J Med.* 2010;363(10):930–1942.

22. Wiviott SD, Braunwald E, Mccabe CH et al. Prasugrel versus clopidogrel in patients with acute coronary syndromes. *N Eng J Med.* 2007;357(20):2001–2015.

23. Wallentin L, Becker RC, Budaj A et al. Ticagrelor versus clopidogrel in patients with acute coronary syndromes. *N Eng J Med.* 2009;361(11):1045–1057.

24. Brener SJ, Moliterno DJ, Lincoff AM, Steinhubl SR, Wolski KE, Topol EJ. Relationship between activated clotting time and ischemic or hemorrhagic complications: Analysis of 4 recent randomized clinical trials of percutaneous coronary intervention. *Circulation.* 2004;110(8):994–998.

25. Aguirre FV, Topol EJ, Ferguson JJ, Anderson K, Blankenship JC, Heuser RR, Sigmon K, Taylor M, Gottlieb R, Hanovich G. Bleeding complications with the chimeric antibody to platelet glycoprotein IIb/IIIa integrin in patients undergoing percutaneous coronary intervention. EPIC Investigators. *Circulation.* 1995;91(12):2882.

26. De Luca G, Suryapranata H, Stone GW, Antoniucci D, Tcheng JE, Neumann F-J, Van de Werf F, Antman EM, Topol EJ. Abciximab as adjunctive therapy to reperfusion in acute ST-segment elevation myocardial infarction: A meta-analysis of randomized trials. *JAMA.* 2005;293(14):1759–1765.

27. Stone GW, McLaurin BT, Cox DA et al. Bivalirudin for patients with acute coronary syndromes. *N Eng J Med.* 2006;355(21):2203–2216.

28. Shahzad A, Kemp I, Mars C et al. Unfractionated Heparin Versus Bivalirudin in Primary Percutaneous Coronary Intervention (HEAT-PPCI): An open-label, single centre, randomised controlled trial. *Lancet.* 2014;384(9957):1849–1858.

29. Dewilde WJ, Oirbans T, Verheugt FWA et al. Use of clopidogrel with or without aspirin in patients taking oral anticoagulant therapy and undergoing percutaneous coronary intervention: An open-label, randomised, controlled trial. *Lancet.* 2013;381(9872):1107–1115.

30. Cannon CP, Bhatt DL, Oldgren J et al. Dual antithrombotic therapy with dabigatran after PCI in atrial fibrillation. *N Eng J Med.* 2017;377(16):1513–1524.

31. Gibson CM, Mehran R, Bode C et al. Prevention of bleeding in patients with atrial fibrillation undergoing PCI. *N Eng J Medicine.* 2016;375(25):2423–2434.

32. Moraes AA, Chammas AZ, Melo NJ, Mendes LC, Aguiar YS, Ramos RF. Bleeding in non-ST-segment elevation acute

coronary syndrome. *Revista Brasileira de Terapia Intensiva.* 2012;24(3):284.

33. Rao SV, Jollis JG, Harrington RA et al. Relationship of blood transfusion and clinical outcomes in patients with acute coronary syndromes. *JAMA.* 2004;292(13):1555–1562.

34. Bhatt DL, Scheiman J, Abraham NS et al. ACCF/ACG/AHA 2008 expert consensus document on reducing the gastrointestinal risks of antiplatelet therapy and NSAID use: A report of the American College of Cardiology Foundation Task Force on Clinical Expert Consensus Documents. *J Am Coll Cardiol.* 2008;52(18):1502–1517.

35. Alexander KP, Chen AY, Roe MT et al. Excess dosing of antiplatelet and antithrombin agents in the treatment of non–ST-segment elevation acute coronary syndromes. *JAMA.* 2005;294(24):3108–3116.

18

Statins in acute coronary syndrome

SS IYENGAR

INTRODUCTION

When one appreciates the pathophysiological process and various players in the field of acute coronary syndrome (ACS) on one side and the pharmacological actions of statins on the other side, it is intuitive to initiate the use of statins in patients with ACS (Figure 18.1).

ACUTE CORONARY SYNDROME

When an underlying vulnerable coronary atheromatous plaque is disrupted, which is driven partly by the influence of inflammation, blood is exposed to the tissue, platelets are activated, coagulation cascade sets in and an occlusive or subocclusive thrombus is formed, leading to ACS. Other factors like coronary constriction, progressive narrowing of coronary arterial lumen and demand-supply mismatch also play an important and a variable role in the pathogenesis of ACS [1].

Three forms of disruptions of coronary artery plaques can precipitate thrombosis: plaque rupture, plaque erosion and disruptive nodular calcification protruding into the lumen [2]. The vulnerable plaque that ruptures is characterised by poor collagen content, thin fibrous plaque, abundant inflammatory cells, smooth muscle cell apoptosis and high levels of LDL-C.

STATINS AND THEIR ACTIONS

The role of LDL cholesterol in the causation of atherosclerosis, and that of statins in lowering LDL-C with consequent mortality and morbidity benefit in atherosclerotic cardiovascular disease (ASCVD), are well established. In a prospective meta-analysis of 90,056 individuals from 14 randomised trials of statins it was seen that statin therapy reduced the 5-year incidence of major cardiovascular events by about 20% with each 38 mg% reduction in LDL-C safely and irrespective of the baseline lipid profile. These benefits increased with time – significantly within the first year and greater in the following years [3].

Statins significantly reduce total cholesterol (TC), LDL-cholesterol and triglyceride levels, and increase high-density lipoprotein (HDL) cholesterol levels. A number of non-lipid actions have been attributed to statins and are referred to as 'pleiotropic effects.' These non-lipid actions of statins have been shown to influence several mechanisms that are involved in the pathogenesis of a vulnerable plaque. The pleiotropic effects lend support to the use of statins for the treatment of ACS.

CLINICAL TRIALS

There are studies specifically looking at the benefit of early and intensive statin therapy in acute coronary syndrome (ACS).

MIRACL study [4]: In this study, 3086 adults aged 18 years or older with unstable angina or non-Q-wave acute myocardial infarction were randomly assigned to atorvastatin (80 mg per day) or placebo between 24 and 96 hours after hospitalisation for ACS. Lipid lowering with atorvastatin, 80 mg daily, reduced recurrent ischaemic events in the first 16 weeks.

PROVE IT TIMI 22 [5]: 4162 patients who had an acute coronary syndrome within the preceding 10 days were randomised to 40 mg of pravastatin daily or 80 mg of atorvastatin daily (intensive therapy). The follow-up period was for a mean period of 24 months. The authors concluded that patients of acute coronary syndrome, among patients who had recently had an acute coronary syndrome, derived greater protection against death or major cardiovascular events with an intensive lipid-lowering statin regimen than with a standard regimen. So, patients with ACS benefitted from early and continued lowering of LDL cholesterol.

Meta-analysis: In a meta-analysis of 13 randomised controlled trials (RCTs) involving 17,963 patients with ACS (a mixture of STEMI

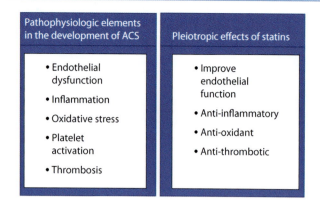

Pathophysiologic elements in the development of ACS	Pleiotropic effects of statins
• Endothelial dysfunction • Inflammation • Oxidative stress • Platelet activation • Thrombosis	• Improve endothelial function • Anti-inflammatory • Anti-oxidant • Anti-thrombotic

Figure 18.1 Pathophysiologic mechanisms involved in ACS provides a reasonable role for pleiotropic statins.

and NSTE-ACS), early (within 4 days of the event), intensive statin therapy compared to control, usually placebo, decreased the rate of death and CV events over 2 years of follow-up by 19% [6]. The benefit began to emerge between 4 and 12 months, achieving statistical significance by 12 months.

These were the studies where statins were administered after the event and percutaneous intervention. Patients with acute coronary syndrome (ACS) experience a high rate of recurrent cardiovascular events in the first 6 months and this risk recedes over time. An early use of statins in patients with ACS at the time of first diagnosis and before intervention reduces the risk of further clinical events [7].

ARMYDA ACS trial [8]: This was a randomised, prospective, double-blind, clinical trial to study the possible beneficial effect of high-dose atorvastatin in statin-naïve patients with ACS undergoing early PCI. 171 patients were randomised to placebo (n = 85) or atorvastatin (n = 86). 80 mg of atorvastatin was administered a mean of 12 hours before coronary angiography and a 40 mg dose approximately 2 hours before intervention. The primary composite end point of 30-day major adverse cardiac events (e.g. death, MI and target vessel revascularisation) was significantly reduced in the atorvastatin arm versus the placebo arm (5% vs. 17%. p = 0.01), and the outcome was mainly driven by periprocedural MI (5 vs. 15%; p = 0.04). On measuring CRP, it was seen that the average percentage increase of CRP levels from baseline was significantly lower in the statin arm. After multivariate analysis, pre-treatment with atorvastatin was associated with 88% and 70% relative risk reduction of 30-day events and periprocedural MI, respectively. The post-procedural elevation of CK-MB and Tn I above ULN was also significantly lower in the atorvastatin arm.

ARMYDA RECAPTURE trial [9]: Patients undergoing PCI while on chronic statin therapy; a similar dosage schedule (80 mg reload administered at a mean of 12 hours before coronary angiography, with a further 40 mg dose administered approximately 2 hours before intervention) was followed in this study, with significant reduction in the primary end point of death, MI and target vessel revascularisation. Subgroup analysis showed that the benefit of atorvastatin reload was confined to patients with ACS (82% reduction of 30-day events); the number needed to treat was 17 in the overall cohort, whereas it was 9 in the ACS subgroup.

The procedural early cardio-protection by the high-dose statin therapy is probably related to the 'pleiotropic effects,' the

long-term beneficial effect coming in addition from reduction in LDL-C levels.

Statin administration before intervention has also been shown to offer protection against contrast-induced nephropathy (CIN) [10].

A multi-centre, randomised, double-blind, placebo-controlled trial studied the effect of fluvastatin therapy initiated as first-line therapy of ACS (Fluvastatin in the Therapy of Acute Coronary Syndrome [FACS] trial) [11]. 156 hospitalised ACS patients were randomised to fluvastatin 80 mg or placebo. Fluvastatin therapy was associated with a significant reduction in the cardiovascular event rate at 1 year (11.5% vs. 24.4%; OR 0.40 [95% CI 0.17–0.95]; p = 0.038).

In the STATIN STEMI trial [12], a favourable effect of 80 mg of atorvastatin administered as first-line treatment of ACS in patients with ST-elevation MI was reported. 171 patients were randomly assigned to 80 mg of atorvastatin or 10 mg of atorvastatin before primary PCI. There was improved coronary flow, faster ST-segment resolution and a trend toward a lower cardiovascular event rate in the intensive atorvastatin group.

CIN prevention may be explained by pleiotropic actions of statin. Statins may modulate the renal perfusion after contrast media administration by downregulating angiotensin receptors and by decreasing synthesis of endothelin and anti-inflammatory effect [13].

Administering statins early in ACS has also a favourable influence on adherence to therapy [14].

GUIDELINES

Guidelines generally recommend early and high intensity statin in patients presenting with ACS, though some are not very specific about the timing of statin administration.

The position statement from the Cardiological Society of India recommends administration of statins as an initial treatment [15]:

A. Position Statement for the Management of STEMI in India (2017)

- Statins are routinely administered in high doses (high intensity statins: atorvastatin 40–80 mg and rosuvastatin 20–40 mg daily) for their LDL-lowering action as well as pleotropic effects.
- Statins are continued indefinitely to achieve and maintain LDL levels less than 70 mg/dL.

ACC/AHA guidelines for percutaneous coronary interventions recommend statins before PCI [16].

B. ACCF/AHA/SCAI Guideline for Percutaneous Coronary Intervention (2011)

CLASS IIa

Administration of a high-dose statin is reasonable before PCI to reduce the risk of periprocedural MI.

- *Level of evidence*: A for statin-naïve patients
- *Level of evidence*: B for those on chronic statin therapy

European guidelines recommend high-intensity statin therapy as early as possible, in patients with STEMI [17] and non-ST ACS [18].

C. ESC Guidelines (STEMI) (2018)

- It is recommended to start high-intensity statin therapy as early as possible, unless contraindicated, and maintain it long term. I A
- An LDL-C goal of <1.8 mmol/L (70 mg/dL) or a reduction of at least 50% if the baseline LDL-C is between 1.8 and 3.5 mmol/L (70–135 mg/dL) is recommended. I B
- It is recommended to obtain a lipid profile in all STEMI patients as soon as possible after presentation. I C
- In patients with LDL-C 1.8 mmol/L (70 mg/dL) despite a maximally tolerated statin dose who remain at high risk, further therapy to reduce LDL-C should be considered.

D. ESC Guidelines (NSTE-ACS) (2015)

- Lipid-lowering treatment is recommended to initiate high-intensity statin therapy (i.e. statin regimens that reduce low-density lipoprotein [LDL] cholesterol by 50%) as early as possible after admission in all NSTE-ACS patients (in the absence of contraindications).
- The intensity of statin therapy should be increased in those receiving a low- or moderate-intensity statin treatment at presentation, unless they have a history of intolerance to high-intensity statin therapy or other characteristics that may influence safety.

Suggested protocol for statin administration in a patient with ACS:

1. High-intensity statin should be administered as soon as possible and positively before PCI.
2. Obtain a lipid profile as soon as possible after presentation.
3. LDL-C goal to be achieved is < 70 mg%.
4. If LDL-C is 70 mg/dL or more despite a maximally tolerated statin dose after 8–12 weeks of high intensity statin, further therapy to reduce LDL-C with non-statin drugs should be considered.

CONCLUSION

It is an unequivocally established fact that statins reduce mortality and morbidity in ASCVD. Early use and their administration before percutaneous coronary intervention are beneficial in reducing post-intervention cardiovascular events, the short-term benefits being ascribed to pleiotropic actions and long-term favourable outcomes due to the additional LDL cholesterol-lowering effects.

REFERENCES

1. Libby P. Mechanisms of acute coronary syndromes and their implications for therapy. *N Engl J Med.* 2013;368(21):2004–2013.
2. Falk E, Nakano M, Bentzon JF et al. Update on acute coronary syndromes: The pathologists' view. *Eur Heart J.* 2013;34(10):719–728.
3. Baigent C, Keech A, Kearney PM et al. Cholesterol treatment trialists collaborators. Efficacy and safety of cholesterol-lowering treatment: Prospective meta-analysis of data from 90,056 participants in 14 randomised trials of statins. *Lancet.* 2005;366(9493):1267–1278.
4. Schwartz GG, Olsson AG, Ezekowitz MD, Ganz P, Oliver MF, Waters D, Zeiher A, Chaitman BR, Leslie S, Stern T. Myocardial ischemia reduction with aggressive cholesterol lowering study investigators. Effects of atorvastatin on early recurrent ischemic events in acute coronary syndromes: The MIRACL study: A randomized controlled trial. *JAMA.* 2001;285(13):1711–1718.
5. Cannon CP, Braunwald E, McCabe CH, Rader DJ, Rouleau JL, Belder R, Joyal SV, Hill KA, Pfeffer MA, Skene AM. Pravastatin or atorvastatin evaluation and infection therapy-thrombolysis in myocardial infarction 22 investigators. intensive versus moderate lipid lowering with statins after acute coronary syndromes. *N Engl J Med.* 2004;350(15):1495–1504.
6. Hulten E, Jackson JL, Douglas K et al. The effect of early, intensive statin therapy on acute coronary syndrome: A meta-analysis of randomized controlled trials. *Arch Intern Med.* 2006;166(17):1814–1821.
7. Cohen M, Antman EM, Murphy SA, Radley D. Mode and timing of treatment failure (recurrent ischemic events) after hospital admission for non-ST segment elevation acute coronary syndrome. *Am Heart J.* 2002;143(1), 63–69.
8. Patti G, Pasceri V, Colonna G et al. Atorvastatin pretreatment improves outcomes in patients with acute coronary syndromes undergoing early percutaneous coronary intervention: Results of the ARMYDA-ACS randomized trial. *J Am Coll Cardiol* 2007;49:1272–1278.
9. Di Sciascio G, Patti G, Pasceri V, Gaspardone A, Colonna G, Montinaro A. Efficacy of atorvastatin reload in patients on chronic statin therapy undergoing percutaneous coronary intervention. *J Am Coll Cardiol.* 2009;54:558–565.
10. Khanal S, Attallah N, Smith DE et al. Statin therapy reduces contrast-induced nephropathy: An analysis of contemporary percutaneous interventions. *Am J Med.* 2005;118:843–849.
11. Ostadal P, Alan D, Vejvoda J et al. Fluvastatin in the first-line therapy of acute coronary syndrome: Results of the multicenter, randomized, double-blind, placebo-controlled trial (the FACS trial). *Trials.* 2010;11:61.
12. Kim JS, Kim J, Choi D et al. Efficacy of high-dose atorvastatin loading before primary percutaneous coronary intervention in ST-segment elevation myocardial infarction: The STATIN STEMI trial. *JACC Cardiovasc Interv.* 2010;3:332–339.
13. Bonetti PO, Lerman LO, Napoli C, Lerman A: Statin effects beyond lipid lowering – are they clinically relevant? *Eur Heart J.* 2003;24:225–248.
14. Fonarow GC, Gawlinski A, Moughrabi S, Tillisch JH. Improved treatment of coronary heart disease by implementation of a Cardiac Hospitalization Atherosclerosis Management Program (CHAMP). *Am J Cardiol.* 2001;87:819–822.
15. Guhaa S, Sethib R, Rayc S et al. Cardiological Society of India: Position statement for the management of ST

elevation myocardial infarction in India. *Indian Heart J.* 2017;69:S63–S97.

16. Levine GN, Bates ER, Blankenship JC et al. 2011 ACCF/AHA/SCAI guideline for percutaneous coronary intervention. *J Am Coll Cardiol.* 2011;58:e44–e122.

17. Ibanez B, James S, Agewall S et al. 2017 ESC Guidelines for the management of acute myocardial infarction in patients presenting with ST-segment elevation. *Eur Heart J.* 2018;39:119–177.

18. Roffi M, Patrono C, Collet JP et al. 2015 ESC Guidelines for the management of acute coronary syndromes in patients presenting without persistent ST-segment elevation. *Eur Heart J.* 2016;37:267–315.

19

Intravenous anti-platelet therapy—GP IIb/IIIa blockers and cangrelor
What has changed recently?

SHRADDHA RANJAN AND GAGANDEEP SINGH WANDER

INTRODUCTION

Anti-platelets are an integral part in the management of coronary artery disease (CAD) considering the fact that pathogenesis of atherothrombotic events is strongly mediated by platelets. The pathophysiology of atherosclerosis starts with narrowing of the arterial lumen by formation of cholesterol laden plaques, which ultimately results in complete obliteration of lumen through erosion or rupture of these lipid-laden and highly inflammatory plaques along with thrombus formation. Platelet adhesion to the subendothelial matrix exposed at sites of plaque rupture results in platelet activation and the release of secondary agonists. This starts a cascade of signalling resulting in platelet aggregation and adhesion with subsequent thrombosis [1]. This justifies the use of anti-platelet agents, especially in secondary prevention of recurrent cardiovascular events whereas for primary prevention, the potential benefit of anti-platelets is debatable. As understanding of the mechanisms by which platelets participate in atherothrombotic processes has increased, new drugs have been developed with a goal of maintaining a perfect balance of efficacy and safety [2]. This chapter will deal with parenterally administered anti-platelet therapy, which although sparsely used in the past 2 decades has gained a renewed interest due to the advent of cangrelor, an intravenous P2Y12 inhibitor.

ORAL ANTI-PLATELETS

a. *Acetylsalicylic acid (aspirin)*: Aspirin has been known to have antithrombotic and anti-inflammatory properties. It is a cyclooxygenase (COX) inhibitor that irreversibly inhibits COX-1 and, in higher doses, COX-2. Inhibition of COX-1 is the main antithrombotic mechanism; the formation of prostaglandin H2 is blocked, thus thromboxane A2, which activates platelets and stimulates their aggregation, cannot be synthesised. The effect lasts for the lifetime of platelets, which ranges from 7–10 days.

b. *P2Y12 receptor antagonists*: P2Y12 receptors are adenosine diphosphate (ADP)-binding receptors expressed on the surface of platelets, which if blocked reduce platelet aggregation and platelet interaction with other cellular or plasma components. The currently available oral P2Y12 receptor blockers are the irreversible thienopyridines (clopidogrel and prasugrel) and reversible triazolopyrimidine ticagrelor. The thienopyridines are prodrugs that require activation by cytochrome system and thus can have drug interactions.

In view of the synergistic mechanism of the ADP-P2Y12 and thromboxane A2 pathways in amplifying platelet activation, dual anti-platelet therapy (DAPT) with a P2Y12 inhibitor in combination with aspirin is the most widely used strategy in acute coronary syndromes (ACS) and post-coronary stent implantation [3]. The classification of anti-platelets and their mechanism of action has been briefly explained in Table 19.1 and Figure 19.1.

NEED FOR IV AGENT

Oral anti-platelets have been well studied and have proven to be of utmost benefit in management of CAD. However, there are a few limitations associated with oral P2Y12 receptor inhibitors that stimulated the search for an intravenous agent. First and foremost is the delayed onset of action as thienopyridines require *in vivo* conversion to an active metabolite. These drugs are also irreversible and have a fairly long duration of action. Even the more potent oral P2Y12 inhibitors, prasugrel and ticagrelor, are associated with delayed platelet inhibition, particularly in patients with ACS. This is due to many factors which impair absorption of oral

Table 19.1 Classification of anti-platelets [2]

Oral anti-platelets	Intravenous anti-platelets
Acetylsalicylic acid-aspirin (non-steroidal anti-inflammatory drug)	Cangrelor (non-thienopyridine, ATP analogue)
Clopidogrel (thienopyridine, P2Y12 receptor antagonist)	Abciximab (glycoprotein IIb/IIIa inhibitor)
Prasugrel (thienopyridine, P2Y12 receptor antagonist)	Tirofiban (glycoprotein IIb/IIIa inhibitor)
Ticagrelor (triazolopyrimidine, P2Y12 receptor antagonist)	Eptifibatide (glycoprotein IIb/IIIa inhibitor)
Vorapaxar (protease-activating receptor-1 antagonist)	

anti-platelets, like acute stress causing stress ulcers, stimulation of intestinal motility, alteration of intestine mucine secretion and use of opioids for pain [4,5].

Secondarily, in a few instances, there is a decision to pre-treat a patient with an ADP-receptor antagonist for a possible immediate angioplasty following angiography. The advantage to this proactive treatment approach is that by the time the patient is ready for angioplasty an oral ADP-receptor antagonist is fully absorbed and platelet inhibition is optimal. The disadvantage is that if the coronary anatomy demands surgical revascularisation, it becomes a problem for surgeons to operate on a patient freshly dosed with an anti-platelet agent. These patients have to be hospitalised for a few days until the drug clears out of the system. An intravenous agent with quick onset and offset of action can be utilised in these scenarios, leading to significant reduction in hospital admission time and financial burden. Less commonly, it is seen that patients with STEMI are cardiopulmonary resuscitation (CPR) survivors and

are unconscious during an initial evaluation, with many proceeding to primary PCI. These patients and any patient who cannot take a dosage orally would be a potential candidate for intravenous anti-platelet therapy.

INTRAVENOUS ANTI-PLATELETS AND THEIR EVIDENCE

CANGRELOR

Cangrelor was approved in 2015 in the United States and Europe as the first intravenous, non-thienopyridine, reversible P2Y12-blocking agent and to this date remains the only intravenous P2Y12 inhibitor available for clinical use. It does not require a loading dose and platelet inhibition is >90%. Platelet inhibition is rapid and potent, occurring immediately within seconds after administration with a short half-life of 3–6 minutes. Cangrelor is reversible as it is inactivated by plasma enzymes in approximately 1 hour and also does not require renal dose modification. These favourable pharmacokinetic properties put cangrelor on the map as a promising agent in management of ACS and for bridging of high-risk patients in the peri-operative setting [6]. The approved indications of cangrelor are discussed in brief along with their supporting evidence.

Adjunct to PCI

CHAMPION PCI (Cangrelor Versus Standard Therapy to Achieve Optimal Management of Platelet Inhibition – PCI) and CHAMPION PLATFORM (Clopidogrel versus Standard Therapy to Achieve Optimal Management of Platelet Inhibition – PLATFORM) were two randomised clinical trials that evaluated the efficacy and safety of cangrelor in patients across a broad spectrum of CAD undergoing percutaneous coronary intervention (PCI) [7,8]. CHAMPION PCI randomly assigned 8716 CAD

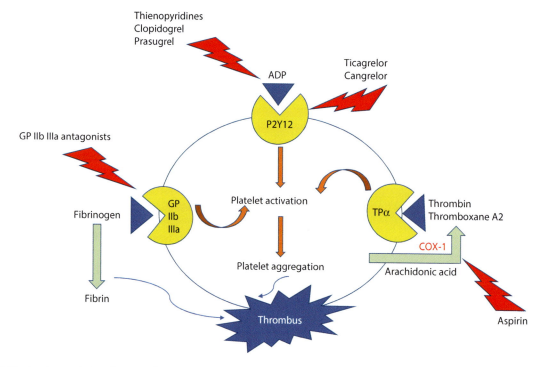

Figure 19.1 Mechanism and site of action of anti-platelets.

patients undergoing PCI to receive either a bolus and infusion of cangrelor followed by 600 mg clopidogrel or only a clopidogrel 600-mg loading dose within 30 minutes of the start of PCI. CHAMPION PLATFORM randomly assigned 5362 NSTE-ACS patients who had not received any thienopyridine in the previous 7 days, or any fibrinolytic agents or GP IIb/IIIa inhibitors within the previous 12 hours, to receive a bolus and infusion of cangrelor followed by a 600 mg of clopidogrel at the end of the infusion or to receive only a clopidogrel 600-mg loading dose immediately after the procedure. Cangrelor was not found to be superior to clopidogrel in either of the two trials with respect to the primary end point of death from any cause, MI or revascularisation at 48 hours, and both trials were terminated prematurely on grounds of futility. However, a post hoc analysis of the pooled CHAMPION PCI and CHAMPION PLATFORM trial data demonstrated a significant reduction in the primary end point of death, MI and ischaemia-driven revascularisation with cangrelor when the universal definition of MI was used instead of trial protocol definition [9]. CHAMPION PHOENIX (Cangrelor Versus Standard Therapy to Achieve Optimal Management of Platelet Inhibition) [10] evaluated the safety and efficacy in reducing acute ischaemic events with addition of cangrelor to dual anti-platelet therapy (aspirin plus clopidogrel) in P2Y12 inhibitor-naive patients undergoing PCI for any of CAD indications. In this trial, 11,145 patients were randomised in a double-blind, placebo-controlled fashion. The primary end point was a composite of death, MI, revascularisation or stent thrombosis at 48 hours. Cangrelor significantly reduced the primary end point compared with the clopidogrel plus aspirin group and the effect of cangrelor was consistent across subgroups regardless of the indication for PCI (stable angina or ACS). The primary safety end point (severe bleeding according to GUSTO criteria) was infrequent and almost similar in both groups. Overall, the net benefit in reduction of adverse clinical events (ischaemic plus bleeding events) was significantly reduced in the cangrelor group and this effect was consistent at 30 days. It cannot be remarked on that the results would have been the same if the more potent oral anti-platelets prasugrel or ticagrelor had been used instead of clopidogrel. Recently a small study (CANgrelor and Crushed TICagrelor in STEMI Patients Undergoing Primary Percutaneous Coronary Intervention – CANTIC [11]) assessed the safety and efficacy of cangrelor compared with a crushed ticagrelor among patients with STEMI undergoing PCI. The results of this trial indicated that cangrelor lowers platelet reactivity rapidly in less than 5 minutes and is maintained throughout the duration of infusion, whereas the incidence of high platelet reactivity was higher in the arm that received only crushed ticagrelor. Although this is a small trial and no end points were studied, it shows the better efficacy of cangrelor compared with even crushed ticagrelor, which is the fastest-acting formulation of oral platelet inhibitors. These studies may mark a path for intravenous cangrelor in establishing it as an alternative strategy for anti-platelet therapy during PCI in the recent future.

Bridge therapy: For cardiac surgery

Cangrelor has also been studied in the phase II clinical trial BRIDGE (Maintenance of Platelet Inhibition With Cangrelor After Discontinuation of Thienopyridines in Patients Undergoing Surgery) [12]. This double-blind study evaluated the use of cangrelor with placebo in 210 patients with ACS or those treated with a coronary stent who had received a thienopyridine and were awaiting coronary artery bypass grafting (CABG) (within 48 hours to 7 days). Patients were randomised to receive a cangrelor 'bridge' intravenous infusion or placebo infusion for at least 48 hours, which was discontinued 1–6 hours before CABG surgery. The primary outcome of the BRIDGE trial was measurement of levels of platelet reactivity, which was assessed daily. It showed that a greater proportion of patients treated with cangrelor had low levels of platelet reactivity i.e. better maintenance of platelet inhibition throughout the treatment period and bleeding was not significantly different between the cangrelor and placebo groups. This study was, however, small and underpowered for hard outcomes, but its results support the role of cangrelor for bridging therapy in patients who are awaiting CABG and are off oral anti-platelets.

Bridge therapy: For non-cardiac surgery

In preparation for any non-cardiac surgery, P2Y12 inhibitors are commonly discontinued 5–7 days before surgery to minimise bleeding risk during the procedure. Though this is a common practise, it can be really disastrous in patients who have undergone recent drug-eluting stenting and are at high ischaemic risk if anti-platelet therapy is interrupted. GP IIb/IIIa inhibitors have sometimes been used as an anti-platelet bridge to surgery but the safety and efficacy of this approach is not known [13]. Now that cangrelor has been shown to be of some benefit in bridging for CABG, it can be used with a similar concept in non-cardiac surgeries as well. An international expert consensus on switching platelet P2Y12 receptor-inhibiting therapies recommends starting cangrelor bridging without a bolus after 3–4 days of prasugrel discontinuation and 2–3 days of clopidogrel and ticagrelor discontinuation and to continue until a few hours before the surgery [14].

GLYCOPROTEIN IIB/IIIA INHIBITORS

The activation of the GP IIb/IIIa receptor is one of the final steps in platelet activation, building platelet–fibrinogen complexes. Glycoprotein IIb/IIIa inhibitors block the adhesion of fibrinogen to the activated platelet by competing with the von Willebrand factor and fibrinogen, preventing the platelet aggregation and adhesion. Abciximab, tirofiban and eptifibatide are intravenous GP IIb/IIIa inhibitors that are available for use [15].

Abciximab is a humanised monoclonal mouse antibody approved only for patients undergoing PCI. It reversibly binds to thrombocytes immediately after administration. A loading dose is required to achieve optimal receptor blockage. It shows the highest affinity to the GP IIb/IIIa receptor among these three drugs. Tirofiban and eptifibatide are synthetic GP IIb/IIIa inhibitors that reversibly bind and rapidly dissociate (10–15 seconds) from the GP IIb/IIIa receptor. Compared with cangrelor, these agents inhibit the platelet response to all agonists and are therefore more potent anti-platelet agents than cangrelor. Though these drugs have a theoretical advantage over slower-acting oral P2Y12 drugs, the clinical benefits of GP IIb/IIIa inhibitors were impressive back in the era of balloon angioplasty before the routine use of dual anti-platelet therapy, potent oral P2Y12 inhibitors and new less thrombogenic stent technologies. More recent trials and systematic reviews, specifically in patients pre-treated with thienopyridines, have shown contradicting evidence in the benefit of routine use of GP IIb/IIIa inhibitors [16]. In a meta-analysis of 10,123 patients undergoing primary PCI, non-fatal MI at 30 days was reduced with use of GP IIb/IIIa inhibitors but there was a significant increase in the risk of minor bleeding and thrombocytopenia. There were no differences in 30-day or 1-year mortality rates [17]. Presently, the administration of GP IIb/IIIa inhibitors is an accepted treatment option for patients undergoing primary PCI and patients with visible thrombus burden as a bailout strategy [1,18]. GP IIb/IIIa inhibitors can also be used through the intracoronary route of delivery. This leads to a higher local concentration and thus better thrombus resolution. It may also limit the risk of myocardial damage due to reperfusion injury caused by thromboembolism in the microvasculature. Intracoronary administration of GP IIb/IIIa inhibitors has been tested in some small studies and has been shown to be safe and probably better than intravenous administration, but these results have not been confirmed in large-scale clinical trials [19].

TIMING AND METHOD OF ADMINISTRATION

It has been proven that shorter GP IIb/IIIa inhibitor infusions and the use of a radial approach may significantly improve the safety profile of GP IIb/IIIa inhibitors and restore interest in their use. If high-risk patients are targeted who have been not adequately preloaded with clopidogrel and have a low risk of bleeding, the net clinical benefit of these drugs increases a lot. These drugs are usually started at the time of PCI as bailout or before PCI if the patient has not been adequately preloaded with P2Y12 inhibitors. Eptifibatide and tirofiban have renal clearance and need dose modification in renal dysfunction. Intracoronary administration of abciximab has been shown to be safe and effective with favourable effects on TIMI flow.

Cangrelor is administered in recommended doses as a diluted IV bolus (less than 1 minute) followed immediately by infusion. The bolus should be completely administered prior to the start of the PCI procedure and continued for at least 2 hours or for the duration of the PCI, whichever is longer. Recommended dose of intravenous anti-platelets is similar for all practical indications and is given in Table 19.2. An oral P2Y12 receptor antagonist (i.e. clopidogrel, ticagrelor or prasugrel) should be started after

Table 19.2 Dose of intravenous anti-platelets [22]

Abciximab	0.25 mg/kg bolus followed by infusion of 0.125–10 mcg/kg/min for 12–24 hrs
Eptifibatide	Double bolus of 180 mcg/kg at an interval of 10 min followed by infusion of 2.0 mcg/kg/min for 18 hrs
Tirofiban	25 mcg/kg bolus for 3 min followed by infusion of 0.15 mcg/kg/min for 18 hrs
Cangrelor	30 mcg/kg diluted IV bolus (less than 1 min) followed immediately by a 4 mcg/kg/min IV infusion

Table 19.3 Recent guideline recommendations on intravenous anti-platelets [1,20–23]

Class I	In NSTE-ACS patients with high-risk features not treated with bivalirudin and not adequately pre-treated with clopidogrel, it is useful at the time of PCI to administer a GP IIb/IIIa inhibitor in patients treated with UFH.
Class IIa	GP IIb/IIIa inhibitors to be used at the time of primary PCI (abciximab, double-bolus eptifibatide or high-bolus-dose tirofiban) in selected patients with STEMI with high thrombus burden receiving unfractionated heparin (regardless of stenting or clopidogrel pre-treatment).
Class IIa	GP IIb/IIIa inhibitors should be considered for bailout if there is evidence of no-reflow or a thrombotic complication during PCI for any indication.
Class IIb	Cangrelor may be considered in patients undergoing PCI for either ACS or stable ischaemic disease who have not received P2Y12 receptor inhibitors.
Class IIb	If both oral anti-platelets have to be discontinued pre-operatively, a bridging strategy with intravenous anti-platelets may be considered, especially if surgery has to be performed within 1 month after stent implantation.

discontinuation of the cangrelor infusion to maintain platelet inhibition. Timing of administration of P2Y12 inhibitors in patients receiving cangrelor infusion at the time of PCI is drug-specific. While ticagrelor can be given anytime before or after cangrelor infusion, clopidogrel or prasugrel should be given at the time of or before cangrelor infusion discontinuation. No dosage adjustment is required for patients with any type of renal or liver impairment [14].

RECENT GUIDELINES

GP IIb/IIIa inhibitors have the greatest role in the treatment of patients who are clinically high risk and those with high-risk angiographic features, i.e. visible thrombus and high-risk anatomy along with a low risk of bleeding. ACC/AHA(2014) and ESC(2015) NSTEMI, ESC(2017) STEMI, ESC(2017) DAPT and ESC(2018) myocardial revascularisation guideline recommendations about IV anti-platelets are summarised in Table 19.3 [1,20–23].

CONCLUSION

It is true that with the increasing complexity of PCI in the high-risk patient, parenteral anti-platelet agents theoretically have an important therapeutic role and to utilise them in clinical practice without compromising safety is the need of the time. GP IIb/IIIa inhibitor use is expected to continue in bailout/rescue scenarios and in those admitted for PCI without effective DAPT and with low bleeding risk. Cangrelor, with its rapid and reversible action, is becoming an option as an adjunct to PCI in patients not loaded with anti-platelets and also for bridging in cardiac and non-cardiac surgeries. However, lack of evidence exists on both grounds as there are no randomised clinical trials comparing the utility of cangrelor and GP IIb/IIIa inhibitors. On the other hand, the clinical role of cangrelor in the era of the potent newer anti-platelets prasugrel or ticagrelor, which have ample evidence to back them up, remains unclear. Current evidence seems favourable for use of intravenous anti-platelets in certain scenario; further real-life experience along with randomised trials are needed to establish their role in adjunctive pharmacotherapy.

REFERENCES

1. Amsterdam EA, Wenger NK, Brindis RG et al. 2014 AHA/ACC guideline for the management of patients with Non-ST-elevation acute coronary syndromes: A report of the American College of Cardiology/American Heart Association task force on practice guidelines. *J Am Coll Cardiol*. 2014;64:e139–e228.

2. Majithia A, Bhatt DL. Novel antiplatelet therapies for atherothrombotic diseases. *Thromb Vasc Biol*. 2019;39: 546–557.

3. Valgimigli M, Bueno H, Byrne RA et al. 2017 ESC focused update on dual antiplatelet therapy in coronary artery disease developed in collaboration with EACTS: The Task Force for dual antiplatelet therapy in coronary artery disease of the European Society of Cardiology (ESC) and of the European Association for Cardio-Thoracic Surgery (EACTS). *Eur Heart J*. 2018;39:213–260.

4. Soderholm JD, Perdue MH. Stress and gastrointestinal tract. II. Stress and intestinal barrier function. *Am J Physiol Gastrointest Liver Physiol*. 2001;280:G7–G13.

5. Fuller EE, Alemu R, Harper JF, Feldman M. Relation of nausea and vomiting in acute myocardial infarction to location of the infarct. *Am J Cardiol*. 2009;104:1638–1640.

6. Angiolillo DJ, Schneider DJ, Bhatt DL et al. Pharmacodynamic effects of cangrelor and clopidogrel: The platelet function substudy from the cangrelor versus standard therapy to achieve optimal management of platelet inhibition (CHAMPION) trials. *J Thromb Thrombolysis*. 2012;34:44–55.

7. Bhatt DL, Lincoff AM, Gibson CM et al. Intravenous platelet blockade with cangrelor during PCI. *The N Engl J Med*. 2009;361:2330–2341.

8. Harrington RA, Stone GW, McNulty S et al. Platelet inhibition with cangrelor in patients undergoing PCI. *N Engl J Med*. 2009;361:2318–2329.

9. White HD, Bhatt DL, Gibson CM et al. Outcomes with cangrelor versus clopidogrel on a background of bivalirudin: Insights from the CHAMPION PHOENIX (a clinical trial comparing cangrelor to clopidogrel standard therapy in subjects who require percutaneous coronary intervention [PCI]). *JACC Cardiovasc Interv*. 2015;8:424–433.

10. Abtan J, Steg PG, Stone GW et al. Efficacy and safety of cangrelor in preventing periprocedural complications in patients with stable angina and acute coronary syndromes undergoing percutaneous coronary intervention: The CHAMPION PHOENIX trial. *JACC Cardiovasc Interv*. 2016;9:1905–1913.

11. Franchi F, Rollini F, Rivas A et al. Platelet inhibition with cangrelor and crushed ticagrelor in patients with ST-segment-elevation myocardial infarction undergoing primary percutaneous coronary intervention. *Circulation*. 2019;139:1661–1670.

12. Angiolillo DJ, Firstenberg MS, Price MJ et al. Bridging antiplatelet therapy with cangrelor in patients undergoing cardiac surgery: A randomized controlled trial. *JAMA*. 2012;307:265–274.

13. Warshauer J, Patel VG, Christopoulos G, Kotsia AP, Banerjee S, Brilakis ES. Outcomes of preoperative bridging therapy for patients undergoing surgery after coronary stent implantation: A weighted meta-analysis of 280 patients from eight studies. *Catheter Cardiovasc Interv: Off J Soc Card Angiography Interv*. 2015;85:25–31.

14. Angiolillo DJ, Rollini F, Storey RF et al. International expert consensus on switching platelet P2Y12 receptor-inhibiting therapies. *Circulation*. 2017;136:1955–1975.

15. Angiolillo D, Giugliano G. Antiplatelet and anticoagulant therapy in acute coronary syndrome. *Hurst's The Heart*. 2017. 14th Ed. The McGraw-Hill.

16. Muniz-Lozano A, Rollini F, Franchi F, Angiolillo DJ. Update on platelet glycoprotein IIb/IIIa inhibitors: Recommendations for clinical practice. *Ther Adv Cardiovasc Dis*. 2013;7:197–213.

17. Winchester DE, Wen X, Brearley WD, Park KE, Anderson RD, Bavry AA. Efficacy and safety of glycoprotein IIb/IIIa inhibitors during elective coronary revascularization: A meta-analysis of randomized trials performed in the era of stents and thienopyridines. *J Am Coll Cardiol*. 2011;57:1190–1199.

18. Bhatt DL, Topol EJ. Current role of platelet glycoprotein IIb/IIIa inhibitors in acute coronary syndromes. *JAMA*. 2000;284:1549–1558.

19. Gurbel PA, Tantry US. Delivery of glycoprotein IIb/IIIa inhibitor therapy for percutaneous coronary intervention: Why not take the intracoronary highway? *Circulation*. 2010;121:739–741.

20. Ibanez B, James S, Agewall S et al. 2017 ESC Guidelines for the management of acute myocardial infarction in patients presenting with ST-segment elevation. *Rev Esp Cardiol*. 2017;70:1082.

21. Roffi M, Patrono C, Collet JP et al. 2015 ESC Guidelines for the management of acute coronary syndromes in patients presenting without persistent ST-segment elevation: Task force for the management of acute coronary syndromes in patients presenting without persistent ST-segment elevation of the European Society of Cardiology (ESC). *Eur Heart J*. 2016;37:267–315.

22. Neumann FJ, Hochholzer W, Siepe M. ESC/EACTS guidelines on myocardial revascularization 2018: The most important innovations. *Herz*. 2018;43:689–694.

23. Schafer A, Bauersachs J. Focused update on dual antiplatelet treatment: ESC guidelines 2017. *Herz*. 2017;42:739–745.

CABG in acute coronary syndrome

OP YADAVA

Acute coronary syndrome (ACS) is an 'operational term' [1] comprising a spectrum ranging from unstable angina (UA), non-ST-elevation myocardial infarction (NSTEMI) to ST-elevation myocardial infarction (STEMI). NSTEMI and UA are the most prevalent types of ACS in contemporary practise. Though early attempts at myocardial revascularisation following ACS were surgical – starting from Keon who first described his experience with emergency coronary artery bypass graft (CABG) surgery for acute myocardial infarction (AMI), followed by extensive experience of DeWood and Philips – pharmaco-invasive therapies have superseded CABG in AMI, essentially for reasons of logistics. Pi et al. from Duke University found CABG in STEMI to be decreasing from 8.3% in 2007 to 5.4% in 2014 (P < 0.001). In their experience, 45.8% of those undergoing CABG for STEMI were primary reperfusion therapies, 38.7% had CABG after percutaneous coronary intervention (PCI) and 8.2% after fibrinolytic therapy [2].

Patients with ACS are a very heterogenous group and should be risk stratified using various risk assessment scores and clinical prediction algorithms like the TIMI score, the PURSUIT risk score, the GRACE risk score and the NCDR-ACTION registry score to assist in the selection of treatment options (Cl 1; LOE 'B') [1].

CABG IN NON-ST-ELEVATION MI ACS

In-hospital CABG is performed in 7%–13% of patients with NSTEMI [3]. Indications for CABG in stabilised NSTEMI are the same as in stable coronary artery disease (CAD), albeit with a stronger impetus for revascularisation in the former. Significant left main or left main equivalent disease, patients unresponsive to optimum guideline directed medical treatment (Cl I; LOE 'A') and patients with proximal left anterior descending (LAD) stenosis, complex coronary lesions and those unsuitable for PCI form an indication for CABG [1].

'Factors that influence the choice of revascularization procedure include the extent and complexity of CAD; short-term risk and long-term durability of PCI; operative mortality, which can be estimated by the Society of Thoracic Surgeons (STS) score; diabetes mellitus (DM); chronic kidney disease (CKD); completeness of revascularisation; left ventricular (LV) systolic dysfunction; previous CABG; and the ability of the patient to tolerate and comply with dual anti-platelet therapy (DAPT). In general, the greater the extent and complexity of the multi-vessel disease, the more compelling the choice of CABG over multi-vessel PCI' [3]. The 'Heart Team' approach, informed by calculation of the SYNTAX score, is strongly recommended. However, there is some evidence from the FREEDOM study lately that the SYNTAX score should not be used to guide the choice of coronary revascularisation in diabetics with complex multi-vessel CAD [4]. Even fractional flow reserve (FFR) needs validation [5].

CABG IN ST-ELEVATION MI

For STEMI, pharmaco-invasive strategy is the accepted first line treatment. However, CABG may be indicated in complicated or failed angioplasty; persistent, refractory ischaemia; mechanical complications of AMI; cardiogenic shock or life-threatening ventricular arrhythmias [6] (Figure 20.1). European guidelines [5] recommend CABG in patients with ongoing ischaemia and large areas of jeopardised myocardium, if PCI of the infarct-related artery cannot be performed (Cl IIa; LOE 'C').

TIMING OF SURGERY

NON-ST-ELEVATION MI

The timing of CABG in NSTEMI is debatable. There seems to be a shift recently towards earlier surgery, if indicated, rather than waiting for the conventional 3–5 days, as proposed in earlier studies. Approximately one-third of patients with NSTEMI undergo CABG within 48 hours of hospital admission (median 73 hours). In-hospital mortality in these patients is approximately 3.7% [3]. Ha et al. [8], in a propensity score matched analysis, compared clinical outcomes between early CABG (less than 48 hours) and delayed CABG (more than 48 hours of admission), and found that the mortality was the same (2% vs. 1.8%; P-0.695), thereby showing that early surgery was safe. The incremental risk factors for mortality were age more than 70 years (OR 3.42%, 95% CI 1.85–6.34; P < 0.001), cardiogenic shock (OR 3.22%, 95% CI-1.35–7.67; P-0.008) and use of mechanical circulatory support with balloon counter pulsation (OR 2.93%, 95% CI-1.45–5.90; P-0.003). Even Davierwala et al. [9] from Leipzig, Germany, found no difference either in early or late mortality between NSTEMI patients operated on in less than 24 hours, 24–72 hours or more than 72 hours to 21 days after AMI, and they were further corroborated by Parikh et al. [3]. However, NSTE-ACS practice guidelines advocate urgent revascularisation for cardiogenic shock, refractory ischaemia despite optimal medical therapy, sustained ventricular arrhythmias, or dynamic ST-segment changes accompanying ischaemic symptoms.

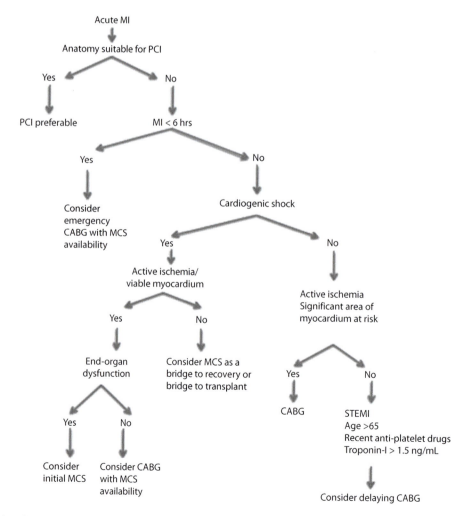

Figure 20.1 Algorithm showing surgical management of acute myocardial infarction [7].

ST-ELEVATION MI

In the experience of Pi et al. [2], the median time interval from coronary angiography to CABG was 23.3 hours in CABG only group, 49.7 hours in CABG after PCI and 56.6 hours in CABG after fibrinolytic therapy. Patients receiving DAPT had the longest delay of a median of 73.0 hours, thereby suggesting that the surgeons do have concerns of bleeding in these patients [2]. Unfortunately, due to the lack of authentic data, there are no LOE 'A' recommendations for optimal timing of CABG in AMI. Timing of surgery may even be guided by anti-platelet therapy (discussed later).

Though the optimal timing for CABG in STEMI has no LOE 'A', Nichols et al. [10] found that the majority of their patients underwent CABG within 3–7 days of AMI (64.3%), followed by 8–21 days (20.5%), 1–2 days (12.1%) and within 24 hours of AMI in 3.2%. The adjusted in-hospital mortality was highest in those patients operated within 24 hours (5.4%), 2.7% in those operated between 8 and 21 days and was the lowest in those operated between 1–2 days and 3–7 days (1.8% and 1.9%, respectively). A large study by Weiss et al. [11] noted a similar 'U'-shaped relationship between timing and outcomes, with early surgery, especially within the first 24 hours, having maximum mortality (0–2 days vs. ≥3 days). We found surgery within 48 hours after AMI as an independent predictor of 30 day mortality [12]. However, Parikh et al. [3] found no difference in mortality between patients undergoing CABG within 48 hours versus more than 48 hours after AMI. Rohn et al. [13] found that it was the haemodynamic state which was more important than the timing of the operation. Overall there was no difference in mortality (8.1% at 30 days) between CABG within 6 hours and 6–24 hours after AMI.

ANTI-PLATELET/FIBRINOLYTIC THERAPY

Guidelines link the timing of surgery in NSTEMI to the time of stoppage of anti-platelet drugs [1]. CABG performed 1–4 days after discontinuation of clopidogrel lead to increase in blood transfusions, but not to higher incidence of life-threatening bleeding [1]. In the TRITON-TIMI 38 trial, CABG-related major bleeding was higher in patients treated with prasugrel than clopidogrel [14]. In the PLATO trial, the rates of major bleeding and transfusion were similar between ticagrelor and clopidogrel [15].

Pi et al. [2] compared STEMI patients who underwent CABG within 5 days of receiving P2Y12 receptor antagonist and those receiving CABG after 5 days, and found that the mortality (5.2% vs. 3.4%), incidence of bleeding (83.5% vs. 79.8%) and blood transfusion rates (53.7% vs. 46.5%) were higher in the former. However, there was no difference in cardiogenic shock (13.6% vs. 13.3%) and stroke (1.9% each) between them. On the flip side, those receiving CABG within 5 days had less reinfarction (1.9% vs. 3.7%) and a shorter hospital stay (median 8 vs. 14 days) than the latter group [2]. Hansson et al. [16] showed that waiting 3 days, as opposed to 5, did not increase CABG-related major bleeding for patients on ticagrelor.

Clinical situation permitting, guidelines recommend that clopidogrel and ticagrelor should be discontinued for at least 5 days (Cl I; LOE 'B') and prasugrel for 7 days before surgery (Cl I; LOE 'C'). However, in patients referred for urgent CABG, clopidogrel and ticagrelor should be discontinued for 24 hours to reduce major bleeding (Cl I; LOE 'B') [1]. To obviate this delay exposing these high-risk patients to adverse cardiac events, the patient is anti-coagulated with unfractionated heparin (UFH) or bivalirudin. To further address this issue, an ongoing CABG-TIME study is looking at the optimum timing of CABG in ACS patients on ticagrelor. However, non–enteric-coated aspirin (81 mg–325 mg daily) should be continued (Cl I; LOE 'B') [1].

Short-acting intravenous GP IIb/IIIa inhibitors (eptifibatide or tirofiban) should be discontinued at least 2–4 hours before surgery and abciximab for 12 hours, to limit blood loss and transfusion (Cl I; LOE 'B'). Emergency CABG after failed thrombolysis can be performed with acceptable outcomes, albeit with higher re-exploration rates [12].

We believe that the use of anti-platelet therapy is not an absolute contraindication to surgery, and if benefits outweigh the risks of bleeding, one can proceed for surgery, totally oblivious to the administration of anti-platelet or fibrinolytic therapies.

PRE-OPERATIVE MANAGEMENT

Critically ill patients should be adequately resuscitated and stabilised before surgery by use of pharmacotherapy like nitrates, inotropes, vasopressors and vasodilators, guided by invasive monitoring and cardiac indices. Diuretics and anti-arrhythmics may also be required. Pre-operative beta-blockers may reduce peri-operative mortality (controversial), and post-operative atrial fibrillation [17]. Guidelines recommend the continuation of beta-blockers peri-operatively for patients taking them pre-operatively.

Judicious use of ventilation and intra-aortic balloon pump (IABP) counter-pulsation can be life-saving. Even though the SHOCK II trial showed that IABP does not improve survival and should not be used routinely, but if the patient is having evidence of persistent and recurrent ischaemia, infarct extension or cardiogenic shock, then short term extra corporeal membrane oxygenation (ECMO), left ventricular assist devices (LVAD) or IABP may be used, depending on the logistics. Mechanical circulatory support when indicated should be used early rather than late in these patients.

TECHNICAL CONSIDERATIONS

1. *Cardiopulmonary bypass (CPB)*: If the decision is to do on-pump CABG, then normothermic CPB should be instituted early to attenuate the infarct process in patients with ongoing ischaemia or haemodynamic and electrical instability. However, if the patient is stable, CPB should be instituted after harvesting of the conduits.
2. *Centrifugal versus roller pump*: Because centrifugal pumps are less damaging to the formed elements of the blood and plasma protein and can also be used for up to 6 hours, they are preferred over roller pumps.
3. *Modified ultra filtration*: This may be indicated in patients with cardiac failure, pulmonary oedema or impairment of

renal functions. It also helps filter out harmful inflammatory mediators.

4. *Myocardial protection*: Cold blood, hyperkalaemic, antegrade, intermittent cardioplegia initially, followed by retrograde cardioplegia through the coronary sinus, is probably the best method of myocardial protection [18]. Buckberg et al. have described various protocols to actively 'resuscitate' severely ischaemic heart undergoing emergency surgery and various elements of these protocols can be incorporated into the myocardial protection strategy depending on operating surgeons philosophy and logistics of availability. Using his own protocol, Buckberg reported an in-hospital mortality of 7% for patients operated within 18 hours of AMI with restoration of LV function [19]. Similarly, Sintek et al. [20] reported in-hospital mortality of 4.4% using Buckberg's protocol.

5. *Order of grafting in acute evolving MI*: The infarct-related vessel should be grafted first to attenuate the infarct process by regional hypothermia and selective perfusion. Allen et al. [19] recommend placing the first graft on the vessel supplying the largest area of contractile viable myocardium, with immediate reperfusion of the same through a side arm cannula, and the last graft should be placed on the vessel supplying the infarcted area. During proximal anastomoses, the graft supplying largest segment of viable myocardium should be anastomosed last to ensure as much perfusion as possible during systemic warming, by graft perfusion. However, the most commonly used strategy is expeditious distal grafting in a single aortic cross clamp and all proximal anastomoses in a single episode of side biting of aorta.

6. *Use of arterial grafts*: At least LIMA-LAD should be a default strategy even in unstable patients. IMA can be harvested on CPB, if the patient is unstable.

OUTCOMES OF CABG IN ACS

Outcomes for CABG are worse in patients with ACS than without ACS. Pre-operative troponin I level is the strongest independent predictor of short-term death [1]. Risk factors for mortality are Killip Class, cardiogenic shock, pre-operative use of catecholamines, ventilation and LV dysfunction [13].

Khaladj et al. [21] found significantly higher in-hospital mortality of 15% for CABG following STEMI, as opposed to 6% in NSTEMI. Mortality for NSTEMI peaked if the operation was performed within 6 hours of AMI and then decreased precipitously. On the other hand, mortality for STEMI remained high during the first 24 hours after AMI before trending downwards [22]. To the contrary, Grothusen et al. [23] from Germany compared results of CABG in STEMI versus NSTEMI within 48 hours of infarct, and found that stable STEMI patients had lesser peri-operative complications and better survival (30 days mortality 2.7% vs. 6.6%, P-0.018), especially when CABG was performed within 6 hours (1.8 vs. 7.1%; P-0.04). Even 10-year survival of STEMI patients was better than non-STEMI (74% vs. 57%; P-<0.001). Independent predictors of early and long-term mortality were increased lactate, age, atrial fibrillation and LV dysfunction.

CABG VERSUS PCI IN ACS

There are no randomised trials comparing CABG with PCI specifically for NSTE-ACS. Data from outdated trials also enrolling UA patients, reveal either no difference in the rate of death, stroke, or MI at 1 year or a marginal increase in survival with PCI [24].

To the contrary, Ruivo et al. [25] compared PCI versus CABG in NSTEMI in a propensity score matched analysis and found that in high-risk NSTEMI patients with multi-vessel CAD, there was a numerically higher incidence of in-hospital events in the PCI group (P-non-significant), but CABG appeared to confer survival benefit. Chang et al. [26] pooled data from the BEST, PRECOMBAT and the SYNTAX trials and found that primary composite end points of death, MI and CVA were lower with CABG than PCI at 5 years (HR 0.74; CI 0.56–0.98; p-0.036). Similarly, Ramanathan et al. [27] from Canada compared surgery versus PCI in diabetic patients with multi-vessel CAD, and found that at 30 days, the odds ratio for major adverse cardiac and cerebral events (MACCE) favoured CABG (0.49%, 95% CI - 0.34–0.71).

Even Caggegi et al. [28] reported that PCI was associated with a statistically higher risk of MACCE through 1 year compared with CABG in NSTEMI. DM and chronic kidney disease may tilt the balance towards CABG to ensure more complete and durable revascularisation [29]. Older patients with NSTEMI appear to have improved outcomes with CABG compared with PCI (5-year mortality – 24.2 vs. 33.5%) [30]. The best revascularisation strategy for female patients remains controversial [31].

In the absence of LOE 'A' data on the subject, the functional SYNTAX score II, though not evaluated for ACS, may inform this decision of CABG versus PCI.

CARDIOGENIC SHOCK: RECOMMENDATIONS

Early revascularisation is a mainstay in the treatment of cardiogenic shock (Cl 1; LOE 'B') as it improves mortality and provides 13% absolute mortality reduction at 6 years [32]. Urgent revascularisation with CABG may be indicated for failed PCI, coronary anatomy not suitable for PCI, and mechanical defects (acute mitral regurgitation, infarct VSD, free-wall rupture).

Recommendations regarding use of inotropes are debatable and need to be customised to the needs of an individual patient. However, dopamine may be associated with increased mortality compared with norepinephrine [33].

OPCAB IN ACS

Limited data regarding primary off-pump CABG (OPCAB) in ACS show lower mortality in off-pump versus on-pump procedures (5% vs. 24%, P = 0.015 [34] and 3.5% vs. 5.4%, P = 0.690 [35]). Mohr et al. [36] demonstrated a low operative mortality of 1.7% using OPCAB in AMI with 1 and 5 year actuarial survival of 94.7% and 82.3%, respectively. Kaya et al. [34] showed that

OPCAB performed within 6 hours from the onset of chest pain has a low incidence of conversion to CPB and is safe.

However, with the recent debate on efficacy of OPCAB, it is the operating surgeon's prerogative to make a call based on his familiarity and comfort with the two techniques, especially due to lack of any high quality, randomised data in favour of any technique. We at the National Heart Institute, use OPCAB as a default strategy in all cases of ACS and resort to pump only if there is haemodynamic or electrical instability.

MECHANICAL CIRCULATORY SUPPORT IN ACS

The randomised IABP-SHOCK II trial was neutral for mortality with and without IABP, albeit with higher complication rates with use of IABP [37]. Therefore, prophylactic use of IABP is not recommended. In heart failure, which cannot be managed pharmacologically, the use of extracorporeal support (VAD/ECMO), with a view to increasing peripheral tissue perfusion, remains the treatment of choice [38,39].

POST-OPERATIVE PHARMACOTHERAPY

Early initiation of high-intensity statin therapy for cholesterol-lowering and anti-inflammatory effects is mandatory following CABG [40] as it reduces cardiac mortality [41]. Similarly, post-operative beta-blocker use is associated with decreased long-term mortality after CABG [42]. Angiotensin converting enzyme inhibitors or angiotensin receptor blockers are also indicated after CABG especially for DM, LV dysfunction, recent MI and/or CKD, unless the patient has hypotension, hyperkalemia and worsening renal function, as they improve long-term outcomes [43].

Dual anti-platelet therapy (aspirin plus a P2Y12 inhibitor) should be used for 12 months for all patients [44]. However, the impact of DAPT on saphenous vein graft patency is controversial with some studies showing no benefit and a few suggesting increased patency. A 2015 AHA Scientific Statement, and the ACC/AHA 2016 DAPT-focussed update give 'soft' Class IIb recommendation for DAPT for 1 year post-CABG to improve vein graft patency [45].

FUTURE

Robotically assisted CABG, totally endoscopic CABG (TECAB) and hybrid strategies have not yet been formally studied, but may offer exciting prospects for the future for treatment of ACS [46].

CONCLUSION

Though pharmaco-invasive therapies are the current gold standard for ACS, CABG when indicated has salutary outcomes. The timing of CABG is strongly influenced by the upstream use of oral P2Y12 inhibitors, but it should not be considered prohibitive, if indications exist. Integrated decision-making by a heart team is mandatory.

REFERENCES

1. Amsterdam EA, Wenger NK, Brindis RG et al. 2014 AHA/ACC guideline for the management of patients with non–ST-elevation acute coronary syndromes. *J Am Coll Cardiol.* 2014;64(24):e139–e228.
2. Pi Y, Roe MT, Holmes DN et al. Utilization, characteristics, and in-hospital outcomes of coronary artery bypass grafting in patients with ST-segment–elevation myocardial infarction. *Circ Cardiovasc Qual Outcomes.* 2017;10:e003490.
3. Parikh SV, de Lemos JA, Jessen ME et al. Timing of in-hospital coronary artery bypass graft surgery for non-ST-segment elevation myocardial infarction patients: Results from the National Cardiovascular Data Registry ACTION Registry-GWTG (acute coronary treatment and intervention outcomes network registry-get with the guidelines). *JACC Cardiovasc Interv.* 2010, 3:419–427.
4. Esper RB, Farkouh ME, Ribeiro EE et al. SYNTAX score in patients with diabetes undergoing coronary revascularization in the FREEDOM Trial. *J Am Coll Cardiol.* 2018;72(23 Part A):2826–2828.
5. Neuman FJ, Uva MS, Ahlsson A et al. 2018 ESC/EACTS guidelines on myocardial revascularization. *Eur Heart J.* 2018. https://doi.org/10.1093/eurheartj/ehy394
6. O'Gara PT, Kushner FG, Ascheim DD et al. 2013 ACCF/AHA guidelines for the management of ST-elevation myocardial infarction: A report of the American College of Cardiology Foundation/American Heart Association Task Force on Practice Guidelines. *J Am Coll Cardiol.* 2013;61:e78–140.
7. Caceres M, Weiman DS. Optimal timing of coronary artery bypass grafting in acute myocardial infarction. *Ann Thorac Surg.* 2013; 95:365–372.
8. Ha LD, Ogunbayo G, Elbadawi A et al. Early versus delayed coronary artery bypass graft surgery for patients with non-ST elevation myocardial infarction. *Coron Artery Dis.* 2017;28(8):670–674.
9. Davierwala PM, Verevkin A, Leontyev S et al. Does timing of coronary artery bypass surgery affect early and long-term outcomes in patients with myocardial infarction? *Circulation.* 2015;132:731–740.
10. Nichols EL, McCullough JN, Ross CS et al. For the Northern New England Cardiovascular Disease Study Group. Optimal timing from myocardial infarction to coronary artery Bypass grafting on hospital mortality. *Ann Thorac Surg.* 2017;103:162–171.
11. Weiss ES, Chang DD, Joyce DL et al. Optimal timing of coronary artery bypass after acute myocardial infarction: A review of California discharge data. *J Thorac Cardiovasc Surg.* 2008;135:503–511.
12. Bana A, Yadava OP, Ghadiok R et al. Myocardial revascularisation after acute myocardial infarction. *Int J Cardiol.* 1999;69:209–216.

13. Rohn V, Grus T, Belohlavek J, Horak J. Surgical revascularisation in the early phase of ST-segment elevation myocardial infarction: Haemodynamic status is more important than the timing of the operation. *Heart Lung Circ.* 2017;26(12):1323–1329.

14. Wiviott SD, Braunwald E, McCabe CH et al. Prasugrel versus clopidogrel in patients with acute coronary syndromes. *N Engl J Med.* 2007;357:2001–2015.

15. James SK, Roe MT, Cannon CP et al. Ticagrelor versus clopidogrel in patients with acute coronary syndromes intended for non-invasive management: Substudy from prospective randomised PLATelet inhibition and patient Outcomes (PLATO) trial. *BMJ.* 2011;342:d3527.

16. Hansson EC, Jidéus L, Åberg B et al. Coronary artery bypass grafting-related bleeding complications in patients treated with ticagrelor or clopidogrel: A nationwide study. *Eur Heart J.* 2016;37:189–197.

17. Khan MF, Wendel CS, Movahed MR. Prevention of post-coronary artery bypass grafting (CABG) atrial fibrillation: Efficacy of prophylactic beta-blockers in the modern era: A meta-analysis of latest randomized controlled trials. *Ann Noninvasive Electrocardiol.* 2013;18:58–68.

18. Bhayana JH, Kalmbach T, Booth FVM et al. Combined antegrade/retrograde cardioplegia for myocardial protection: A clinical trial. *J Thorac Cardiovasc Surg.* 1989;98:956–960.

19. Allen BS, Rosen Kranz E, Buckberg GD et al. Myocardial infarction with left ventricular power failure: A medical surgical emergency requiring urgent revascularisation with maximal protection of remote muscle. *J Thorac Cardiovasc Surg.* 1989;98:691–703.

20. Sintek F, Pfeffer TA, Khonsari S. Surgical revascularisation after acute myocardial infarction: Does timing make a difference? *J Thorac Cardiovasc Surg.* 1994;107:1317–1322.

21. Khaladj N, Bobylev D, Peterss S et al. Immediate surgical coronary revascularisation in patients presenting with acute myocardial infarction. *J Cardiothorac Surg.* 2013; 8:167.

22. Lee DC, Oz MC, Weinberg AD et al. Optimal timing of revascularisation: Transmural versus non-transmural acute myocardial infarction. *Ann Thorac Surg.* 2001;71:1198–1204.

23. Grothusen C, Friedrich C, Loehr J et al. Outcome of stable patients with acute myocardial infarction and coronary artery bypass surgery within 48 hours: A single-center, retrospective experience. *Am Heart Assoc.* 2017;6(10):e005498.

24. Rodriguez A, Bernardi V, Navia J et al. Argentine randomized study: Coronary angioplasty with stenting versus coronary bypass surgery in patients with multiple-vessel disease (ERACI II): 30-day and one-year follow-up results. *J Am Coll Cardiol.* 2001;37:51–58.

25. Ruivo C, Sa FM, Santos LG et al. On behalf of Portuguese National Registry of Acute Coronary Syndromes. PCI or CABG in NSTEMI patients with multivessel disease: Which has more in-hospital events? https://academic.oup.com/eurheartj/article-abstract/38/Suppl_1/ehx493.P6478/4087497

26. Chang M, Lee CW, Ahn JM et al. Comparison of outcome of coronary artery bypass grafting versus drug-eluting stent implantation for non-ST-elevation acute coronary syndrome. *Am J Cardiol.* 1 Aug 2017;120(3):380–386.

27. Ramanathan K, Abel JG, Park JE et al. Surgical versus percutaneous coronary revascularization in patients with diabetes and acute coronary syndromes. *J Am Coll Cardiol.* 19 Dec 2017;70(24):2995–3006.

28. Caggegi A, Capodanno D, Capranzano P et al. Comparison of one-year outcomes of percutaneous coronary intervention versus coronary artery bypass grafting in patients with unprotected left main coronary artery disease and acute coronary syndromes (from the CUSTOMIZE Registry). *Am J Cardiol.* 2011;108:355–359.

29. Patel MR, Dehmer GJ, Hirshfeld JW et al. ACCF/SCAI/STS/AATS/AHA/ASNC/HFSA/SCCT 2012 Appropriate use criteria for coronary revascularization focused update. *J Am Coll Cardiol.* 2012;59:857–881.

30. Roe MT, Li S, Thomas L et al. Long-term outcomes after invasive management for older patients with non-ST-segment elevation myocardial infarction. *Circ Cardiovasc Qual Outcomes.* 2013;6:323–332.

31. Clemmensen P, Roe MT, Hochman JS et al. TRILOGY ACS Investigators. Long-term outcomes for women versus men with unstable angina/non-ST-segment elevation myocardial infarction managed medically without revascularization: Insights from the TaRgeted platelet Inhibition to cLarify the Optimal strateGy to medicallY manage Acute Coronary Syndromes trial. *Am Heart J.* 2015;170:695.e5–705.e5.

32. Hochman JS, Sleeper LA, Webb JG et al. Early revascularization and long-term survival in cardiogenic shock complicating acute myocardial infarction. *JAMA.* 2006;295:2511–2515.

33. De Backer D, Biston P, Devriendt J et al. Comparison of dopamine and norepinephrine in the treatment of shock. *N Engl J Med.* 2010:362:779–789.

34. Kaya K, Cavolli R, Telli A et al. Off-pump versus on-pump coronary artery bypass grafting in acute coronary syndrome: A clinical analysis. *J Cardiothorac Surg.* 2010;5:31.

35. Jasinski MJ, Wos S, Olszowka P et al. Primary OPCAB as a strategy for acute coronary syndrome and acute myocardial infarction. *Heart Surg Forum.* 2003;6:31–35.

36. Mohr R, Moshkovitch Y, Shapira I et al. Coronary artery bypass without cardiopulmonary bypass for patients with acute myocardial infarction. *J Thorac and Cardiovasc Surg.* 1999;118(1):50–56.

37. Thiele H, Schuler G, Neumann FJ et al. Intraaortic balloon counterpulsation in acute myocardial infarction complicated by cardiogenic shock: Design and rationale of the Intraaortic Balloon Pump in Cardiogenic Shock II (IABP-SHOCK II) trial. *Am Heart J.* 2012;163:938–945.

38. Caceres M, Esmailian F, Moriguchi JD et al. Mechanical circulatory support in cardiogenic shock following an acute myocardial infarction: A systematic review. *J Card Surg.* 2014;29(5):743–751.

39. Khan MH, Corbett BJ, Hollenberg SM. Mechanical circulatory support in acute cardiogenic shock F1000Prime Reports [Internet]. 2014;6. Available from: http://www.scopus.com/inward/record.url?eid=2-s2.0-84908255982&partnerID=40&md5=20800b84a7a8c81cc91a86b7a39db05

40. Sodha NR, Sellke FW. The effect of statins on perioperative inflammation in cardiac and thoracic surgery. *J Thorac Cardiovasc Surg.* 2015;149:1495–1501.

41. Collard CD, Body SC, Shernan SK et al. Preoperative statin therapy is associated with reduced cardiac mortality after coronary artery bypass graft surgery. *J Thorac Cardiovasc Surg.* 2006;132:392–400.

42. Hillis LD, Smith PK, Anderson JL et al. 2011 ACCF/AHA Guideline for Coronary Artery Bypass Graft Surgery: Executive summary: A report of the American College of Cardiology Foundation/American Heart Association Task Force on Practice Guidelines. *Circulation.* 2011;124:2610–2642.

43. Kulik A. Ruel M. Jneid H. Secondary prevention after coronary artery bypass graft surgery: A scientific statement from the American Heart Association. *Circulation.* 2015; 131:927–964.

44. Levine GN, Bakaeen FG. Adding CABG to the dual antiplatelet salad. *J Am Coll Cardiol.* 2017;69(2):128–130.

45. Levine GN, Bates ER, Bittl JA et al. 2016 ACC/AHA Guideline focused update on duration of dual antiplatelet therapy in patients with coronary artery disease: A report of the American College of Cardiology/American Heart Association Task Force on Clinical Practice Guidelines. *J Am Coll Cardiol.* 2016;68:1082–1115.

46. Joo JH, Liao JM, Bakaeen FG, Chu D. Surgical revascularization for acute coronary syndromes: A narrative review. *Vessel Plus.* 2018;2:2.

21

Acute coronary syndrome with haemodynamic instability

DAVINDER SINGH CHADHA AND KESHAVAMURTHY GANAPATHY BHAT

INTRODUCTION

Acute coronary syndrome (ACS) is the most common cardiac emergency which includes unstable angina (UA), non-ST-elevation myocardial infarction (NSTEMI) and ST-segment elevation myocardial infarction (STEMI). It is often accompanied by haemodynamic instability which is seen in up to 10% of patients and carries worse prognoses.

Sudden onset myocardial ischaemia may result in systolic and diastolic dysfunction, thereby causing inadequate tissue perfusion failure and elevated filling pressure leading to a state of cardiogenic shock (CS). CS is characterised by persistent hypotension (systolic blood pressure <80–90 mmHg or mean arterial pressure 30 mmHg lower than baseline) with severe reduction in the cardiac index (<1.8 L/min per m² without support or <2 to 2.2 L/min per m² with support) and adequate or elevated filling pressures [1,2]. CS in ACS carries a mortality of 50% [1,2]. The outcome is directly related to the severity of haemodynamic compromise and multi-organ dysfunction due to ongoing organ hypoperfusion. In this review we discuss the causes and contemporary management of ACS with haemodynamic instability.

CAUSES OF HAEMODYNAMIC INSTABILITY IN ACS

Impaired cardiac performance is the most frequent mechanism of haemodynamic instability. The most common aetiology of CS in ACS is an acute myocardial infarction (usually ST-elevation myocardial infarction) with left ventricular failure (less commonly right ventricular failure), but it can also be caused by mechanical complications, such as acute mitral regurgitation or rupture of either the ventricular septal or free walls [2,3].

CS is noted in 7.5% of ST-elevation MI and in approximately 2.5% of patients with a non-ST-elevation MI [1,2,4,5]. It generally develops after a median interval of 6.2 hours post MI. Severe dysfunction is often associated with an anterior MI, but may result from an infarct in any location, particularly in patients who have had a prior infarct.

The predictors of the early shock include extensive ischaemia due to left main or multi-vessel coronary artery stenosis, multiple infarct locations, chest pain at the onset of shock, inferior wall MI and ST elevation in >2 leads. While recurrent ischaemia, left anterior artery stenosis and Q wave in >2 leads predicts late onset of CS, autopsy studies in patients dying with CS due to acute MI have revealed that ≥40% of the LV myocardium is infarcted (old and new) [6]. Most patients have severe three vessel coronary disease on coronary angiography. Severe right ventricular (RV) failure is a cause of, or a major contributor to, CS in 5% of cases and is typically seen with an inferior MI [1,2].

Mechanical complications causing CS include:

- Acute, severe mitral regurgitation due to rupture of a papillary muscle or chordae tendineae or severe papillary muscle dysfunction. This is more common in the setting of infero-posterior infarction [2,7].
- Ventricular septal rupture after either an anterior or inferior infarction, with an acute left-to-right shunt, which is associated with the highest risk of in-hospital mortality (87%) [8].
- Cardiac tamponade which occurs after rupture of the LV free wall or a haemorrhagic pericardial effusion.

Contributing factors: In the setting of acute MI, other factors may contribute to hypotension:

- Severe bradycardia, due either to complete heart block or sinus bradycardia.
- Bradycardia can cause a low cardiac output and hypotension in the setting of an acute MI with impaired ventricular function.
- Haemorrhagic shock due to treatment with fibrinolytic agents and anti-coagulants.
- Septic shock in patients with indwelling catheters or suspected infectious foci. Hypovolemia from any cause including diuretic therapy.
- Severe valvular heart disease with limited cardiac reserve, such as in critical aortic stenosis. These patients can present with CS with even a small infarction.
- The excessive use of anti-hypertensive and/or negative inotropic medications.
- Rapid atrial arrhythmias, such as atrial fibrillation with rapid ventricular response or ventricular tachycardia.

Risk factors: Older age, anterior myocardial infarction (MI), history of hypertension, diabetes mellitus, multi-vessel coronary artery disease, prior MI, systolic blood pressure <120 mmHg, heart rate >90 beats per minute, diagnosis of heart failure on admission, ST-elevation MI and left bundle branch block on the electrocardiogram are risk factors and predictors of CS complicating acute MI [1,2,9].

PATHOPHYSIOLOGY

Acute MI, due to acute occlusion of one or more coronary arteries, is the most common clinical entity leading to CS. This results in failure of the left or right ventricle to pump an adequate amount of blood (<2.2 L/min/m^2) and elevated filling pressures of the ventricular chambers. Hypotension, tissue hypoperfusion and pulmonary and systemic venous congestion follows [1,2,10,11]. The reduction in tissue perfusion results in decreased oxygen and nutrient delivery to the tissues and, if prolonged, potentially end-organ damage and multi-system failure sets in.

The systemic vascular resistance is often high, but it may be in the normal or low range. The fall in blood pressure may in part be moderated by a marked elevation in systemic vascular resistance (SVR), a response that is mediated by increased release of endogenous vasopressors such as norepinephrine and angiotensin II.

The combination of a low cardiac output and elevated SVR may result in a marked reduction in tissue perfusion. Individuals with the associated decrease in coronary perfusion pressure can lead to a vicious cycle of ischaemia, further myocardial dysfunction and a downward spiral with progressive end-organ hypoperfusion and ultimately death [12,13].

In addition, the acute inflammatory response in MI is associated with elevated serum cytokine concentrations [14,15]. Cytokine activation leads to induction of nitric oxide (NO) synthase and increased levels of NO, which can cause inappropriate vasodilation with reduced systemic and coronary perfusion pressure [10,16]. These are individuals with normal or low range of systemic vascular resistance who represent a group of patients with more profound hypoperfusion and inflammatory response and carry worse prognoses [11].

CLINICAL FEATURES

The classic picture of CS is hypotension, signs of systemic hypoperfusion (e.g. cool extremities, oliguria and/or alteration in mental status) and respiratory distress due to pulmonary congestion. However, not all patients present with these classic features. The majority of patients have new or worsening hypotension, tachycardia and tachypnea. The following signs are variable [2,17,18]: distended neck veins, coolness of the skin, rales, gallop rhythm or new heart murmur and decreased volume and intensity of the distal pulses. Right ventricular MI and shock is characterised by the absence of pulmonary congestion and the presence of jugular venous distension.

The development of late CS may be related to recurrent ischaemia or reinfarction or to mechanical complications, such as rupture of the ventricular septum, ventricular free wall, or papillary muscle. Some cases of late CS are in part iatrogenic due to medications [19].

Recently, SCAI clinical expert group has described five stages of cardiogenic shock from A to E [20]. Stage A is 'at risk' for CS, stage B is 'beginning' of CS, stage C is 'classic' CS, stage D is 'deteriorating' and E is 'extremis'. Features of hypoperfusion are present in stages C and higher. Stage D implies deteriorating clinical status despite initial interventions and 30 minutes of observation. Stage E is the extremis where the patient is highly unstable, often with cardiovascular collapse and cardiopulmonary resuscitation (CPR).

INVESTIGATIONS AND DIAGNOSIS

The diagnostic evaluation in these patients should be carried out in conjunction with resuscitative efforts. ECG is generally the first investigation which confirms ACS by fresh ST-T changes and Q waves or new onset LBBB.

CS is suspected in patients with ACS if they have worsening of chest pain or dyspnoea accompanied by hypotension and features of other organ hypoperfusion, suggested by cold clammy skin, altered sensorium, diminished urine output, etc.

The diagnosis of CS is established when the haemodynamic profile shows arterial hypotension (a persistent systolic blood pressure below 90 mmHg or a mean blood pressure 30 mmHg lower than the patient's baseline level), a severe reduction in the cardiac index (<1.8 L/min per m^2 without support or <2.2 L/min per m^2 with support) and an elevated pulmonary capillary wedge pressure (PCWP) above approximately 15 mmHg.

Laboratory testing including complete blood count, biochemistry (including blood sugar, renal function and electrolyte status), prothrombin and partial thromboplastin times, quantitative troponin measurements, acid base gas (ABG) analysis and a chest radiograph should be done in all patients. Patients who present with acute MI with electrocardiographic abnormalities should undergo a quick echocardiogram to determine the ventricular function and also to detect any associated mechanical complications (tamponade, severe mitral regurgitation, ventricular septal or free-wall rupture). The diagnosis of right ventricular MI is suspected in patients with inferior MI, clear lung fields and shock. Placement of a Swan-Ganz catheter to confirm diagnosis, guide management and assess the need for more aggressive mechanical cardiac support if the patient has not responded to initial resuscitative efforts [2,13,21,22] is recommended.

Coronary angiography (or repeat coronary angiography) should be performed in all patients with CS and ACS. They are candidates for revascularisation with either percutaneous coronary intervention (PCI) or coronary artery bypass graft surgery (CABG) [21]. All patients who have undergone reperfusion with fibrinolytic therapy should be evaluated emergently for failure of reperfusion if they exhibit new or persistent signs of CS.

DIFFERENTIAL DIAGNOSIS

The diagnosis of CS in ACS is usually confirmed with typical clinical and haemodynamic profile and a bedside echocardiogram. However, other clinical scenarios at times may mimic this presentation, for example acute MI with shock due to non-cardiac causes such as sepsis from an indwelling catheter or hypovolemia caused by overaggressive diuresis. The haemodynamic profile of patients with shock due to sepsis or hypovolemia generally differs from that of patients with CS.

Cardiovascular diseases in which the primary problem is not acute MI are:

- Stress-induced cardiomyopathy (Takotsubo cardiomyopathy) with characteristic finding of apical ballooning as seen on left ventriculography accompanied with ST-elevation on ECG and may present with CS in 20% patients [23].
- Hypertrophic cardiomyopathy or acute myopericarditis. These may present with any combination of chest pain, ST or T wave changes on ECG and hypotension.
- Pulmonary embolism.
- Acute MI due to ascending aortic dissection. Shock in this setting can result from the infarction caused by occlusion of one or more coronary arteries, acute aortic insufficiency and/or cardiac tamponade.

MANAGEMENT

A summary of various treatment options is given in Table 21.1.

General principles: Correction of hypoxemia and lactic acidosis is important since they lead to myocardial depression and decrease the responsiveness to vasopressors and inotropes. In addition, shock in the setting of ACS may also be caused by overzealous use of diuretics, beta-blockers or anti-hypertensives. Haemodynamic management options comprise fluid resuscitation to increase preload (in RVMI), administration of vasopressors to maintain systemic blood pressure, administration of inotropes to increase contractility and cardiac output and early revascularisation with or without mechanical circulatory support (MCS) devices.

MEDICATIONS

Oral anti-platelet therapy: All patients should receive soluble/chewable aspirin (150–325 mg). If patient is intubated without a nasogastric tube, alternative options include crushing a tablet for absorption through the buccal mucosa or administration of a rectal suppository.

P2Y12 inhibitors should be deferred until after angiography, as many with MI and CS will require urgent CABG. When P2Y12 inhibitors are deferred, glycoprotein (GP) IIb/IIIa inhibitors should be used as soon as possible after the decision has been made to proceed to angiography. GP IIb/IIIa inhibitors improve the outcome of patients with non-ST-elevation acute coronary syndrome (ACS). A possible mechanism of benefit is relief of microvascular obstruction.

Glucose control: Very tight glycemic control is not warranted. Glucose level should be maintained between 120–180 mg/dl.

Heparin: Intravenous heparin infusion, especially in conjunction with reperfusion therapy, reduces mortality in acute MI. The dosage of heparin is given in Table 21.1 [20].

Vasopressors and inotropes: Sympathomimetic inotropic and vasopressor agents remain the mainstay of first-line therapy. However, all these agents increase cardiac work and raise the PCWP, hence the minimum required dose should be used [21]. The indication and dosage of various vasopressors is given in Table 21.2.

- Norepinephrine is a potent vasopressor with some positive inotropic properties that may be used for rapid initial circulatory support for CS.
- Dopamine has its effects based upon the dose administered. At low doses, it has primarily positive inotropic effects but at higher doses it stimulates alpha adrenergic receptors, resulting in vasoconstriction and increased systemic vascular resistance. High dosage results in undesirable elevation in pulmonary capillary wedge pressure (PCWP). While historically dopamine has been chosen before norepinephrine, some evidence suggests that outcomes may be better with norepinephrine.
- Dobutamine may be used in less sick patients with a low cardiac index and high PCWP but without severe hypotension (e.g. systolic blood pressure >80 mmHg).

Repeat haemodynamic assessment with insertion of haemodynamic (PCWP) catheter is done to guide therapeutic intervention (fluid replacement and vasopressor dosage). However, reperfusion therapy should not be delayed for the sake of insertion of a haemodynamic catheter [17,21,22]. Optimal PCWP for each patient is the lowest value that results in the highest cardiac output as long as the SaO2 is above 90%. The usual value in acute MI-related CS is between 18 and 25 mmHg [25].

- Assessment of cardiac filling pressures so that hypovolemia and volume overload can be identified and corrected. Right ventricular (RV) MI often seen with inferior wall MI when complicated with CS may require more volume support as filling pressures are increased. Intravenous (IV) fluid replacement in these patients is indicated even if jugular

Table 21.1 Treatment options for patients with cardiogenic shock

S. No.	Treatment option	Remarks
1.	**General measures**	
	Ventilator support	This should be in the form of non-invasive or endotracheal intubation in order to correct hypoxemia and accompanying acidosis.
	Optimise intravascular volume	Use pulmonary wedge catheter to guide the fluid therapy. Use sodium bicarbonate only for severe metabolic acidosis (arterial pH less than 7.10 to 7.15).
	Pharmacotherapy	Anti-platelet agents – aspirin 75–150 mg, withhold a thienopyridine until after diagnostic coronary angiography. Glycoprotein (GP) IIb/IIIa inhibitor should be added coronary intervention is planned.
		Heparin as a 60 units/kg bolus (maximum 4000 units) followed by an intravenous infusion of 12 units/kg per hour (maximum 1000 units per hour) adjusted to target aPTT of 50 to 70 seconds should be given as indicated.
		Vasopressors are used for hypotension (systolic blood pressure <80 mmHg). Norepinephrine is preferred as the initial agent.
2.	**Mechanical support**	
	Intra-aortic balloon pump	Used in patients who do not stabilise on initial pharmacotherapy usually combined with percutaneous coronary intervention or coronary artery bypass graft surgery or possible thrombolytic therapy who are not fit for transfer to facility capable of performing urgent revascularisation.
	Extra-corporeal membrane oxygenator	
	Left ventricular or biventricular assist devices	Patients whose haemodynamic parameters and clinical status are rapidly deteriorating while on vasopressor and inotropic support after revascularisation, and are candidates for bridge to transplantation or wearable ventricular assist device.
3.	**Reperfusion/ Revascularisation**	All patients with CS complicating MI should undergo an attempt at reperfusion. An open infarct-related artery in patients with CS and ACS correlates strongly with in-hospital survival.
	Fibrinolytic therapy	Fibrinolysis is recommended if PCI is not possible or if it is significantly delayed.
	Primary percutaneous coronary intervention (PCI)	For patients with ST-elevation MI, revascularisation as opposed to fibrinolytic therapy should be attempted. Fibrinolytic therapy should be used only when PCI is not possible. In absence of mechanical complications, PCI is preferred in patients with double or triple vessel or left main disease.
	Coronary artery bypass graft (CABG)	CABG is preferred in patients with mechanical complications.

Table 21.2 Vasopressors and inotropes in treatment of cardiogenic shock

Agent	Dose	Remarks
Norepinephrine (noradrenaline)	8–12 mcg/min (0.1–0.15 mcg/kg/min) Refractory cases – 35–100 mcg/min (0.5–0.75 mcg/kg/min)	Initial vasopressor of choice in septic, cardiogenic and hypovolemic shock.
Epinephrine (adrenaline)	1–10 mcg/min (0.014–0.14 mcg/kg/min) Refractory cases – 10–35 mcg/min (0.14–0.5 mcg/kg/min)	Typically, an add-on agent to norepinephrine, however, increases heart rate; may induce tachyarrhythmias and cause ischemia.
Dopamine	5–20 mcg/kg/min Refractory cases – 20 to >50 mcg/kg/min	An alternative to norepinephrine in patients with compromised systolic function or absolute or relative bradycardia. More adverse effects at doses ≥20 mcg/kg/min and less effective than norepinephrine for reversing hypotension in septic shock.
Dobutamine	5–20 mcg/kg/min	Initial agent of choice in cardiogenic shock with low cardiac output and maintained blood pressure. Add-on to norepinephrine for cardiac output augmentation in patients with myocardial dysfunction.
Vasopressin (arginine-vasopressin)	0.01–0.03 units/min	Add-on to norepinephrine to raise blood pressure to target mean arterial pressure. Pure vasoconstrictor; may decrease stroke volume and cardiac output in myocardial dysfunction or precipitate ischaemia in coronary artery disease.
Milrinone	0.125–0.75 mcg/kg/min Dose adjustment in renal impairment needed.	Alternative for short-term cardiac output augmentation to maintain organ perfusion in cardiogenic shock refractory to other agents. May cause peripheral vasodilation, hypotension and/or ventricular arrhythmia.

(central) venous pressure is not elevated. Excess fluid replacement may, however, lead to RV dilatation with septal shift into the left ventricular and compromise its filling [26]. An early echocardiogram can be performed in this setting to guide clinical management.

- Evaluation of the response of cardiac output to therapeutic interventions, including volume management, sympathomimetics and mechanical support.
- Detection and quantification of intracardiac shunting in ventricular septal defect complicating acute MI.
- Calculation of systemic vascular resistance and discrimination of vasoconstrictive from vasodilatory shock.

Ventilatory support: This is indicated in patients of CS with the following conditions:

- Patients with deterioration of consciousness or cardiac arrest to protect the airway and maintain oxygen supply.
- Patients with acute respiratory failure most often due to cardiogenic pulmonary oedema.
- Patients with metabolic acidosis to ease the work of breathing and correct the pH.

MECHANICAL CIRCULATORY SUPPORT (MCS)

Intra-aortic balloon pump: Routine use of an intra-aortic balloon pump (IABP) in patients with ACS complicated by CS is not recommended. However, patients with mechanical defects (such as mitral regurgitation or a ventricular septal defect) and selected other patients who are rapidly deteriorating may benefit from MCS devices. The role of IABP in MI patients treated with fibrinolytic therapy who will be transferred for possible revascularisation is not well established.

The use of the IABP for AMI shock failed to demonstrate a significant difference in mortality over standard therapy at either 30 days or 1 year and this has led to its use in AMI being downgraded to class IIa from class I [27–29].

Other mechanical devices: Patients with AMI and CS have significant amounts of stunned myocardium that could potentially recover over time post-revascularisation. There was a need for a mechanical support device other than IABP which could provide better support. This led to the development and rapid evolution of entirely new types of mechanical devices which could provide greater support.

These include:

- Percutaneous transvalvular left ventricular assist device (Impella LP 2.5 or Impella CP). This is placed via the femoral artery, retrograde across the aortic valve into the left ventricle. It decompresses the left ventricle and delivers a maximum flow of 2.5 to 4.0 L/min into the ascending aorta, thereby leading to reduction of ventricular workload and oxygen consumption. The device has been approved for use in AMI-related CS based on circulatory support effect. The Impella RP System (Abiomed, United States) is a right ventricular assist device (RVAD) that provides peripherally-placed circulatory support in patients with refractory RV shock.

- Left ventricular and biventricular assist devices. In the setting of CS, these surgically placed devices are usually placed as a bridge to recovery or as a bridge to transplantation. The other device which can be used is a percutaneous left atrial-to-femoral arterial ventricular assist device (Tandem Heart).
- Percutaneous cardiopulmonary bypass support with use of an extracorporeal membrane oxygenator (ECMO) may be utilized when oxygenation is severely impaired to stabilise the patient and allow organ function recovery, followed by a delayed CABG.

Most of the studies with the mechanical support devices have been non-randomised and underpowered to demonstrate a survival benefit. The lack of clinical trials to demonstrate superiority of these devices over IABP in AMI is due to the fact that patients with the diagnosis of AMI and CS are a heterogeneous group. These patients are often very unstable with varying degrees of shock, previous infarction and have variable potential for improvement hence are challenging to enroll in clinical trials.

REPERFUSION/REVASCULARISATION

The high mortality associated with CS has improved over time [2,30–33]. This benefit is predominantly due to increased use of coronary reperfusion strategies which limit infarct size as well as interrupt the vicious spiral that characterises CS [2,30,31,34]. Outcomes are better when successful reperfusion can be delivered early in the course of myocardial infarction (MI). The short-term and long-term mortality in patients with CS is significantly lower among those who underwent revascularisation [35].

Fibrinolysis: Fibrinolysis is recommended if PCI is not possible. The choice of agent should probably not be different from patients without CS. The window period is 12 hours, however, it may be administered post 12 hours in patients who develop shock late due to recurrent coronary artery occlusion and urgent angiography and revascularisation is not possible.

Percutaneous coronary intervention (PCI): If the facilities exist, PCI is preferred to fibrinolysis [2,34,35]. Immediate PCI should be performed on the culprit lesion(s) of the infarct-related artery, while PCI of severe disease in other vessels should be deferred [36,37].

The clinical response to primary PCI is highly variable. In-hospital mortality after PCI is related to the degree of reperfusion achieved in the infarct-related artery [38]. Among 276 patients undergoing PCI, the mortality for TIMI grade 3 (normal), grade 2, or grade 0/1 flow was 33%, 50% and 86%, respectively. The time from symptom onset to PCI may be another determinant of outcome. However, late presenters should not be denied emergency revascularisation based upon timing alone. PCI is efficacious in LMCA occlusion and stenting fares better than POBA alone [24]. Although emergent CABG is a revascularisation option, it appears to be seldom utilised in contemporary clinical practice [31].

Coronary artery bypass surgery: The majority of patients with CS after MI have significant left main or three vessel disease (16% and 53%, respectively, in the SHOCK trial registry) [34]. In such patients, the ability to achieve complete revascularisation makes CABG a potentially critical therapeutic strategy. A surgical approach also permits the correction of concomitant severe

Risk stratification of patient in emergency department by multi-disciplinary team

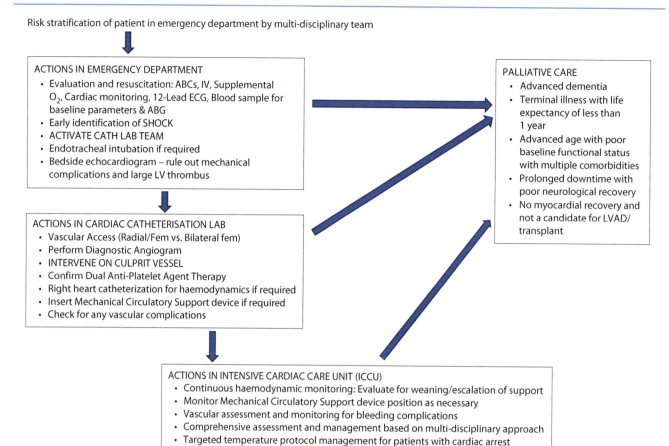

ACTIONS IN EMERGENCY DEPARTMENT
- Evaluation and resuscitation: ABCs, IV, Supplemental O_2, Cardiac monitoring, 12-Lead ECG, Blood sample for baseline parameters & ABG
- Early identification of SHOCK
- ACTIVATE CATH LAB TEAM
- Endotracheal intubation if required
- Bedside echocardiogram – rule out mechanical complications and large LV thrombus

PALLIATIVE CARE
- Advanced dementia
- Terminal illness with life expectancy of less than 1 year
- Advanced age with poor baseline functional status with multiple comorbidities
- Prolonged downtime with poor neurological recovery
- No myocardial recovery and not a candidate for LVAD/ transplant

ACTIONS IN CARDIAC CATHETERISATION LAB
- Vascular Access (Radial/Fem vs. Bilateral fem)
- Perform Diagnostic Angiogram
- INTERVENE ON CULPRIT VESSEL
- Confirm Dual Anti-Platelet Agent Therapy
- Right heart catheterization for haemodynamics if required
- Insert Mechanical Circulatory Support device if required
- Check for any vascular complications

ACTIONS IN INTENSIVE CARDIAC CARE UNIT (ICCU)
- Continuous haemodynamic monitoring: Evaluate for weaning/escalation of support
- Monitor Mechanical Circulatory Support device position as necessary
- Vascular assessment and monitoring for bleeding complications
- Comprehensive assessment and management based on multi-disciplinary approach
- Targeted temperature protocol management for patients with cardiac arrest

Figure 21.1 Management of cardiogenic shock in acute coronary syndrome.

mitral regurgitation, which is often present. Pooled data on 370 patients in 22 studies revealed an in-hospital mortality rate of 36% when CABG was performed during the hospitalisation for acute MI with CS [38]. Despite this benefit, CABG is underutilised in the community setting.

An algorithmic approach to CS in ACS is depicted in Figure 21.1.

CONCLUSION

The mortality of CS patients is still unacceptably high at around 50%. The incidence of CS, however, is slightly declining, due to more rapid and efficient reperfusion. A multi-disciplinary team at a specialised centre may improve the clinical outcome of these patients. Currently, there are many unsettled issues, such as the type of reperfusion (culprit-lesion-only PCI vs. multi-vessel PCI), the optimal inotrope or vasopressor support, treatment of bleeding complications, and the optimal timing, type and role of different mechanical support devices. If patients are treated according to guidelines with an early reperfusion and an optimal intensive care treatment the outcomes of CS may improve further.

REFERENCES

1. Reynolds HR, Hochman JS. Cardiogenic shock: Current concepts and improving outcomes. *Circulation* 2008;117:686.

2. van Diepen S, Katz JN, Albert NM et al.; on behalf of the American Heart Association Council on Clinical Cardiology; Council on Cardiovascular and Stroke Nursing; Council on Quality of Care and Outcomes Research; and Mission: Lifeline. Contemporary management of cardiogenic shock: A scientific statement from the American Heart Association. *Circulation* 2017;136:e232–e268.

3. Hochman JS, Boland J, Sleeper LA et al. Current spectrum of cardiogenic shock and effect of early revascularization on mortality. Results of an International Registry. SHOCK Registry Investigators. *Circulation* 1995;91:873.

4. Holmes DR Jr, Berger PB, Hochman JS et al. Cardiogenic shock in patients with acute ischemic syndromes with and without ST-segment elevation. *Circulation* 1999;100:2067.

5. Hasdai D, Harrington RA, Hochman JS et al. Platelet glycoprotein IIb/IIIa blockade and outcome of cardiogenic shock complicating acute coronary syndromes without persistent ST-segment elevation. *J Am Coll Cardiol.* 2000;36:685.

6. Alonso DR, Scheidt S, Post M, Killip T. Pathophysiology of cardiogenic shock. Quantification of myocardial necrosis, clinical, pathologic and electrocardiographic correlations. *Circulation* 1973;48:588.

7. Picard MH, Davidoff R, Sleeper LA et al. Echocardiographic predictors of survival and response to early revascularization in cardiogenic shock. *Circulation* 2003;107:279.

8. Menon V, Webb JG, Hillis LD et al. Outcome and profile of ventricular septal rupture with cardiogenic shock after

myocardial infarction: A report from the SHOCK Trial Registry. SHould we emergently revascularize Occluded Coronaries in cardiogenic shocK? *J Am Coll Cardiol.* 2000;36:1110.

9. Hasdai D, Califf RM, Thompson TD et al. Predictors of cardiogenic shock after thrombolytic therapy for acute myocardial infarction. *J Am Coll Cardiol.* 2000;35:136.

10. Hochman JS. Cardiogenic shock complicating acute myocardial infarction: Expanding the paradigm. *Circulation* 2003;107:2998.

11. Kohsaka S, Menon V, Lowe AM et al. Systemic inflammatory response syndrome after acute myocardial infarction complicated by cardiogenic shock. *Arch Intern Med.* 2005;165:1643.

12. Hollenberg SM, Kavinsky CJ, Parrillo JE. Cardiogenic shock. *Ann Intern Med.* 1999;131:47.

13. Califf RM, Bengtson JR. Cardiogenic shock. *N Engl J Med.* 1994;330:1724.

14. Frangogiannis NG, Smith CW, Entman ML. The inflammatory response in myocardial infarction. *Cardiovasc Res.* 2002;53:31.

15. Neumann FJ, Ott I, Gawaz M et al. Cardiac release of cytokines and inflammatory responses in acute myocardial infarction. *Circulation* 1995;92:748.

16. Wildhirt SM, Dudek RR, Suzuki H, Bing RJ. Involvement of inducible nitric oxide synthase in the inflammatory process of myocardial infarction. *Int J Cardiol.* 1995;50:253.

17. Menon V, White H, LeJemtel T et al. The clinical profile of patients with suspected cardiogenic shock due to predominant left ventricular failure: A report from the SHOCK Trial Registry. SHould we emergently revascularize Occluded Coronaries in cardiogenic shocK? *J Am Coll Cardiol.* 2000;36:1071.

18. Menon V, Slater JN, White HD et al. Acute myocardial infarction complicated by systemic hypoperfusion without hypotension: Report of the SHOCK Trial Registry. *Am J Med.* 2000;108:374.

19. Nguyen HL, Yarzebski J, Lessard D et al. Ten-year (2001–2011) trends in the incidence rates and short-term outcomes of early versus late onset cardiogenic shock after hospitalization for acute myocardial infarction. *J Am Heart Assoc.* 2017;6.

20. Baran DA, Grines CL, Bailey S et al. SCAI clinical expert consensus statement on the classification of cardiogenic shock. *Catheter Cardiovasc Interv.* 2019;94(1):29–37.

21. Levine GN, O'Gara PT, Bates ER et al. 2015 ACC/AHA/SCAI focused update on primary percutaneous coronary intervention for patients with ST-elevation myocardial infarction: An update of the 2011 ACCF/AHA/SCAI guideline for percutaneous coronary intervention and the 2013 ACCF/AHA guideline for the management of ST-elevation myocardial infarction: A report of the American College of Cardiology/American Heart Association Task Force on Clinical Practice Guidelines and the Society for Cardiovascular Angiography and Interventions. *J Am Coll Cardiol.* 2016;67:1235–1250.

22. Mueller HS, Chatterjee K, Davis KB et al. ACC expert consensus document. Present use of bedside right heart catheterization in patients with cardiac disease. American College of Cardiology. *J Am Coll Cardiol.* 1998;32:840.

23. Chockalingam A, Tejwani L, Aggarwal K, Dellsperger KC. Dynamic left ventricular outflow tract obstruction in acute myocardial infarction with shock: Cause, effect, and coincidence. *Circulation* 2007;116:e110.

24. Marso SP, Steg G, Plokker T et al. Catheter-based reperfusion of unprotected left main stenosis during an acute myocardial infarction (the ULTIMA experience). Unprotected Left Main Trunk Intervention Multi-center Assessment. *Am J Cardiol.* 1999;83:1513.

25. Hochman JS, Ohman EM. Cardiogenic shock (AHA Clinical Series, 2009).

26. O'Gara PT, Kushner FG, Ascheim DD et al. 2013 ACCF/AHA guideline for the management of ST-elevation myocardial infarction: Executive summary: A report of the American College of Cardiology Foundation/American Heart Association Task Force on Practice Guidelines: Developed in collaboration with the American College of Emergency Physicians and Society for Cardiovascular Angiography and Interventions. *Catheter Cardiovasc Interv.* 2013;82:E1.

27. Task Force on the management of ST-segment elevation acute myocardial infarction of the European Society of Cardiology (ESC), Steg PG, James SK, Atar D et al. ESC Guidelines for the management of acute myocardial infarction in patients presenting with ST-segment elevation. *Eur Heart J.* 2012;33:2569.

28. Roffi M, Patrono C, Collet JP et al. 2015 ESC Guidelines for the management of acute coronary syndromes in patients presenting without persistent ST-segment elevation: Task Force for the Management of Acute Coronary Syndromes in Patients Presenting without Persistent ST-Segment Elevation of the European Society of Cardiology (ESC). *Eur Heart J.* 2016;37:267.

29. Goldberg RJ, Gore JM, Thompson CA, Gurwitz JH. Recent magnitude of and temporal trends (1994–1997) in the incidence and hospital death rates of cardiogenic shock complicating acute myocardial infarction: the second national registry of myocardial infarction. *Am Heart J.* 2001;141:65.

30. Goldberg RJ, Samad NA, Yarzebski J et al. Temporal trends in cardiogenic shock complicating acute myocardial infarction. *N Engl J Med.* 1999;340:1162.

31. Babaev A, Frederick PD, Pasta DJ et al. Trends in management and outcomes of patients with acute myocardial infarction complicated by cardiogenic shock. *JAMA* 2005;294:448.

32. Zeymer U, Vogt A, Zahn R et al. Predictors of in-hospital mortality in 1333 patients with acute myocardial infarction complicated by cardiogenic shock treated with primary percutaneous coronary intervention (PCI); Results of the primary PCI registry of the Arbeitsgemeinschaft Leitende Kardiologische Krankenhausärzte (ALKK). *Eur Heart J.* 2004;25:322.

33. Meinertz T, Kasper W, Schumacher M, Just H. The German multicenter trial of anisoylated plasminogen streptokinase activator complex versus heparin for acute myocardial infarction. *Am J Cardiol.* 1988;62:347.

34. Wong SC, Sanborn T, Sleeper LA et al. Angiographic findings and clinical correlates in patients with cardiogenic shock complicating acute myocardial infarction: A report from the SHOCK Trial Registry. SHould we emergently revascularize Occluded Coronaries for cardiogenic shocK? *J Am Coll Cardiol.* 2000;36:1077.

35. Berger PB, Holmes DR Jr, Stebbins AL et al. Impact of an aggressive invasive catheterization and revascularization strategy on mortality in patients with cardiogenic shock in the Global Utilization of Streptokinase and Tissue Plasminogen Activator for Occluded Coronary Arteries (GUSTO-I) trial. An observational study. *Circulation* 1997;96:122.

36. de Waha S, Jobs A, Eitel I et al. Multivessel versus culprit lesion only percutaneous coronary intervention in cardiogenic shock complicating acute myocardial infarction: A systematic review and meta-analysis. *Eur Heart J Acute Cardiovasc Care.* 2018;7:28.

37. Thiele H, Akin I, Sandri M et al. PCI strategies in patients with acute myocardial infarction and cardiogenic shock. *N Engl J Med.* 2017;377:2419.

38. Webb JG, Sanborn TA, Sleeper LA et al. Percutaneous coronary intervention for cardiogenic shock in the SHOCK Trial Registry. *Am Heart J.* 2001;141:964.

22

Acute coronary syndrome in special populations
Women, the elderly, chronic kidney disease and the young

PB JAYAGOPAL AND SAKALESH PATIL

INTRODUCTION

Coronary artery disease (CAD) is currently the most common, non-communicable disease in India and worldwide and will affect more than 65 million Indians by the year 2015. 'Time is muscle' is an old adage. Despite advances in the management of coronary artery disease especially in acute coronary syndrome, the Global Burden of Diseases study reported the estimated mortality from coronary artery disease in India as 1.6 million in the year 2000. It has been predicted that by the year 2020 there will be an increase by almost 75% in the global CVD burden [1]. Acute coronary syndrome encompasses ST-segment elevation and non-ST-segment elevation myocardial infarction (MI) and unstable angina. STEMI continues to be a challenge for treating physicians due to its varied presentations and complications on arrival.

The CREATE registry from India found that median pre-hospital delay was 600 minutes and was similar in both STEMI and NSTEMI. Only 33% reached within 6 hours from symptom onset. This focussed chapter discusses the presentations, problems and managing ACS in special populations, namely women, the elderly, patients with CKD and the young [2].

ACS IN WOMEN

It is a well-known fact that women are protected from coronary artery disease due to the protective oestrogen effect, hence their presentation with heart disease is at least 10 years later than in men. However, women often underestimate their symptoms, and therefore presentation is late. Absence of typical chest pain in many women or symptoms like arm pain, dizziness, fatigue sweating or jaw pain were often non-specific or less severe. The national registry of MI found the difference of symptom perception compared to men was 37% versus 27%. In the same study they found 42% of female patients had no chest pain. In a study of 82196 of which 21071 (25.6%) were women, women with ACS were older than men (69.0 vs. 61.1 yrs P < 0.001) and were found to have more comorbidities. Men were more likely to present with STEMI. Women were more likely to present with heart failure (9.1% vs. 5.7%, p<0.001) (probably an underestimation of symptoms as mentioned earlier). Cardiogenic shock (3.1% vs. 2.8% P = 0.004) was also more common in women [3].

In the Kerala ACS Registry of 5825 women out of 25748, women at presentation were 5 years older than men. However, in this registry outcome of death, stroke, heart failure, reinfarction and cardiogenic shock were statistically insignificant [4].

In the INTERHEART study, nine major risk factors were attributed to cardiovascular events, of which 94% of women were found with such risk factors. Diabetes mellitus and psychosocial risk factors had a greater impact on acute myocardial infarction in women. Eligible women were less likely to receive early oral anti-platelet therapy, heparin, diuretics, hospitalisation and reperfusion therapy for STEMI as compared to men [5].

STEMI in younger women is uncommon, but in pregnant women the incidence is found to be high compared to non-pregnant women. Probable aetiologies are atherosclerosis, coronary dissection, coronary artery spasm, APLA, Kawasaki disease and coronary thrombosis without atherosclerosis. Roth and Elkayam studied 96 women (angiogram/autopsy) and found atherosclerosis with or without coronary thrombosis in 40%. Their study found that atherosclerotic disease was more prevalent in the ante-partum period (54%) and coronary dissection as the primary cause in the peri-partum period (50%) [6].

Coronary spasm is often normal in pregnancy. Around 13% of coronary arteries in angiogram are found to be normal. Enhanced vascular reactivity, endothelial dysfunction, use of cigarettes and cocaine attributes to it. There is a higher prevalence of stress cardiomyopathy in women than men, comprising 90% of patients presenting with this condition. This unusual form of ACS usually occurs with acute emotional stress and is frequently accompanied by ECG ST-segment elevation and a rise in troponin levels.

The diagnosis of STEMI in pregnancy is often overlooked, probably due to rarity of the condition, symptoms of dyspnea, palpitation and chest discomfort attributed to pregnancy. CAG is warranted when other diagnostic tests are highly suggestive of STEMI. Coronary angiogram should be performed cautiously due to the fragile nature of the coronary vasculature. Risk of radiation to the fetus can be minimised by shielding the abdomen properly. Reperfusion therapy for STEMI in pregnancy is primary angioplasty (class I C) and the standard care is the same as in non-pregnant women, as use of thrombolytic is a relative contraindication due to chances of maternal haemorrhage, spontaneous abortion, vaginal bleed and sub-chorionic haematoma.

ACS IN THE ELDERLY

Age is a strong and independent risk factor for the development of coronary atherosclerosis [7]. Atherosclerosis is more severe in older patients, with higher prevalence of LMCA, MVD and impaired LV function. Age is one of the strongest predictors of ACS outcome, hence in many ACS risk scores, age is the important prognostic risk factor. Only a minority of elderly patients present with typical angina/chest pain. More often presentation is with fatigue, exertional dyspnoea, lack of energy, epigastric or back discomfort. Chest pain is reported in approximately 40% in aged >85 years and 80% in those <65 years. History may be mistaken or diagnosis of ACS is often overlooked due to declining activity level, comorbid conditions and cognitive impairment. Silent MI is more common. The diagnosis of ACS is often confounded due to baseline ECG abnormalities. Hence serial ECGs and cardiac biomarkers are required for correct diagnosis. NSTE-ACS and type 2 MI is more common than STEMI. Mortality in elderly women is higher than in men.

Twenty percent of community dwelling adults over 70 years of age have troponin levels above the 99th percentile normal baseline. The EMMACE & GRACE registry found 85% deaths, 32%–43% were NSTEMI, 24%–28% STEMI in ACS age group were 68–75 yrs.

Managing ACS in the elderly is a real-world challenge due to multiple comorbid conditions, renal impairment being the most common. Age-related changes in coronary and great vessel anatomy and physiology, tortuosity of vessels, multi-vessel involvement and increased calcium burden are also problematic. The choice of anti-platelets is also limited (age >75 years prasugrel is contraindicated).

The value of statin in elderly individuals may be limited due to CKD, uncontrolled hypertension, AF and poor compliance with medications. Primary PCI is always preferred over thrombolysis in the elderly, with reasons being less intracranial haemorrhage, decreased reinfarction and need for repeat revascularisation.

Also, increased risk of myocardial rupture with thrombolysis was found when compared to PCI. Beta-blockers have greater benefit in morbidity and mortality in elderly individuals in preventing subsequent myocardial infarctions and heart failure. However, a correct diagnosis of ACS in the elderly leads to a delay in therapy.

ACS IN CKD PATIENTS

Presence of CKD itself poses a great risk for ischaemic heart disease and ACS. Risk increases with the severity of renal insufficiency, especially for those who are on dialysis. CKD is an independent and incremental predictor of adverse cardiovascular outcome following ACS. CKD patients are often found to have multi-vessel disease and increased calcium burden which hinders complete revascularisation. CKD patients are found to have a 2-year mortality of 50%. It was also noted that ST depression is higher compared to patients with normal renal function and high TIMI risk score [8]. It is always mandatory to check renal function in patients who have taken metformin before angiography and to withhold metformin if renal function deteriorates (class I LOE A).

CONTRAST-INDUCED NEPHROPATHY (IN)

CKD patients are unlikely to get the usual revascularisation strategy in ACS due to fear of CI-AKI. The risk of contrast-induced nephropathy (CIN) depends on multiple factors like age, GFR, DM, HTN female gender, volume of contrast and hemodynamic instability. Adequate hydration remains the mainstay of CIN prevention. High-dose statins are also found to be beneficial in the secondary prevention (Tables 22.1 and 22.2). It is strongly recommended to keep total contrast volume GFR ration < 3.7 for better outcome [9].

ACS IN THE YOUNG

The incidence of coronary artery disease has been rising in the last two decades. The reasons being modifiable risk factors like smoking (56.8%), dyslipidemia (51.7%) and hypertension (49.8%). In a study between 18 and 44 years, 90.3% of patients were found to have more than one risk factor. Haematologic disorders (cyanotic CHD, TTP, DIC, polycythemia), situations like increased oxygen demand (thyrotoxicosis, cocaine use) and anomalous coronaries are other predisposing factors.

Table 22.1 ESC/EACTS guidelines for myocardial revascularisations

Recommendations	Class	Level
Patients undergoing coronary angiography or multi-slice CT		
It is recommended that all patients are assessed for the risk of contrast-induced nephropathy	I	C
Adequate hydration is recommended	I	C

Table 22.2 ESC/EACTS guidelines for myocardial revascularisations

Patients with moderate or severe CKD			
Use of low-osmolar or iso-osmolar contrast media is recommended		I	A
It is recommended that the volume of contrast media be minimised	Total contrast volume/GFR	I	B
In statin-native patients, pre-treatment with high-dose statins should be considered	Rosuvastatin 40/20 mg or atorvastatin 80 mg	IIa	A
Pre- and post-hydration with isotonic saline should be considered if the expected contrast volume is >100 mL	1 mL/kg/hr 12 hrs before and continued for 24 hrs after the procedure (0.5 mL/kg/hr if LVEF ≤3 5% or NYHA >2)	IIa	C

Patients with myocardial infarction with non-obstructive coronary arteries (MINOCA) compared to atherosclerotic mediated myocardial infarction tend to be younger individuals and often females. Coronary spasm, plaque erosion and spontaneous coronary dissection are proposed mechanisms in MINOCA. One-third of patients with MINOCA presents as MI and one-half of them on coronary angiogram are found to have smooth vessels.

Managing ACS poses many challenges in young individuals. CAG in these individuals are often ectatic with high thrombus burden.

Young individuals are often found to have large thrombus burden with minimal or no disease. Jayagopal P.B et al. (Figure 22.1) found that low-dose intracoronary thrombolysis is a safe and effective method for improving epicardial flow and tissue level perfusion by dissolving thrombus [10]. In this study series, STEMI patients who were taken up for PPCI with large thrombus burden were treated successfully with low-dose intracoronary thrombolysis. The study found intracoronary thrombolysis with tenecteplase is a good option in young patients with large thrombus burden and with ectatic coronaries and obviates the need for stenting in these patients [10].

PRE-HOSPITAL THROMBOLYSIS

The aim of treatment regimes for AMI is to open the infarct-related artery at the earliest. 'Time is muscle', so reperfusion should be

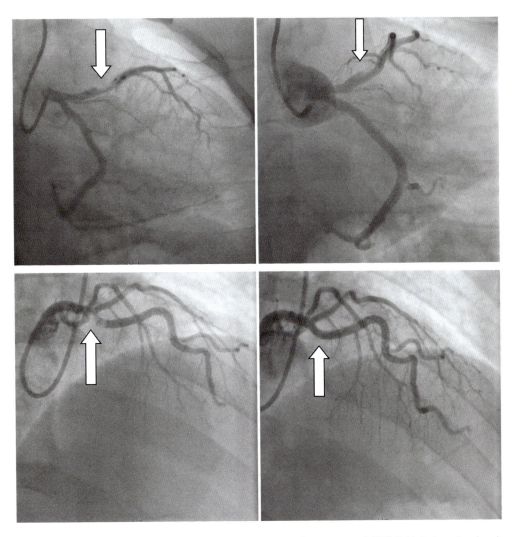

Figure 22.1 Coronary angiogram of two individual patients who presented with anterior wall STEMI, high thrombus burden with minimal or no lesion, was successfully managed with intracoronary tenecteplase alone.

initiated as soon as possible. Reperfusion delays in AMI are often noted in developing countries like India, with reasons being delay from onset of symptoms—recognition and call for aid, delay in out-of-hospital transport, delay in in-hospital evaluation and treatment. Nearly three-fourths of the 'total ischaemic time' in STEMI is in the pre-hospital phase and only less than one-fourth accounts for the DBT/DNT in-hospital. Pre-hospital thrombolysis (PHT) constitutes one of the means to shorten the delay from symptom onset to the delivery of reperfusion therapy.

Trials like CAPTIM, PRAGUE 2, GREAT, MITI and EMIP showed patients presenting earlier (within 2–3 hours) had similar or lower mortality with lysis than with primary PCI. In all trials, a trend towards lower mortality in the pre-hospital lysis group was noted. Meta-analysis of all trials showed a 17% reduction in mortality in the PHT group. A 1-hour gain by PHT translated into 20 lives saved/1000 patients treated. For patients presenting within 1 hour of symptom onset there were 65 fewer deaths/1000 as compared to longer duration of symptoms. Thrombolytics recommended were tenecteplase and reteplase.

In India, with a dominant rural population, PPCI for all STEMI in the time frame mandated is extremely difficult and PHT is a reasonable and feasible alternative. It depends on multiple factors:

- Availability of organised fully trained EMS
- Easy accessibility to EMS
- Trained paramedics and emergency physicians
- Thrombolytics-bolus
- Role of telemedicine
- Legislative support to providers

CONCLUSION

Women hospitalised for ACS were less likely to receive acute treatment and strategies for secondary prevention than men. In elderly individuals, diagnosis and management may be delayed due to baseline ECG abnormality, delayed diagnosis and delayed presentation due to cognitive impairment. CKD patients may not receive optimal revascularisation due to fear of contrast-induced nephropathy and complexity and multi-vessel disease. Young individuals found with large thrombus burden with minimal lesion may be managed effectively with intracoronary thrombolysis.

Lack of awareness about the disease, limited resources and lack of political will towards the health sector, especially in countries like India, are major challenges when discussing the need to strengthen the care in managing emergency situations like ACS with better care and primary prevention with the help of international support.

REFERENCES

1. Gupta R, Joshi P, Mohan V, Reddy KS, Yusuf S. Epidemiological and causation of coronary heart disease and stroke in India. *Heart*. 2008;94(1):16–26.
2. Xavier D, Pais P, Deveraux PJ et al. Treatment and outcomes of acute coronary syndromes in India (CREATE): A prospective analysis of registry data. *Lancet*. 26 Apr 2008;371(9622):1435–1442.
3. Every NR, Frederick PD, Robinson M et al. A comparison of the national registry of myocardial infarction 2 with the cooperative cardiovascular project. *J Am Coll Cardiol*. 1999 Jun;33(7):1886–1894.
4. Mohanan PP, Mathew R, Harikrishnan S et al. Presentation, management, and outcomes of 25 748 acute coronary syndrome admissions in Kerala, India: results from the Kerala ACS Registry. *Eur Heart J*. Jan 2013;34(2):121–129. doi: 10.1093/eurheartj/ehs219. Epub 2012 Sep 7.
5. Yusuf S, Hawken S, Stephanie O et al. Effect of potentially modifiable risk factors associated with myocardial infarction in 52 countries (the INTERHEART study): case-control study. *Lancet*. 11–17 Sep 2004;364(9438):937–952.
6. Roth A, Elkayam U. Acute myocardial infarction associated with pregnancy. *J Am Coll Cardiol*. 15 Jul 2008;52(3):171–180.
7. Eagle KA, Lim MJ, Omar HD et al. GRACE investigators. A validated prediction model for all forms of acute coronary syndrome: Estimating the risk of 6 month postdischarge death in an international registry. *JAMA*. 2004;291:2727–2733.
8. Asim M, Jeffrey RF. Management of acute coronary syndrome in patients with chronic kidney disease; If we don't risk anything, we risk even more. *Nephron Clin Pract*. 2011;119:c333–c337.
9. Mueller C, Buerkle G, Buettner HJ et al. Prevention of contrast media-associated nephropathy: Randomized comparison of 2 hydration regimens in 1620 patients undergoing coronary angioplasty. *Arch Intern Med*. 2002;162:329–336.
10. Jayagopal PB, Sarjun Basha KM. Intracoronary tenecteplase in STEMI with massive thrombus. *Indian Heart J*. May–Jun 2018;70(3):446–449.

23

Short-term rehabilitation after an acute coronary event

MANISH BANSAL AND RAJEEV AGARWALA

In patients presenting with acute coronary syndrome (ACS), the time period encompassing early convalescence to next few days/weeks is crucial for guiding their long-term care and to transfer guideline-directed medical therapy driven benefits to the community. This is the time period during which the patients resume physical activity and return to their daily routine. Hence, it is important to assess their residual risk for cardiac decompensation and provide appropriate guidance for safe resumption of the normal physical routine. At the same time, as ACS represents only an acute worsening in an otherwise chronic, life-long disease, appropriate secondary prevention strategies need to be instituted to prevent further cardiac events in future. Early convalescence is the ideal time window to address this issue as the patients are likely to be most receptive during this period and are more like to adhere to the advice given. Accordingly, the secondary prevention prescription during this period sets the tone for the long-term care of these patients. A cardiac rehabilitation programme is therefore an integral component of the overall management of ACS.

BENEFITS OF CARDIAC REHABILITATION AFTER ACS

A formal, structured cardiac rehabilitation programme permits effective integration of various components of the care of post-ACS patients, including pharmacological management, lifestyle modification and physical and emotional rehabilitation. It also allows an opportunity to titrate and monitor various pharmacotherapies, educate patients about various aspects of their disease and the ways to prevent future events, introduce risk reduction lifestyle changes and to monitor adequacy of the risk factor control. A supervised cardiac rehabilitation programme enhances patients' confidence, improves their psychological status and leads to more effective risk factor control, translating eventually into better clinical outcomes.

Previous studies have demonstrated significant benefits with participation in structural cardiac rehabilitation programmes.

Suaya et al. analysed data on 601099 US Medicare beneficiaries who were hospitalised for coronary conditions or revascularisation procedures [1]. They found that participation in a cardiac rehabilitation programme was associated with 21%–34% lower mortality rates. Similarly, Taylor et al. performed a systematic review and meta-analysis of 48 randomised controlled trials of cardiac rehabilitation involving 8940 patients with at least 6 months of follow-up [2]. It was found that compared with usual care, cardiac rehabilitation was associated with a 20% relative reduction in all-cause mortality and 26% reduction in cardiac mortality. This beneficial effect was independent of type and dose of cardiac rehabilitation as well as trial publication date. Similar findings were noted in a more recent Cochrane review and meta-analysis of 63 studies with 14,486 participants with a median follow-up of 12 months [3]. The participation in cardiac rehabilitation resulted in 26% reduction in cardiovascular mortality and 18% reduction in the rate of rehospitalisations. Once again, the benefits were seen regardless of the patient type, intervention performed and the study quality, setting and publication date. These analyses demonstrate that cardiac rehabilitation is beneficial, even in the era of contemporary, effective medical management of ACS.

Given this encouraging evidence, there has been an increasing emphasis in the guidelines on formal cardiac rehabilitation for all patients with ACS. Referral to a structured cardiac rehabilitation programme is assigned class I recommendation in the latest American Heart Association (AHA)/American College of Cardiology (ACC) guidelines for management of both ST-segment elevation myocardial infraction (STEMI) and non-ST-elevation myocardial infarction (NSTEMI) [4,5]. Similarly, the European Society of Cardiology (ESC) guidelines provide class I and class IIa recommendations, respectively, for referral to cardiac rehabilitation for patients with STEMI and NSTEMI [6,7]. It is further recommended that the referral should take place either prior to hospital discharge or during the first follow-up office visit. For low-risk patients, a home-based cardiac rehabilitation programme is recommended as a reasonable alternative to a supervised, centre-based programme.

Unfortunately, despite the documented beneficial effect on clinical outcomes and the current practice recommendations encouraging cardiac rehabilitation, the utilisation of such services remains poor due to inertia and ignorance by the practitioners as well as infrastructure/logistic constraints.

COMPONENTS OF CARDIAC REHABILITATION AFTER ACS

Cardiac rehabilitation is generally offered as an outpatient programme of 8–24-weeks duration, depending on the underlying illness and the patient requirements. Following are the key components of a structured cardiac rehabilitation programme for patients recovering from an ACS:

- Risk assessment and determining the need for further cardiac intervention (for complete revascularisation)
- Pharmacological intervention for secondary prevention
- Physical activity counselling, exercise training and sexual rehabilitation
- Other lifestyle changes, psychosocial counselling

Risk assessment and determining the need for further cardiac intervention

ASSESSMENT OF LEFT VENTRICULAR SYSTOLIC FUNCTION

All patients who present with an ACS should have an estimation of left ventricular ejection fraction (LVEF) during the hospital stay. Echocardiography should be performed early after hospitalisation and should preferably be repeated on the day of discharge (class I, both AHA/ACC and ESC) [5,7]. For the patients who have LV systolic dysfunction (LVEF <40%) and have undergone coronary revascularisation, a repeat assessment of LVEF is recommended ≥40 days after revascularisation to determine the need for an automated implantable cardioverter defibrillator for primary prevention of sudden cardiac death (class I, both AHA/ACC and ESC) [5,7].

CARDIAC STRESS TESTING

Keeping with the current practice recommendations, most patients with an ACS these days undergo coronary angiography and revascularisation during the index hospitalisation itself. In patients with STEMI, coronary angiography is advisable in most patients who present within first 24–48 hours of symptom onset, regardless of whether they have received fibrinolytic therapy or not (class I as part of primary percutaneous intervention [PCI] or in case of failed fibrinolysis; IIa as routine invasive strategy within 3–24 hours after successful fibrinolysis) [5,7]. Coronary angiography is also recommended in all those who have clinical features of recurrent ischaemia, reduced LVEF (<40%), mechanical complication of myocardial infarction (MI) and/or ongoing haemodynamic or electrical instability (class I, both AHA/ACC and ESC) [5,7]. Similarly, in patients with NSTEMI, coronary angiography and revascularisation are recommended in all patients during the initial hospitalisation,

though the exact timing would differ depending on whether an immediate invasive, early invasive or delayed invasive approach is adopted [4,6].

Thus, most patients with ACS would get discharged after having undergone coronary angiography and some form of coronary revascularisation. Therefore, additional testing for further coronary risk stratification is needed only in a select group of patients:

- STEMI patients who have undergone successful pharmacological reperfusion but could not undergo further invasive evaluation (as a routine) due to logistic reasons or in whom conservative approach was adopted because of perceived low risk,
- STEMI patients who presented late after symptom onset did not receive reperfusion therapy and did not have any high-risk feature and
- STEMI patients who have multi-vessel coronary artery disease (CAD) and have undergone only the culprit-vessel revascularisation during the initial stay.

Two different approaches have been used for early exercise testing following an MI-submaximal exercise test achieving a pre-specified target heart rate or metabolic equivalent (MET) level or a symptom-limited exercise test [5]. Pharmacological stress testing is an alternative in patients who are unable to exercise for some reason.

A submaximal exercise test is usually performed at 3 to 5 days after ACS in patients who are stable and free of complications [5]. The objectives of performing a pre-discharge submaximal stress test include: (1) recognition of easily inducible ischaemia or other high-risk features that could be associated with early post-discharge cardiac events and would warrant early intervention, (2) to guide exercise prescription in the first few days after discharge, before the patient is enrolled in a formal cardiac rehabilitation programme.

In contrast, a symptom-limited stress test is typically performed at 2–3 weeks after discharge [5]. It allows more complete assessment of functional capacity and inducible ischaemia. It is the preferred approach for assessment of non-infarct artery stenosis identified at initial coronary angiography. A symptom-limited exercise test performed at 2 weeks or later also forms the basis for a formal cardiac rehabilitation programme. Although a symptom-limited stress test can also be performed early after MI (at around 5 days), safety of such an approach is not fully established. Therefore, clinical judgment must be used when an early symptom-limited stress test is required [5].

The 2013 AHA/ACC guidelines for STEMI [5] management recommend the following:

i. The patients without complications who have not undergone coronary angiography and who might be potential candidates for revascularisation should undergo provocative testing before hospital discharge,
ii. On the other hand, in patients with non-infarct artery disease who have undergone successful PCI of the infarct artery and have an uncomplicated course, it is reasonable to proceed with discharge and plans for close clinical follow-up with stress imaging within 3 to 6 weeks.

PHARMACOLOGICAL INTERVENTION FOR SECONDARY PREVENTION

ANTI-PLATELET THERAPY

Dual anti-platelet therapy, which refers to a combination of aspirin and one of the P2Y12 inhibitors (clopidogrel, prasugrel or ticagrelor), for 1 year is recommended to all patients presenting with an ACS (class I, both AHA/ACC and ESC) [8,9]. This recommendation is regardless of the management strategy and the type of stent used (if the patient underwent PCI).

The recommended dose of aspirin is 75–100 mg/d, especially if the patient is on ticagrelor [8]. Aspirin should be continued lifelong (class I) [8,9]. Among the three P2Y12 inhibitors, prasugrel or ticagrelor are the preferred agents for the patients undergoing PCI. Prasugrel is not recommended in medically-managed patients, in whom ticagrelor is the preferred agent. Prasugrel should also not be used in patients with previous stroke or transient ischaemic attack (class III) [8]. Clopidogrel is to be used only as an alternative when more effective agents such as prasugrel or ticagrelor cannot be used for some reason (AHA/ACC class IIa [8], also supported by the ESC guideline [9]).

STATINS

High-intensity statin therapy (rosuvastatin 20–40 mg/d or atorvastatin 40–80 mg/d) is recommended for all patients presenting with an ACS with age <75 yrs (class I), irrespective of the management strategy [4–7]. The goal of the treatment is to reduce low-density lipoprotein cholesterol (LDL-C) to <70 mg/dL (preferably <50 mg/dL) or bring about at least 50% reduction in LDL-C from the baseline (when the baseline LDL-C is not too high). Statin therapy has been convincingly shown to reduce cardiovascular events, cardiovascular death, and total mortality and may delay progression and even lead to regression in the long term [10].

The duration of high-intensity statin therapy remains debatable, particularly in Indian patients. The long-term studies conducted in the Western populations have not shown any appreciable safety concern with the prolonged use of high-intensity statin therapy [11]. However, similar long-term studies in Indian subjects are lacking, though the preliminary evidence from short-term studies does not suggest any major safety issue [12,13]. Nonetheless, it is a common practise among Indian cardiologists to reduce the dose of statin to a maximum 40 mg/d of atorvastatin or 20 mg/d of rosuvastatin at 3 months after an ACS. Such a strategy is reasonable if LDL-C is <40 mg/dL on two consecutive occasions. However, if the LDL-C remains elevated, it is preferable to continue with the maximum tolerated dose of statin. In patients who are unable to tolerate the required dose of statin or have any safety concerns, the dose of statin should be reduced, and ezetimibe should be added [10]. If LDL-C remains >70 mg/dL despite a combination of maximum-tolerated statin and ezetimibe, a proprotein convertase subtilisin/kexin type 9 (PCSK9) inhibitor should be used [10]. One of the PCSK9 inhibitors (evolocumab) is now available in India. A lower-intensity statin therapy is acceptable in elderly individuals above 75 years of age.

ANGIOTENSIN CONVERTING ENZYME INHIBITORS/ANGIOTENSIN RECEPTOR BLOCKERS

An angiotensin converting enzyme inhibitor (ACEI) is recommended, unless contraindicated, in all patients with ACS who have any of the following comorbid conditions: systemic hypertension, LVEF <40%, diabetes or stable chronic kidney disease (class I, both ACC/AHA and ESC) [4–7]. The ACEI should be used cautiously in patients with underlying renal dysfunction. In such patients, serum creatinine and potassium levels need to be monitored closely, especially during the initial one week after initiation or dose up-titration of ACEI. If the patient is unable to tolerate ACEI for some reason (e.g. cough), then an angiotensin receptor blocker (ARB) should be prescribed in place of ACEI (class I) [4–7].

Angiotensin receptor-neprilysin inhibitor (ARNI) is another class of drug which acts on the renin angiotensin system (RAS). Its use has been shown to result in significant mortality reduction in comparison to enalapril in patients with heart failure (HF) with reduced EF (HFrEF) [14]. Accordingly, it is recommended that ARNI should be substituted for ACEI/ARB in all those patients with HFrEF who remain symptomatic despite optimum doses of ACEI/ARB, beta-blocker and a mineralocorticoid receptor antagonist (class I, both AHA/ACC and ESC) [15,16]. In fact, the 2017 ACC/AHA focussed update on HF management even recommends ARNI as the first line therapy, alongside ACEI/ARB, in HFrEF (class I, level of evidence B) [15]. Although ARNI has not been specifically tested in ACS patients, two studies have recently been published demonstrating safety of early administration of ARNI in acute decompensated HF [17,18]. Addition of ARNI once the patients became haemodynamically stable or at the time of discharge was not only safe but also led to greater reduction in natriuretic peptides over a follow-up of 4–8 weeks [17].

MINERALOCORTICOID RECEPTOR ANTAGONIST

Mineralocorticoid or aldosterone receptor antagonists are effective yet vastly underutilised drugs in post-MI patients. In the EPHESUS (Eplerenone Post-Acute Myocardial Infarction Heart Failure Efficacy and Survival) study, 6632 patients with acute MI complicated by LV systolic dysfunction or HF were randomly assigned to eplerenone (25 mg per day initially, titrated to a maximum of 50 mg per day) or placebo in addition to optimal medical therapy [19]. After a mean follow-up of 16 months, the eplerenone group had a 15% reduction in all-cause mortality, 17% reduction in cardiovascular mortality and 21% reduction in the risk of sudden cardiac death. Importantly, these benefits were observed on top of ACEIs/ARBs (prescribed to 87% of patients) and beta-blockers (75% patients).

Based on this evidence, both the ACC/AHA and ESC guidelines for both STEMI and NSTEMI recommend an aldosterone receptor antagonist (preferably eplerenone) in all patients with LVEF <40% and either symptomatic HF or diabetes mellitus, provided there are no contraindications (e.g. renal dysfunction defined as creatinine >2.5 mg/dL in men or >2.0 mg/dL in women; hyperkalemia with K+ >5.0 mEq/L) (class I) [4–7]. The patients should be receiving optimum doses of an ACEI/ARB and a beta-blocker. Renal function, electrolytes and blood pressure need to be monitored in these patients.

BETA-BLOCKERS

Beta-blockers have an undisputed role in the management of the patients with LV systolic dysfunction, with or without symptomatic HF. Therefore, all patients with ACS who have LVEF <40% should be prescribed a beta-blocker. One of the three agents with proven efficacy in HF (bisoprolol, metoprolol succinate and carvedilol) should be used. The therapy should be started within the first 24 hours after presentation, unless contraindicated, and should be continued indefinitely (class I, both AHA/ACC and ESC) [4–7]

In contrast to LV systolic dysfunction, the role of beta-blockers in patients with preserved LVEF and no evidence of HF or angina is rather controversial. In 1999, Freemantle et al. published a meta-regression analysis of 82 randomised trials that examined the effects of beta-blockers compared with control [20]. Of these, 31 trials evaluated long-term (6 to 48 months) benefits of beta-blockade. The analysis showed 23% reduction in the odds of death with beta-blockers. The rates of MI were also reduced significantly. This analysis formed the basis for the current guidelines recommending beta-blockers for at least 3 years in all patients with ACS, unless contraindicated (class IIa, both AHA/ACC and ESC) [5,7,21]. However, it is noteworthy that most of the trials included in this analysis were conducted during the pre-reperfusion era. It remains to be determined whether beta-blockers have similar beneficial effects even in the contemporary era where the patients undergo effective reperfusion/revascularisation early after an ACS. There is no large-scale randomised study to answer this question, but a large-scale registry attempted to address this issue using propensity-matching as the means to eliminate confounding. The registry analysed data on 21860 patients belonging to one of following three clinical groups: stable patients with a prior history of MI, those with CAD but no history of MI and those with only risk factors for CAD [22]. The primary outcome was a composite of cardiovascular death, non-fatal MI, or non-fatal stroke. No benefit on primary outcome was observed with beta-blockers in this registry, even in the prior-MI cohort (6758 patients). Subsequently, a meta-analysis was published that explored beneficial effects of beta-blockers, stratified according to the timing of the study [23]. This analysis which included 60 trials with 102003 patients, demonstrated a significant reduction in mortality in the pre-reperfusion era but not in the reperfusion era. Although beta-blockers reduced recurrent MI and angina (that too only in the short-term), this occurred at the expense of increased rates of HF, cardiogenic shock and drug discontinuation. Similar findings were noted in another meta-analysis of 16 observational studies published between 2000 and 2017 [24]. After eliminating the 'small study effect', no association was seen between beta-blockers and all-cause mortality. Thus, there is insufficient evidence to support routine administration of beta-blockers to all patients with ACS in absence of LV systolic dysfunction or residual myocardial ischaemia. On the contrary, it has been shown that prescription of multiple preventive therapies may even be detrimental by compromising compliance to treatment. Korhonen et al. analysed data on 90,869 US Medicare beneficiaries ≥65 years of age who were prescribed ACEI/ARBs, beta-blockers and statins, and who survived ≥180 days after MI hospitalisation in 2008 to 2010 [25]. Patients adherent only to ACEI/ARBs and statins had similar mortality rates than those adherent to all three therapies, suggesting that there was limited incremental benefit with beta-blockers in patients already receiving statins and ACEIs/ARBs. In contrast, non-adherence to ACEI/ARBs and/or statins was associated with higher mortality. Together, these findings suggest that even though the current guidelines continue to recommend beta-blockers for at least 1–3 years following ACS, there is little justification for this recommendation in patients who have normal LVEF, no evidence of HF and have undergone effective revascularisation.

Beta-blockers should not be used in ACS patients with recent history of cocaine and methamphetamine abuse (class III) [4].

MANAGEMENT OF BLOOD PRESSURE

Effective control of blood pressure is an important treatment goal in all patients with hypertension, even more so in those with previous ACS. Both the latest AHA/ACC and ESC guidelines for management of hypertension recommend a goal blood pressure, <130/80 mmHg in these patients [26,27]. The ESC guidelines further suggest that it is not advisable to lower blood pressure to <120/70 mmHg [27]. Among various classes of anti-hypertensive agents, ACEIs/ARBs and beta-blockers are preferred in post-ACS patients.

AVOID NON-STEROID ANTI-INFLAMMATORY DRUGS

Non-steroid anti-inflammatory drugs (NSAIDs) are known to interfere with infarct healing and are associated with increased risk of major adverse cardiovascular events when administered to patients with ACS. Accordingly, in these patients, NSAIDs should be avoided during hospital stay and early convalescence (class III) [4,5]. If the patient has already been using an NSAID for some non-cardiac indications, it should be discontinued, at least temporarily (class III B) [4,5].

PHYSICAL ACTIVITY COUNSELLING, EXERCISE TRAINING AND SEXUAL ACTIVITY

PHYSICAL ACTIVITY

Return to work after an ACS represents an important indicator of recovery. Apart from being a psychological boost, regular physical activity has several additional benefits. It enhances functional capacity, helps control of various risk factors such as lipids, blood pressure, body weight, blood glucose, etc. and improves overall cardiac outcomes.

Following an ACS, daily walking can be encouraged soon after discharge for most patients. Aerobic exercise training can generally begin 1 to 2 weeks after discharge, whereas mild-to-moderate resistance training can be started 2 to 4 weeks after aerobic training [4,28,29]. Sedentary patients should be strongly encouraged to engage in regular physical activity. They should start with light-intensity exercise, after an adequate exercise-related risk stratification has been performed.

If feasible, regular exercise training ≥3 times a week with each session for 30 minutes is recommended [6]. When performed without supervision, 60%–75% of maximum age-predicted heart rate should be targeted, whereas supervised training may target a higher heart rate (70%–85% of age-predicted maximum) [28]. Eventually (by 6–8 weeks), it is recommended that individuals accumulate at least 30 minutes/day, 5 days/week of moderate intensity physical activity (i.e. 150 min/week) or 15 minutes/day, 5 days/week of vigorous intensity physical activity (75 min/week), or a combination of both, performed in sessions with a duration of at least 10 minutes [30]. Shorter exercise sessions (i.e. 10 min) may also be appropriate, especially in very deconditioned individuals. Longer durations and more intense exercise sessions may be needed for weight reduction.

In addition to detailed instructions for daily exercise, patients should also be given specific instruction about various activities of daily living and driving. The decision to return to work needs to be individualised, based on the overall physical fitness of the individual, symptomatic status, LV systolic function, completeness of revascularisation, presence or absence of arrhythmias and the job characteristics.

SEXUAL REHABILITATION

Resuming sexual activity is an important emotional concern in patients who have been sexually active before suffering the acute coronary event. In such patients, the ability to engage in sexual activity boosts confidence, helps instill a sense of well-being and often translates into completeness and effectiveness of treatment.

Studies have shown that myocardial workload during usual sexual activity is generally equivalent to mild to moderate physical activity in the range of 3 to 5 METs [31]. However, the overall effort and its haemodynamic impact vary according to the patient's physical fitness and emotional state [31,32]. For a healthy, young individual, the effort involved in normal sexual intercourse is comparable to climbing 2 flights of stairs. On the other hand, in older individuals, who are unaccustomed to regular physical activity, sexual intercourse may produce much greater demand on the cardiovascular system [33].

Sexual activity has been shown to be associated with increased risk of MI in individuals who are physically inactive, but not in those who are physically active [34–36]. Even in those leading a sedentary life, the absolute risk of ACS due to sexual activity is very small because the increased workload is only for a brief period and the total cumulative burden is minimal [35,36]. Therefore, it can be safely mentioned that the patients who have resumed their normal physical activity after an ACS, can resume normal sexual life as well.

The AHA has published a scientific statement regarding sexual activity in patients with cardiovascular diseases [37]. It makes the following recommendations for resumption of sexual activity following ACS:

- Sexual activity is reasonable 1 or more weeks after uncomplicated MI if the patient is without cardiac symptoms during mild to moderate physical activity (class IIa, level of evidence C).
- Sexual activity is reasonable for patients who have undergone complete coronary revascularisation (class IIa, level of evidence B) and may be resumed (a) several days after PCI if the vascular access site is without complications (class IIa, level of evidence C) or (b) 6 to 8 weeks after standard coronary artery bypass graft surgery, provided the sternotomy is well healed (class IIa, level of evidence B).

- For patients with incomplete coronary revascularisation, exercise stress testing can be considered to assess the extent and severity of residual ischaemia (class IIb, level of evidence C).
- Sexual activity should be deferred for patients with unstable or refractory angina until their condition is stabilised and optimally managed (class III, level of evidence C).

OTHER LIFESTYLE CHANGES, PSYCHOSOCIAL COUNSELLING AND OTHER MEASURES

- Adhering to healthy lifestyle including a healthy diet is important for secondary prevention of CAD [21,30]. Several different diets are considered heart-healthy, such as AHA diet, DASH (Dietary Approaches to Stop Hypertension) diet, Mediterranean diet, etc. All these diets have similar basic principles and emphasis on intake of vegetables, fruits and whole grains; include low-fat dairy products, poultry, fish, legumes, non-tropical vegetable oils and nuts; and limit intake of sweets, sugar-sweetened beverages and red meats. Intake of saturated fats should also be minimised in lieu of polyunsaturated fats. Trans-fats must be avoided completely.
- All patients must be encouraged to quit smoking completely. A meta-analysis involving 20 observational studies with 12,603 patients with CAD showed a 36% reduction of mortality in those who quit smoking [38]. Another meta-analysis that included cohort studies of patients after acute MI reported a reduction in cardiovascular mortality rate by nearly 50% with smoking cessation [39]. An analysis from the SAVE (Survival and Ventricular Enlargement) study, which evaluated the beneficial effect of captopril in acute MI patients with LV dysfunction, explored the impact of smoking cessation on cardiovascular outcomes [40]. Among baseline smokers (924 subjects), smoking status at 6 months was available for 731 subjects. It was found that smoking cessation at 6-month follow-up was associated with a 43% reduction in all-cause mortality, 32% reduction in death or recurrent MI and 35% reduction in death or HF hospitalisation.

  Initial hospitalisation due to ACS is the best opportunity to provide counselling about smoking cessation. When such counselling is followed by frequent reinforcements over the next few weeks, it is associated with much higher quitting rates than when advised later [41,42]. Referral to a structured cardiac rehabilitation programme enhances quitting rates [42]. Behaviour counselling and appropriate pharmacotherapies such as nicotine replacement therapy, bupropion and varenicline are the mainstay in achieving smoking cessation. Nicotine containing electronic cigarettes also seem to be helpful in reducing smoking rates [43].
- Moderate alcohol consumption (maximum of 2 glasses [20 g of alcohol] daily for men and 1 for women) is permissible but those not consuming alcohol should continue to abstain from it [7].
- An annual influenza vaccination is recommended for all patients with cardiovascular disease (AHA/ACC class I [4,21], ESC class IIb [30]). This recommendation is applicable also to those who have had ACS [4].

CONCLUSION

Short-term cardiac rehabilitation has an important role in the management of patients with ACS. It facilitates safe transition of the patients from in-hospital care to regular life, while also allowing effective introduction and monitoring of secondary prevention therapies. Evidence from clinical trials and registries shows significant improvement in clinical outcomes with participation in formal, structured cardiac rehabilitation programmes. Accordingly, the current management guidelines unanimously recommend referral to cardiac rehabilitation for all patients with ACS. It is high time the clinicians involved in the care of ACS patients recognise these benefits and incorporate formal cardiac rehabilitation in their practiscs. Inertia and ignorance about secondary prevention guidelines remain the two major barriers to effective cardiac rehabilitation, which need to be overcome by clinicians and patients alike.

REFERENCES

1. Suaya JA, Stason WB, Ades PA, Normand SL, Shepard DS. Cardiac rehabilitation and survival in older coronary patients. *J Am Coll Cardiol.* 2009;54:25–33.

2. Taylor RS, Brown A, Ebrahim S et al. Exercise-based rehabilitation for patients with coronary heart disease: Systematic review and meta-analysis of randomized controlled trials. *Am J Med.* 2004;116:682–692.

3. Anderson L, Oldridge N, Thompson DR et al. Exercise-based cardiac rehabilitation for coronary heart disease: Cochrane systematic review and meta-analysis. *J Am Coll Cardiol.* 2016;67:1–12.

4. Amsterdam EA, Wenger NK, Brindis RG et al. 2014 AHA/ACC Guideline for the Management of Patients with Non-ST-Elevation Acute Coronary Syndromes: A report of the American College of Cardiology/American Heart Association Task Force on Practice Guidelines. *J Am Coll Cardiol.* 2014;64:e139–e228.

5. O'Gara PT, Kushner FG, Ascheim DD et al. 2013 ACCF/AHA guideline for the management of ST-elevation myocardial infarction: A report of the American College of Cardiology Foundation/American Heart Association Task Force on Practice Guidelines. *J Am Coll Cardiol.* 2013;61:e78–e140.

6. Roffi M, Patrono C, Collet JP et al. 2015 ESC Guidelines for the management of acute coronary syndromes in patients presenting without persistent ST-segment elevation: Task Force for the Management of Acute Coronary Syndromes in Patients Presenting without Persistent ST-Segment Elevation of the European Society of Cardiology (ESC). *Eur Heart J.* 2016;37:267–315.

7. Ibanez B, James S, Agewall S et al. 2017 ESC Guidelines for the management of acute myocardial infarction in patients presenting with ST-segment elevation: The Task Force for the Management of Acute Myocardial Infarction in patients presenting with ST-segment elevation of the European Society of Cardiology (ESC). *Eur Heart J.* 2018;39:119–177.

8. Levine GN, Bates ER, Bittl JA et al. 2016 ACC/AHA Guideline Focused Update on Duration of Dual Antiplatelet Therapy in Patients with Coronary Artery Disease: A Report of the American College of Cardiology/American Heart Association Task Force on Clinical Practice Guidelines. *J Am Coll Cardiol.* 2016;68:1082–1115.

9. Valgimigli M, Bueno H, Byrne RA et al. 2017 ESC focused update on dual antiplatelet therapy in coronary artery disease developed in collaboration with EACTS: The Task Force for dual antiplatelet therapy in coronary artery disease of the European Society of Cardiology (ESC) and of the European Association for Cardio-Thoracic Surgery (EACTS). *Eur Heart J.* 2018;39:213–260.

10. Grundy SM, Stone NJ, Bailey AL et al. 2018 AHA/ACC/AACVPR/AAPA/ABC/ACPM/ADA/AGS/APhA/ASPC/NLA/PCNA Guideline on the Management of Blood Cholesterol: A Report of the American College of Cardiology/American Heart Association Task Force on Clinical Practice Guidelines. *J Am Coll Cardiol.* 2019; 73:e285–350.

11. Mach F, Ray KK, Wiklund O et al. Adverse effects of statin therapy: Perception vs. the evidence - focus on glucose homeostasis, cognitive, renal and hepatic function, haemorrhagic stroke and cataract. *Eur Heart J.* 2018;39:2526–2539.

12. Agrawal D, Manchanda SC, Sawhney JPS et al. To study the effect of high dose Atorvastatin 40 mg versus 80 mg in patients with dyslipidemia. *Indian Heart J.* 2018;70(Suppl 3):S8–S12.

13. Kaul U, Varma J, Kahali D et al. Post-marketing Study of Clinical Experience of Atorvastatin 80 mg vs 40 mg in Indian Patients with Acute Coronary Syndrome- A Randomized, Multi-centre Study (CURE-ACS). *J Assoc Physicians India.* 2013;61:97–101.

14. McMurray JJ, Packer M, Desai AS et al. Angiotensin-neprilysin inhibition versus enalapril in heart failure. *N Engl J Med.* 2014;371:993–1004.

15. Yancy CW, Jessup M, Bozkurt B et al. 2017 ACC/AHA/HFSA Focused Update of the 2013 ACCF/AHA Guideline for the Management of Heart Failure: A Report of the American College of Cardiology/American Heart Association Task Force on Clinical Practice Guidelines and the Heart Failure Society of America. *J Am Coll Cardiol.* 2017;70:776–803.

16. Ponikowski P, Voors AA, Anker SD et al. 2016 ESC Guidelines for the diagnosis and treatment of acute and chronic heart failure: The Task Force for the diagnosis and treatment of acute and chronic heart failure of the European Society of Cardiology (ESC) Developed with the special contribution of the Heart Failure Association (HFA) of the ESC. *Eur Heart J.* 2016;37:2129–2200.

17. Velazquez EJ, Morrow DA, DeVore AD et al. Angiotensin-neprilysin inhibition in acute decompensated heart failure. *N Engl J Med.* 2019;380:539–548.

18. Wachter R, Senni M, Belohlavek J, Butylin D, Noe A, Pascual-Figal D. Initiation of sacubitril/valsartan in hospitalized patients with heart failure with reduced ejection fraction after hemodynamic stabilization: Primary results of the TRANSITION study. Abstract P6531. *Presented at:*

European Society of Cardiology Congress; Aug. 25–29, 2018; Munich. 2018.

19. Pitt B, Remme W, Zannad F et al. Eplerenone, a selective aldosterone blocker, in patients with left ventricular dysfunction after myocardial infarction. *N Engl J Med.* 2003;348:1309–1321.

20. Freemantle N, Cleland J, Young P, Mason J, Harrison J. beta Blockade after myocardial infarction: Systematic review and meta regression analysis. *BMJ.* 1999;318:1730–1737.

21. Smith SC, Jr., Benjamin EJ, Bonow RO et al. AHA/ACCF secondary prevention and risk reduction therapy for patients with coronary and other atherosclerotic vascular disease: 2011 update: A guideline from the American Heart Association and American College of Cardiology Foundation. *Circulation.* 2011;124:2458–2473.

22. Bangalore S, Steg G, Deedwania P et al. Beta-blocker use and clinical outcomes in stable outpatients with and without coronary artery disease. *JAMA.* 2012;308:1340–1349.

23. Bangalore S, Makani H, Radford M et al. Clinical outcomes with beta-blockers for myocardial infarction: A meta-analysis of randomized trials. *Am J Med.* 2014;127:939–953.

24. Dahl Aarvik M, Sandven I, Dondo TB et al. Effect of oral beta-blocker treatment on mortality in contemporary post-myocardial infarction patients: A systematic review and meta-analysis. *Eur Heart J Cardiovasc Pharmacother.* 2019;5:12–20.

25. Korhonen MJ, Robinson JG, Annis IE et al. Adherence tradeoff to multiple preventive therapies and all-cause mortality after acute myocardial infarction. *J Am Coll Cardiol.* 2017;70:1543–1554.

26. Whelton PK, Carey RM, Aronow WS et al. 2017 ACC/AHA/AAPA/ABC/ACPM/AGS/APhA/ASH/ASPC/NMA/PCNA Guideline for the Prevention, Detection, Evaluation, and Management of High Blood Pressure in Adults: A Report of the American College of Cardiology/American Heart Association Task Force on Clinical Practice Guidelines. *J Am Coll Cardiol.* 2018;71:e127–e248.

27. Williams B, Mancia G, Spiering W et al. 2018 ESC/ESH Guidelines for the management of arterial hypertension. *Eur Heart J.* 2018;39:3021–3104.

28. Thompson PD. Exercise prescription and proscription for patients with coronary artery disease. *Circulation.* 2005;112:2354–2363.

29. Pollock ML, Franklin BA, Balady GJ et al. AHA Science Advisory. Resistance exercise in individuals with and without cardiovascular disease: Benefits, rationale, safety, and prescription: An advisory from the Committee on Exercise, Rehabilitation, and Prevention, Council on Clinical Cardiology, American Heart Association; Position paper endorsed by the American College of Sports Medicine. *Circulation.* 2000;101:828–833.

30. Piepoli MF, Hoes AW, Agewall S et al. 2016 European Guidelines on cardiovascular disease prevention in clinical practice: The Sixth Joint Task Force of the European Society of Cardiology and Other Societies on Cardiovascular Disease Prevention in Clinical Practice (constituted by representatives of 10 societies and by invited experts)Developed with the special contribution of the European Association for Cardiovascular Prevention & Rehabilitation (EACPR). *Eur Heart J.* 2016;37:2315–2381.

31. Bohlen JG, Held JP, Sanderson MO, Patterson RP. Heart rate, rate-pressure product, and oxygen uptake during four sexual activities. *Arch Intern Med.* 1984;144:1745–1748.

32. Hellerstein HK, Friedman EH. Sexual activity and the post-coronary patient. *Arch Intern Med.* 1970;125:987–999.

33. Lindau ST, Schumm LP, Laumann EO, Levinson W, O'Muircheartaigh CA, Waite LJ. A study of sexuality and health among older adults in the United States. *N Engl J Med.* 2007;357:762–774.

34. Moller J, Ahlbom A, Hulting J et al. Sexual activity as a trigger of myocardial infarction. A case-crossover analysis in the Stockholm Heart Epidemiology Programme (SHEEP). *Heart.* 2001;86:387–390.

35. Muller JE, Mittleman MA, Maclure M, Sherwood JB, Tofler GH. Triggering myocardial infarction by sexual activity. Low absolute risk and prevention by regular physical exertion. Determinants of Myocardial Infarction Onset Study Investigators. *JAMA.* 1996;275:1405–1409.

36. Dahabreh IJ, Paulus JK. Association of episodic physical and sexual activity with triggering of acute cardiac events: Systematic review and meta-analysis. *JAMA.* 2011;305:1225–1233.

37. Levine GN, Steinke EE, Bakaeen FG et al. Sexual activity and cardiovascular disease: A scientific statement from the American Heart Association. *Circulation.* 2012;125:1058–1072.

38. Critchley JA, Capewell S. Mortality risk reduction associated with smoking cessation in patients with coronary heart disease: A systematic review. *JAMA.* 2003;290:86–97.

39. Wilson K, Gibson N, Willan A, Cook D. Effect of smoking cessation on mortality after myocardial infarction: Meta-analysis of cohort studies. *Arch Intern Med.* 2000;160:939–944.

40. Shah AM, Pfeffer MA, Hartley LH et al. Risk of all-cause mortality, recurrent myocardial infarction, and heart failure hospitalization associated with smoking status following myocardial infarction with left ventricular dysfunction. *Am J Cardiol.* 2010;106:911–916.

41. Thomson CC, Rigotti NA. Hospital- and clinic-based smoking cessation interventions for smokers with cardiovascular disease. *Prog Cardiovasc Dis.* 2003;45:459–479.

42. Dawood N, Vaccarino V, Reid KJ et al. Predictors of smoking cessation after a myocardial infarction: The role of institutional smoking cessation programs in improving success. *Arch Intern Med.* 2008;168:1961–1967.

43. McRobbie H, Bullen C, Hartmann-Boyce J, Hajek P. Electronic cigarettes for smoking cessation and reduction. *Cochrane Database of Systematic Reviews.* 2014; doi: 10.1002/14651858.CD010216.pub2:CD010216.

24

Acute coronary syndrome
Case-based scenarios

SURAJ KUMAR AND GURPREET S WANDER

INTRODUCTION

In India, the epidemiological transition from predominantly infectious disease conditions to non-communicable diseases has occurred over a rather brief period of time. Premature mortality in terms of years of life lost because of CVD in India increased by 59%, from 23.2 million (1990) to 37 million (2010). Acute coronary syndrome with or without ST-segment elevation (STEMI or NSTEACS) is a common cardiac emergency, with the potential for substantial morbidity and mortality. Most of the deaths in acute STEMI occur within the first 24 hours (80%), of which the first hour is the most critical, contributing to 40%–65% of the mortality.

Though the therapeutic options have improved over the past three decades, patients cannot avail themselves of the full benefits due to delayed presentation to hospitals even in the current era. In this chapter, we will discuss three real-life case scenarios with the goal to find the correct clinical approach and management.

CASE SCENARIO 1

A 42-year-old male school teacher presented to the emergency department of a tertiary care centre with a 40-minute episode of chest pain with diaphoresis. The pain was retrosternal, radiating to both arms and was crushing in nature. He was not aware of any other cardiovascular risk factors. His blood pressure was 106/62 mmHg, the heart rate was 112 bpm and regular and oxygen saturation was 94% on room air. There were no heart murmurs present on cardiac auscultation, and the chest was clear. Electrocardiogram showed ST-elevation in V1-V3, suggesting acute anterior wall ST-elevation MI (Figure 24.1).

DISCUSSION

In this case, we can see an educated patient, who recognised his symptoms early and presented within the window period. The usual initiating mechanism for acute myocardial infarction is rupture or erosion of a vulnerable, lipid-laden, atherosclerotic coronary plaque, resulting in exposure of circulating blood to highly thrombogenic core and matrix materials. A totally occluding thrombus typically leads to STEMI. In the current era of potent lipid-lowering therapy, erosion as an underlying cause is increasing as compared to rupture.

The diagnosis of STEMI starts with symptom assessment: history of chest pain lasting at least 20 minutes or more and not responding to nitroglycerine is typical. A 12-lead ECG must be performed as soon as possible. If the initial ECG is not suggestive of STEMI but the patient continues to have symptoms, repeat ECGs must be obtained (every 15 minutes or so), also considering the addition of posterior (V7–V8–V9) or right leads (V4R–V5R, V6R) in patients with high suspicion, respectively, of posterior or right ventricle infarction. The diagnostic electrographic sign is a new ST-segment elevation measured at the J-point in two contiguous leads with the following thresholds: $\geq$0.25 mV in men below the age of 40 years, $\geq$0.2 mV in men over the age of 40 years, or $\geq$0.15 mV in women in leads V2-V3 and/or $\geq$0.1 mV in other leads [1].

RISK STRATIFICATION

The Killip-Kimball classification is a prognostic classification for STEMI patients according to the presence and severity of heart failure signs:

- Class I: No rales or third sound
- Class II: Rales in <50% of pulmonary field with or without third sound

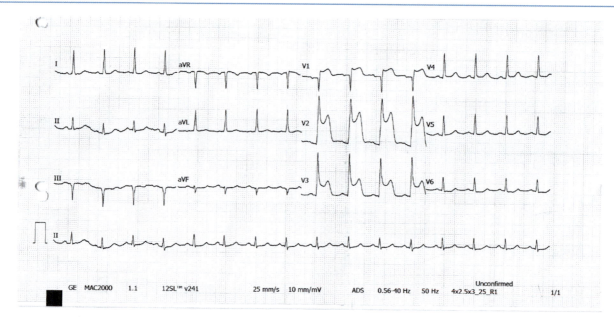

Figure 24.1 12-Lead electrocardiogram shows ST-elevation in leads V1-V3.

- Class III: Rales in >50% of pulmonary field (pulmonary oedema)
- Class IV: Cardiogenic shock

The original data from 1967 shows mortality of patients in Killip Class I-IV is estimated to be around 6%, 17%, 38% and 81%, respectively. With treatment advances, the mortality rates have declined in each class.

All patients with STEMI should have an early assessment of short-term risk, including an evaluation of the extent of myocardial damage, the occurrence of successful reperfusion, and the presence of clinical markers of high risk of further events. The following characteristics have been most consistently associated with adverse outcomes in patients with STEMI:

1. Older age (age ≥75 years)
2. Higher Killip Class (class III or IV)
3. Lower systolic blood pressure (<100 mmHg)
4. Higher heart rate (>100/min)
5. Anterior MI

REPERFUSION

Emergency reperfusion of ischaemic myocardium that is in the process of becoming infarcted is the primary therapeutic goal. Coronary reperfusion is accomplished by means of primary PCI or intravenous fibrinolytic therapy. Primary PCI (with a goal of D2B time ≤90 minutes) is the preferred approach at PCI-capable hospitals for STEMI with onset of symptoms within the previous 12 hours (ACC–AHA class I recommendation) and for STEMI with cardiogenic shock, regardless of the timing [2]. The advantages of primary PCI over fibrinolysis include lower rates of early death, reinfarction and intra-cranial hemorrhage. However, when PCI is delayed by more than 120 minutes, fibrinolytic therapy should be given if it is not contraindicated (ACC–AHA class I recommendation), followed by routine consideration of transfer in the

following 3 to 24 hours to a PCI-capable facility (ACC–AHA class IIa recommendation). With application of reperfusion therapy for STEMI, 30-day mortality rates have declined from more than 20% to less than 5%. The recent evolution in the treatment of acute myocardial infarction largely involves management in the catheterisation laboratory. Second-generation drug-eluting stents have assumed a dominant role in PCI. Cobalt chromium everolimus-eluting stents had the most favourable safety and efficacy profile, with reduced rates of cardiac death, acute myocardial infarction, and stent thrombosis.

Although early data favoured manual thrombus aspiration during primary PCI, data from more recent trials have not. In the largest trial (involving 10732 patients), manual aspiration had no significant effect on the risk of death from cardiovascular causes, myocardial infarction or severe heart failure at 180 days, as compared with conventional PCI (without aspiration thrombectomy), and the risk of stroke at 30 days was higher with manual aspiration. Currently, the routine use of thrombus aspiration during PCI is not indicated (ACC–AHA class IIb recommendation).

The use of IABP during acute myocardial infarction with cardiogenic shock had been present with the paucity of adequately powered randomised controlled trials. In a trial on patients with AMI and cardiogenic shock, in a comparison of IABP with standard therapy, no difference in 30-day mortality or in any key secondary end points (haemodynamic stabilisation, length of stay in the ICU, lactate levels, dose and duration of catecholamine therapy and RFT) was found. Although IABP was safe, there was no evidence that it was associated with haemodynamic improvement.

Fibrinolytic therapy is an important reperfusion strategy in settings where primary PCI cannot be offered in a timely manner, and prevents 30 early deaths per 1000 patients treated within 6 hours after symptom onset. The largest absolute benefit is seen among patients at highest risk, including the elderly, and when treatment is offered <2 hours after symptom onset. Fibrinolytic therapy is recommended within 12 hours of symptom onset if primary PCI cannot be performed within 120 minutes from STEMI diagnosis and there are no contraindications. The later the patient presents (particularly after 3 hours), the more consideration should be given to transfer for primary PCI (as opposed to administering fibrinolytic therapy) because the efficacy and clinical benefit of fibrinolysis decrease as the time from symptom onset increases. Following initiation of lytic therapy, it is recommended to transfer the patients to a PCI centre. In cases of failed fibrinolysis, or if there is evidence of re-occlusion or reinfarction with recurrence of ST-segment elevation, immediate angiography and rescue PCI is indicated. In this setting, re-administration of fibrinolysis has not been shown to be beneficial and should be discouraged. Even if it is likely that fibrinolysis will be successful (ST-segment resolution >50% at 60–90 minutes; typical reperfusion arrhythmia; and disappearance of chest pain), a strategy of routine early angiography (pharmaco-invasive strategy) within 3 to 24 hours is recommended if there are no contraindications.

ANTITHROMBOTIC THERAPY

Non-enteric coated aspirin, at a dose of 325 mg, is recommended at the time of the first medical contact for all patients with an acute coronary syndrome (ACC–AHA class I recommendation). The initial dose is followed by an indefinite daily maintenance dose of 81 to 325 mg of aspirin. A maintenance dose of 81 mg of aspirin is recommended with ticagrelor. In addition to aspirin, an oral P2Y12 inhibitor (clopidogrel, prasugrel, or ticagrelor) is recommended. For patients with STEMI who are undergoing primary PCI, a loading dose should be given as early as possible or at the time of PCI, followed by a daily maintenance dose for at least 1 year (ACC–AHA class I recommendation). Prasugrel and ticagrelor are more potent than clopidogrel and may be preferred with primary PCI who are not at high risk for bleeding (e.g. those without a history of stroke or transient ischaemic attack). Clopidogrel is recommended in association with fibrinolytic therapy and is given after fibrinolytic therapy for a minimum of 14 days and for a maximum of 1 year.

Glycoprotein IIb/IIIa inhibitors are a class of anti-platelet drugs given intravenously, have a more limited role in the treatment of acute coronary syndromes, but when needed, they can provide rapid onset of anti-platelet activity before the patient is taken to the catheterisation laboratory or for prevention and treatment of peri-procedural thrombotic complications. Cangrelor, a short-acting intravenous P2Y12 inhibitor, can also be used adjunct to PCI for reducing the risk of peri-procedural ischaemic events in patients who have not been pre-treated with a P2Y12 or a glycoprotein IIb/IIIa inhibitor.

Administration of a parenteral anti-coagulant agent (i.e. UFH, enoxaparin, bivalirudin, or fondaparinux) is recommended for patients who present with an acute coronary syndrome. Fondaparinux alone does not provide adequate anti-coagulation to support PCI but is useful for medical therapy, especially if the risk of bleeding is high. Enoxaparin is somewhat more effective than unfractionated heparin, particularly in patients who are treated with a non-invasive strategy. During non-invasive management of an ACS, anti-coagulants are administered for at least 2 days and preferably for the duration of hospitalisation, up to 8 days, or until PCI is performed.

CASE SCENARIO 2

A 55-year-old male presented with a history of class II dyspnoea on exertion for the past 6 months and with epigastric pain for the past 2 days. He was known to be diabetic and hypertensive for the past 7 years and has been taking regular medicines. His blood pressure was 130/82 mmHg, the heart rate was 84 bpm and regular. Cardiovascular and respiratory system examination were unremarkable. Electrocardiogram (Figure 24.2) showed T wave inversions in II, III, aVF, V3-V6 and troponin-T was elevated. These findings suggest that the patient is having NSTEACS.

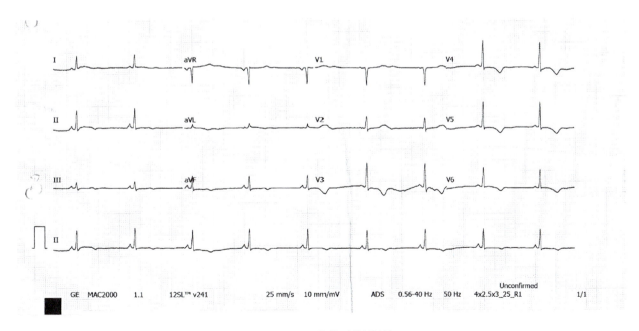

Figure 24.2 12-Lead electrocardiogram shows T wave inversions in II, III, aVF, V3-V6.

DISCUSSION

NSTEACS includes unstable angina and non-ST-elevation MI (NSTEMI) and the two entities are often indistinguishable at presentation. NSTEMI is persistent symptoms with elevated cardiac troponin levels but no ST-segment elevation. Unstable angina produces symptoms suggestive of cardiac ischaemia without elevated cardiac troponin levels. In view of a missed diagnosis (2% patients, approximately) during emergency department evaluation and atypical presentation of ACS patients, a proper approach is very important.

Anginal pain in NSTEACS patients may have the following presentations:

- Prolonged (>20 minutes) anginal pain at rest
- New onset (de novo) angina (CCS class II or III)
- Recent destabilisation of previously stable angina with at least CCS class III angina (crescendo angina)
- Post-MI angina

Prolonged and de novo/crescendo angina are observed in ~80% and ~20% of patients, respectively. Atypical presentations include epigastric pain, indigestion-like symptoms and are more often observed in the elderly, in women and in patients with diabetes, chronic renal disease or dementia. Conditions that may exacerbate or precipitate NSTEACS include anaemia, infection, inflammation, fever and metabolic or endocrine (in particular thyroid) disorders.

The resting 12-lead ECG is the first-line diagnostic tool in the assessment of patients and must be done within 10 minutes of the patient's arrival in the emergency room. ECG in the setting of NSTEACS may be normal in more than one-third of patients. Characteristic abnormalities include ST depression, transient ST-elevation and T wave changes. Comparison with previous tracings is valuable, particularly in patients with pre-existing ECG abnormalities. Biomarkers complement clinical assessment and 12-lead ECG in the diagnosis, risk stratification and treatment of patients with suspected NSTEACS. Cardiac troponins are more sensitive and specific markers of cardiomyocyte injury than CK-MB.

On the basis of the history, ECG and cardiac troponin result, rapid diagnostic triage is performed to address key management decisions (Table 24.1) [3].

Table 24.1 Initial assessment and management decisions in patients presenting with acute coronary syndrome

1. On the basis of the history, examination, ECG and cardiac troponin, patients are classified as either suffering from STEMI or NSTEACS.
2. Using a risk score (e.g. TIMI or GRACE score) to assess risk of cardiovascular death or recurrent ischaemia (high, intermediate, or low risk).
3. The choice of early invasive versus non-invasive strategy is based on risk and the patient's preferences.
4. A second anti-platelet agent is added to aspirin, with selection based on timing of invasive strategy, likelihood of need for surgical revascularisation and risk of bleeding.
5. According to the initial management strategy (invasive or non-invasive), anti-coagulant agent (unfractionated heparin, low molecular weight heparin, fondaparinux, or bivalirudin) is chosen.

RISK STRATIFICATION

The initial risk assessment of a patient in whom an ACS is suspected should address two risks: the risk that the presenting syndrome is in fact an acute coronary syndrome, and if it is, the risk of an early adverse outcome. The risk of an early adverse outcome is more closely linked to presenting features than to risk factors for coronary artery disease. Two validated models have been developed to assess this risk: the thrombolysis in myocardial infarction (TIMI) and Global Registry of Acute Coronary Events (GRACE) models, which are available and can be useful in initial patient care (ACC–AHA class IIa recommendation). Variables used in the GRACE risk calculation include age, history of HF or AMI, systolic blood pressure, pulse rate, serum creatinine, elevated cardiac biomarkers and ST deviation. TIMI risk score discriminative accuracy is inferior to that of the GRACE risk. The TIMI risk score uses seven variables in an additive scoring system: age $\geq$65 years, three or more CAD risk factors, known CAD, aspirin use in the past 7 days, severe angina (two or more episodes within 24 hours), ST change $\geq$0.5 mm and positive cardiac marker.

APPROACH TO MANAGEMENT OF NSTEACS

The initial management includes bed rest with ECG monitoring and prompt initiation of antithrombotic therapy.

Given residual perfusion in the ischaemic zone in acute coronary syndromes without ST-segment elevation, the urgency of and approach to revascularisation differ from that in STEMI. Once a definite or likely diagnosis of an NSTEACS has been made, the patient is triaged to either an invasive strategy or an ischaemia-guided strategy (i.e. an initial medical strategy with angiography reserved for evidence of spontaneous or provoked ischaemia).

An invasive strategy leads to improved outcomes and is favoured for the majority of patients; the urgency of angiography (performed with the goal of revascularization) depends on the presence or absence of high-risk features (Table 24.2) [4]. If initial medical therapy stabilizes the patient's hemodynamic condition and relieves ischemic discomfort, angiography can proceed within 12 to 24 hours. An even more delayed approach (with angiography performed within 25 to 72 hours) is an option for patients at lower immediate risk. In patients whose condition is unstable, urgent PCI is performed, as it is for patients with STEMI. In low-risk patients, a non-invasive stress test (preferably with imaging) for inducible ischaemia is recommended before deciding on an invasive strategy.

Fibrinolytic therapy may be harmful in patients who have an acute coronary syndrome without ST-segment elevation and is therefore contraindicated. At the time of angiography, PCI is the most common intervention, but depending on the coronary anatomy and clinical features, a decision may be made to perform CABG instead of PCI or to forgo an intervention. Indeed, because the culprit artery may be difficult to identify with certainty in patients who have an acute coronary syndrome without ST-segment elevation, simultaneous multi-vessel PCI is often performed if the patient is haemodynamically stable.

Table 24.2 Intervention categories in patients with NSTEACS

| Variable | Invasive intervention | | | Ischaemia-guided intervention |
	Immediate	Early	Delayed	
Timing Indications	Within 2 hrs • Refractory angina • New-onset heart failure • Recurrent angina despite medical treatment	Within 24 hrs • High risk (GRACE score >140) • Rising troponin level • New ST-segment depression	Within 24–72 hrs • Intermediate risk (GRACE score 109–140, TIMI ≥2) • Post-infarction angina • Prior CABG or PCI	Depends on ischemia • Low risk (TIMI score of 0 or 1) • Troponin-negative women • Patient's or physician's preference in absence of high-risk features

CASE SCENARIO 3

A 58-year-old housewife presented with history of epigastric and retrosternal burning, which was of maximum intensity 2 days prior. It was associated with excessive sweating and an episode of vomiting. Now she complains of dyspnoea while lying down but no chest pain. She was a known diabetic for the past 12 years and has been on irregular medicines. Her blood pressure was 130/82 mmHg and her heart rate was 108 bpm. There were bilateral basal crepitations on auscultation. Electrocardiogram showed Q waves with ST-elevation in II, III, aVF, suggesting late presentation of inferior wall myocardial infarction (Figure 24.3).

DISCUSSION

Late presentation is a common case scenario in the Indian setting. Any patient presenting 24 hours after onset of chest pain due to STEMI represents a failure of the prevailing STEMI care system. The 'total ischaemic time' (symptom onset to initiation of reperfusion therapy) has two components: (a) patient delay and (b) system delay (including FMC to diagnosis and diagnosis to initiation of reperfusion therapy). When a patient presents as late as 24 hours after onset of symptoms, patient-related delay accounts for the main reason of delay and system-related delay becomes relatively insignificant. Various Indian ACS registries report that less than 50% of patients with STEMI receive reperfusion therapy and most of the non-reperfusion resulted from late presentation of patients beyond the therapeutic window of reperfusion. Treatment options in India are often dictated by resources, logistics, availability and affordability (Table 24.3). In our country, not many hospitals offer primary PCI services round the clock in the urban areas and this inadequacy is pronounced more in rural areas where penetration of medical care is modest at best.

RISK STRATIFICATION IN LATECOMERS AFTER STEMI

Clinical: In the presence of haemodynamic or electrical instability and/or if the patient continues to experience ischaemic symptoms, a reperfusion-based strategy using PCI is recommended.

ECG: The presence or absence of Q waves by itself is a poor marker of viability or IRA patency. ST-elevation may also be due to aneurysm formation in late presenters.

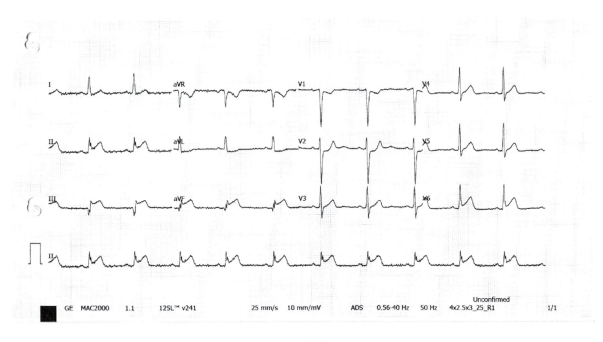

Figure 24.3 12-Lead electrocardiogram shows ST-elevation in leads V1-V3.

Table 24.3 Reasons for delay in STEMI care

- Lack of awareness of symptoms and its attribution to a GI problem
- Family members' inability to appreciate the gravity of the situation
- Self-treatment
- Transportation and inaccessibility to medical care, especially in rural areas
- Delays in call for medical attention/ambulance
- Poorly equipped ambulances
- Poorly trained paramedics/technicians
- Lack of primary PCI facilities
- Lack of 24-hr catheterisation lab access
- Lack of economic affordability and health insurance schemes

Angiographic: There are a few experimental and clinical studies suggesting that an open IRA is of advantage. However, a single large OAT study failed to show any advantage of the routine opening of IRA beyond 72 hours of symptom onset. The importance of an open IRA in patients presenting with a window of 24–72 hours is not known. There exists an important yet unrecognised interplay between time to reperfusion and presence of residual coronary flow within the area at risk. Beyond 4 hours of symptoms, significant salvage only occurred in the presence of well-developed collateral vessels or preserved antegrade flow in the IRA.

Stress testing: Exercise testing is useful in assessing exercise capacity, identifying persistent ischaemia and risk stratification for future cardiac events. Submaximal testing may be done in asymptomatic patients after 3–5 days and symptom-limited testing may be done in the same subset of patients after 5 days. The DANAMI-1 and SWISS trials have demonstrated beneficial effects of PCI performed late after MI in patients with persistent ischaemia on stress testing.

Myocardial viability: In the VIAMI trial, patients not treated with primary or rescue PCI but otherwise in the non-high-risk category were subjected to either invasive (PCI) or a conservative (ischaemia-guided) strategy if the infarct area was proven to be viable. Benefit in terms of composite end points of death, myocardial infarction or unstable angina was seen at follow-up of 1 year and at long-term follow-up of median 8 years with initial in-hospital invasive strategy. Viability early after AMI is associated with improvement in LV function after revascularisation. When a viable myocardium is not revascularised, the LV tends to remodel with increased LV volumes, without improvement of EF. Absence of viability results in ventricular dilatation and deterioration of LVEF, irrespective of revascularisation status. Various modalities that can be used to assess myocardial viability are SPECT (Th-201 or Tc-99), FDG-PET, dobutamine stress ECHO, dobutamine stress cardiac MRI and contrast enhanced MRI.

REPERFUSION PCI IN LATECOMERS WITH STEMI

Open artery hypothesis: This hypothesis was first proposed by Eugene Braunwald in 1989 when he noted that patients with

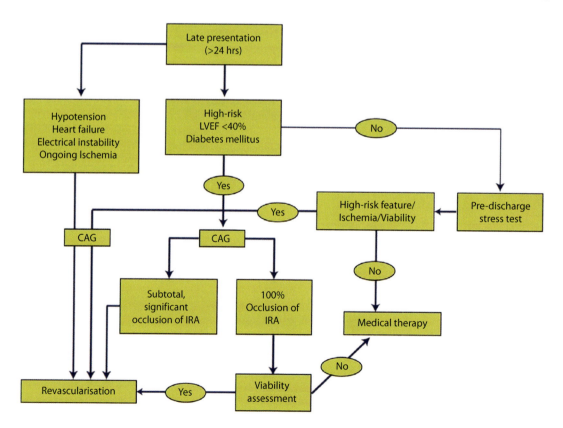

Figure 24.4 Proposed algorithm for management of stable patients of acute myocardial infarction presenting more than 24 hours from symptom onset.

spontaneous recanalisation of the IRA had fewer adverse events during the following weeks and months. These effects are not likely to be attributable to small benefits in infarct salvage and probably arise from limitation of infarct expansion, reduction of LV remodelling development, scaffolding effect of reperfused vessel, a conduit for collateral vessel, improvement of blood supply to hibernating myocardium, increased infarct wound healing, development of contraction band necrosis rather than coagulation necrosis in infarcted myocardium, reduction of myocardial apoptosis, increased baroreceptor sensitivity and vagal activity and reduced ventricular arrhythmia. These mechanisms extended the time window of reperfusion to 12 hours and possibly 24 hours after onset of AMI. However, the period after 24 hours of onset of AMI is more challenging. On the basis of the OAT study (2006), routine PCI 3 days to weeks after AMI is not recommended for persistently occluded IRA in asymptomatic high-risk patients, since higher reinfarction rates were seen in the PCI group and yet, no differences were seen between PCI and conservative groups in terms of event-free survival after median follow-up of 3.2 years or LV systolic function at 1 year. Subsequently, Appelton et al. performed a meta-analysis and systematic review of randomised trials in 2008 comparing late PCI (defined as greater than 12 hours from symptom onset) with medical therapy in haemodynamically stable patients with primary end point of survival. PCI was associated with an overall improvement in survival and further, a greater improvement in LV function was seen in patients assigned to PCI than medically managed patients supporting the concept that late revascularisation may reverse adverse cardiac remodelling over a longer term. Later, Busk et al. also demonstrated in 2009 that substantial myocardial salvage can be obtained beyond the 12 hours limit, even when the infarct-related artery is totally occluded. Thus, 'not so latecomers' (12 to 48 hours) may gain through reperfusion of the hibernating myocardium in the peri-infarct region.

The Cardiology Society of India has published a position statement for the management of ST-elevation myocardial infarction in India in 2017 and has proposed an algorithm for management of patients of acute myocardial infarction presenting more than 24 hours from symptom onset (Figure 24.4) [5].

CHALLENGES OF LATE REVASCULARISATION

Total occlusion of an IRA is commonly associated with a significant thrombotic burden. The thrombus is at least partially organised and thus mechanically more resistant to guidewire recanalisation. On-going micro-vascular damage also interferes with TIMI-3 perfusion grades. When thrombus is angiographically evident, aggressive antithrombotic therapy and thrombosuction prior to stent implantation may be helpful in minimising distal embolisation and recurrent myocardial infarction.

CONCLUSION

Three clinically relevant case scenarios have been described with an aim to provide a more mechanistic approach to the categorisation of ACS and to provide a framework for future tailoring, triage, and therapy for patients in a more personalised and precise manner. It is essential for clinicians to take an individualised approach to the treatment of ACS.

REFERENCES

1. Thygesen K, Alpert JS, Jaffe AS et al. Third universal definition of myocardial infarction. *J Am Coll Cardiol.* 2012;60:1581–1598.
2. O'Gara PT, Kushner FG, Ascheim DD et al. 2013 ACCF/AHA guideline for the management of ST-elevation myocardial infarction: A report of the American College of Cardiology Foundation/American Heart Association Task Force on Practice Guidelines. *J Am Coll Cardiol.* 2013;61(4):e78–e140.
3. Anderson JL, Morrow DA. Acute myocardial infarction-review article. *N Engl J Med.* 2017;376(21):2053–2064.
4. Amsterdam EA, Wenger NK, Brindis RG et al. 2014 AHA/ACC guideline for the management of patients with non-ST-elevation acute coronary syndromes: A report of the American College of Cardiology/American Heart Association Task Force on Practice Guidelines. *J Am Coll Cardiol.* 2014;64(24):e139–e228.
5. Guha S, Sethi R, Ray S et al. Cardiological Society of India: Position statement for the management of ST elevation myocardial infarction in India. *Indian Heart J.* 2017;69:S1–S104.

25

Quality improvement programme for acute coronary syndrome care in India

PP MOHANAN

INTRODUCTION

Cardiovascular diseases (CVDs) have become the leading cause of mortality in India with the turn of century [1]. While the number of CVD deaths has not changed significantly in high-income countries since 1990, the number of deaths has increased by about 66% in low- and middle-income countries (LMICs) over the same interval [2]. While attempting to address the burden of CVD, LMICs face the challenges of limited health care budgets and infrastructure as well as constrained professional health workforce capacity.

In the context of scarce resources available to support health care in LMICs, the imperative of clinical quality improvement is to get the most out of known effective interventions within the limitations of available resources rather than recommending unproven interventions that would require early-phase studies or those that would require substantial financial and human resource investment for implementation. Clinical quality improvement can be implemented within any setting immediately and need not be expensive.

Quality care delivery in low income countries does not necessarily mean dissemination and implementation of a universal set of standards formulated in high income countries. Standards and interventions should be dictated by context and community capacity. Adaptation to local settings is necessary to achieve optimal clinical outcomes and patient satisfaction.

The application of high-quality and safe care can be unevenly distributed within and among regions, hospitals and even physicians. For example, Figure 25.1 shows substantial, hospital-level heterogeneity in the use of the combination of dual anti-platelet therapy, anti-coagulant therapy, beta-blockers and statins for patients with acute coronary syndromes in Kerala [3]. Some of this heterogeneity may be due to physician judgment, patient preference, or contraindication that was not captured or adequately documented, but some of this heterogeneity is unexplained and likely represents an error of omission toward high-quality care.

Errors of commission in cardiovascular care have also been demonstrated. For example, patients with non-ST-segment myocardial infarction in the Kerala Acute Coronary Syndrome Registry received thrombolysis 19% of the time, which was associated with increased risk of an in-hospital adverse event [5].

We cannot doubt the intent of treating physicians to provide the best possible care of each patient, but at times the hectic and rapid pace of cardiovascular medicine in India can make it difficult to implement these intentions. Quantity can, at times, overwhelm quality. On the other hand, high-volume centres can be hubs within a learning health system [6] that aims to continuously improve efficiencies and outcomes using task sharing and audit and feedback mechanisms as demonstrated by Aravind Eye Institute, Narayana Hridayalaya, among others in India.

Data are essential to translate knowledge into action at the clinical level by understanding areas for improving cardiovascular health care quality and patient safety in India, which is poised for major growth, particularly as stakeholders including patients, government and payers push for higher quality care at lower cost.

BRIEF HISTORY OF CARDIOVASCULAR HEALTH CARE QUALITY IMPROVEMENT

Over the past 20 years, there has been considerable emphasis on cardiovascular health care quality improvement programmes. For example, in the United States the American Heart Association's

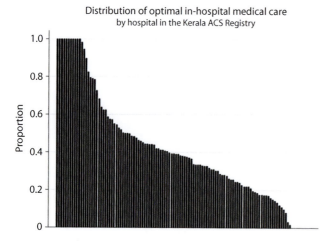

Figure 25.1 Hospital-level distribution of 'optimal' in-hospital medical care, defined as dual anti-platelet therapy, anti-coagulant therapy, beta-blockers and statins for patients with acute coronary syndromes in Kerala [4].

(heart.org) Get With the Guidelines programme and the American College of Cardiology's National Cardiovascular Data Registry (cvquality.acc.org/NCDR) have been key programmes for quality improvement as well as training and infrastructure development since 1997. Hospitals can now voluntarily report data to the public using these data. Cardiovascular professional organisations have led much of these efforts but were preceded by state-level efforts that began in New York, which began collecting data in 1988 and first reported hospital-level data on adult cardiac surgery survival in 1990 [7].

The United States federal government collected and reported hospital-level post-discharge mortality rates even earlier (1986 to 1992) but stopped due to criticisms related to the methods of data collection and analysis [8]. Other national and international organisations such as the Agency for Healthcare Research and Quality (ahrq.gov), United Kingdom's National Institute for Health and Care Excellence (nice.org.uk), or the World Health Organization's (WHO) Patient Safety Programme (who.int/patientsafety) provide guidance on developing, implementing, evaluating and advocating for strategies to improve quality and safety. Other non-governmental quality organisations, such as the Institute for Healthcare Improvement (ihi.org) or National Quality Forum (nqf.org), train and convene wider groups of stakeholders beyond cardiovascular medicine. Still other organisations focus on hospital-level accreditation such as the National Accreditation Board for Hospitals and Healthcare Providers (nabh.co; part of the larger Quality Council of India [qcin.org] founded in 1997), Joint Commission International, among others. While high-quality data demonstrating improvements in clinical outcomes through hospital accreditation have been lacking thus far [9], effects from a complex intervention such as accreditation can be difficult to assess. Nevertheless, the health care quality and patient safety movement seems likely to expand in India, particularly as payment shifts from individuals at the point-of-service to pre-payment through government or private insurance programmes.

FUNDAMENTAL CONCEPTS RELATED TO QUALITY, SAFETY AND QUALITY IMPROVEMENT

The Institute of Medicine defines *quality* as the 'degree to which health services for individuals and populations increase the likelihood of desired health outcomes and are consistent with current professional knowledge' [10]. Six quality aims were identified in the Institute of Medicine's landmark Quality Chasm report: (1) safety, (2) efficiency, (3) patient-centeredness, (4) timeliness, (5) effectiveness and (6) equity. The Institute of Medicine defines safety as 'freedom from accidental injury', whereas others more broadly define patient safety as a 'discipline in the health care professions that applies safety science methods toward the goal of achieving a trustworthy system of health care delivery … (and) an attribute of health care systems that minimizes the incidence and impact of adverse events and maximizes recovery from such events' [11]. *Quality improvement* includes a set of techniques for continuous study and improvement of the processes of delivering health care services and products to meet the needs and expectations of the customers of those services and products. Quality improvement focuses on customer knowledge and experience; processes of health care delivery, and statistical approaches that aim to reduce variations in those processes [12]. Figure 25.2 outlines five typical steps for improving quality, including (1) identifying area(s) of improvement, (2) determining what processes can be modified to improve outcomes, (3) developing and executing strategies to improve quality, (4) tracking performance and outcomes and (5) disseminating results to spur broad quality improvement.

Increasingly there has been an emphasis on the method of evaluating the effect of a quality improvement intervention. For example, in Brazil [13], China [14], Europe [15] and India (acsquik.org), there have been or are studies of cardiovascular quality improvement using randomised controlled trial study designs in contrast with the non-randomised study designs in other settings [16]. However, there are common components across all study designs, including:

1. Empowered, interdisciplinary quality teams including physicians, specialists, nurses and technicians with regular meetings for continuous quality improvement,
2. Standardised admission and discharge order sets, clinical algorithms and patient education materials and
3. Audit and feedback mechanisms.

CARDIOVASCULAR HEALTH CARE QUALITY IMPROVEMENT PROGRAMMES IN ACS IN INDIA

Indian cardiovascular medicine boasts a multitude of local, regional and national registries that report data on presentation, management and outcomes of patients with cardiovascular diseases. However, there are limited numbers of interventional projects and programmes designed to improve health care quality and

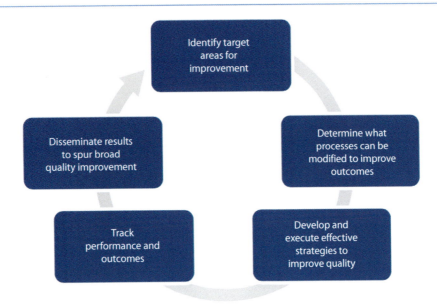

Figure 25.2 Five steps for improving quality. (Analysis by Avalere Health and American Hospital Association.)

patient safety that have been reported since 2010. We outline the major aim(s) and key components of each in the following sections.

TAMIL NADU ST-ELEVATION MYOCARDIAL INFARCTION (TN-STEMI)

The Tamil Nadu ST-Elevation Myocardial Infarction (TN-STEMI) study was a prospective, controlled, multi-centre pretest/post-test quasi-experimental study that aimed to improve the rate and speed of reperfusion therapy in patients with STEMI [17–19]. The trial collected data for at least 12 weeks before (n = 898 participants) and a mean of 32 weeks after the intervention (n = 1522 participants) was implemented and followed patients up for 12 months. The trial employed four clusters of hospitals in a hub-and-spoke model:

Class A hospitals: Hub hospital capable of 24-hour percutaneous coronary intervention (PCI)
Class B hospitals: Hub hospital not capable of 24-hour PCI
Class C hospitals: Spoke hospital within 30 minutes of a hub hospital
Class D hospitals: Spoke hospital beyond 30 minutes of a hub hospital

Key partners in this health system strengthening study include the government of Tamil Nadu, Gunapati Venkata Krishna Emergency Management and Research Institute (GVK-EMRI) public-private ambulance partnership, and STEMI India physician-led health care non-profit organisation. The intervention included the development of this health system to facilitate primary and rescue PCI, pharmaco-invasive management of patients at class D hospitals using the aforementioned ambulance partnership, and mobile clinical technologies to facilitate rapid ECG acquisition and interpretation in the field. The co-primary outcomes included use of reperfusion therapy, timely reperfusion and early invasive risk stratification among individuals initially treated with fibrinolysis. Overall, reperfusion rates were similar before and after the intervention implementation period (89% vs. 90%, p = 0.21), but rates of coronary angiography (35% vs. 61%, p < 0.001) and percutaneous coronary intervention (30% vs. 47%, p < 0.001) were higher in the post-implementation period. In-hospital mortality rates were similar (5.8% vs. 5.6%, p = 0.83) but 1-year mortality was lower in the post-implementation period (17.6% vs. 14.2%, p = 0.04), which persisted after multi-variable adjustment (odds ratio = 0.76, 95% CI 0.58, 0.98).

SECONDARY PREVENTION OF CORONARY EVENTS AFTER DISCHARGE (SPREAD)

The Secondary Prevention of CoRonary Events After Discharge from hospital (SPREAD) trial is a randomised, parallel group trial evaluating the effect of trained community health workers on improving adherence to medication and health behaviours at 12 months compared with usual care among heart attack survivors in 14 hospitals throughout India [20]. This complex intervention includes a combination of facility- and home-based visits between participants and community health workers, the latter who are supported by trial project offers, to encourage self-care behaviours through education, coaching and multiple reminder tools (diary, calendar). The trial enrolled 806 participants (83% men; mean [SD] age 66.4 [11.3] years, 54% ST-segment elevation myocardial infarction) between 2011 and 2012, and results are pending.

MANAGEMENT OF ACUTE CORONARY SYNDROMES IN SECONDARY CARE SETTINGS IN KERALA: IMPACT OF A QUALITY IMPROVEMENT PROGRAMME

A well-defined geographical area comprising the Trichur, Palaghat and Malappuram districts of Kerala, India was identified for the quality improvement programme (QIP). Kerala is well known for the concept of good health at low cost. The identified area has a population of about 300,000 as per the estimates of the 2001 census. A total of 40 secondary care hospitals/nursing homes in this area had basic facilities for the management of patients with ACS. The study was conducted in three different phases—pre-intervention, intervention and post-intervention. The sample size planned for the study was 500 patients with ACS both in the pre- and post-intervention phases to demonstrate significant changes in the treatment pattern. In the pre-intervention phase, all the participating physicians were asked to register consecutive patients with ACS (20 each) presenting to their clinic. The proforma was explained to all the physicians and regular feedback was sent to them on quality and completeness of data collection. The intervention phase mainly involved the use of a service delivery package and formal education of health care professionals in the detection and optimal management of ACS. Continuing medical education (CME) programmes were conducted as panel discussions for the physicians (rate of participation: 90%–100%) who were involved in providing care to patients with ACS. The service delivery package comprised standard admission orders and patient-directed discharge instructions, which were finalised at the beginning of the intervention phase by a focus group discussion among the entire group of participating physicians. Post intervention all participating physicians were again asked to register consecutive cases of ACS (20 each) presenting to their clinic during this period. The same structured proforma used in the pre-intervention phase was used in this phase. Improvements in evidence-based treatment practices were observed after the comprehensive quality improvement programme (QIP). The time to thrombolysis (TTT) dropped significantly (median difference of 54 minutes, $p < 0.05$) after the intervention programme. Additionally, when TTT was stratified into different groups, we observed that 52.1% of STEMI patients received thrombolysis within the first 2 hours of the onset of symptoms in the post-intervention group as compared with 45.3% in the pre-intervention group. Such a significant reduction in TTT has the potential to improve clinical outcomes in patients with ACS [21].

ACUTE CORONARY SYNDROME QUALITY IMPROVEMENT IN KERALA (ACS QUIK; ACSQUIK.ORG)

This project developed from the Kerala ACS Registry and has been supported by the Cardiological Society of India – Kerala Chapter and National Heart, Lung, and Blood Institute. The primary aim was to develop, implement and evaluate the effect of a locally developed quality improvement toolkit on 30-day major adverse cardiovascular event rates among patients with acute coronary syndrome through a cluster randomised, stepped wedge clinical trial across 63 hospitals in Kerala [22]. Other aims included the evaluation of health-related quality of life among acute coronary syndrome patients as well as individual- and household-level, or microeconomic costs to evaluate patients' perspectives more clearly. The toolkit included a monthly audit and feedback

reporting mechanism with support for quality improvement team meetings; admission and discharge checklists; patient behaviour change materials to support healthy diets, physical activity including home-based cardiac rehabilitation and behavioural counselling for tobacco cessation; and support for cardiac arrest and rapid response team development. A total of 21,374 participants from 63 hospitals were recruited between November 2014 and November 2016. The participants' mean age was 60.7 years, 76% were men, and two-thirds presented with ST-segment elevation myocardial infarction. The results are pending.

Other programmes such as the Ministry of Health and Family Welfare's National Programme for Prevention and Control Non-Communicable Diseases and Indian Stroke Association [23] aim to improve quality through detection, treatment and control of cardiovascular diseases, principally acute and chronic manifestations of ischaemic heart disease and cerebrovascular disease, but their status is less clear. Overall, these project the breadth of conditions and populations that are being targeted, albeit generally at early stages, for improving cardiovascular health care quality and safety in India to date.

CHALLENGES, OPPORTUNITIES AND FUTURE DIRECTIONS

CHALLENGES

1. *Stakeholder fragmentation*: Because health is a responsibility of the state in India, national coordination for improving cardiovascular health care quality and improving safety may remain limited amidst stakeholder fragmentation and inequities among states will persist. Professional organisations, such as the Cardiological Society of India, can lead coordinate, and promote quality and safety efforts, including the development of local clinical practice guidelines, but professional organisations must engage other stakeholders including governmental leaders on the state and central levels, private insurers, regulators, administrators, physicians, nurses and other allied health professionals and patient advocacy groups.

2. *Costs*: Most individuals pay out-of-pocket for their medical expenses and cannot use group financial leverage to influence quality and safety. The rise of private insurance coverage and health care regulation through bodies such as the National Accreditation Board of Hospitals may help influence quality of care delivery, particularly on the inpatient level. Private health care organisations are likely to be early adopters to improving quality though government health care organisations who are essential to improve care broadly and for those most vulnerable and with the fewest resources.

3. *Capacity*: Beyond the capacity to care for the large numbers of patients in India with cardiovascular diseases, cardiovascular health care quality and patient safety infrastructure, systems and personnel are under-developed in many parts of the country. For example, while there are many facility-based registries documenting the quality of care at individual, or at times, many institutions, there are few coordinated systems to

link registries to action, let alone link them together to create learning health care systems. Many hospitals rely on paper-based record keeping and many may have limited Internet access, which makes data capture time consuming. Also, few hospitals have dedicated, trained and interdisciplinary quality improvement teams who are empowered to effect change at the local level. Training programmes such as the Institute for Healthcare Improvement (ihi.org) have chapters in India, but the penetrance of these chapters remains relatively low. Further, limited health technology assessment capacity to identify, appraise and synthesise data evaluating the effects of complex quality improvement interventions makes it difficult for stakeholders to know which interventions are most likely to lead to sustained improvements in process of care measures and outcomes. Stakeholder fragmentation means that no one organisation will be responsible for increasing capacity for health care quality and safety, such as the United Kingdom's National Institute for Health and Care Excellence (www.nice.org.uk), which has provided 'national guidance and advice to improve health and social care' for the National Health Service since 1999.

4. *Sustainability*: Each of the quality projects or programmes listed previously has been supported through a sponsor model, meaning that an extramural funding body pays the study teams to carry out their proposed work. However, these projects or programmes may not be sustained without appropriate funding mechanisms such as a subscription-based model wherein hospitals, payers, or both support the infrastructure and training costs for cardiovascular quality improvement and safety activities.

Opportunities

1. *State-level innovations*: Because health is a responsibility of the state, Indian states can serve as innovative health care quality and safety 'laboratories' by testing new interventions that can later be adapted, implemented and evaluated at the national level. This opportunity counterbalances the challenge of stakeholder fragmentation.
2. *Near-term gains are within sight*: Major near-term gains in quality and safety appear possible and within reach for acute and chronic cardiovascular health care based on the ongoing efforts listed previously, particularly if teams are able to develop sustainable funding models. Quality and safety campaigns in other areas, such as maternal mortality highlighted in the Why Women Die campaign that focused on post-partum haemorrhage, have been rapidly scaled up. Similarly, focused activities within cardiovascular medicine could improve outcomes quickly.
3. *Information technology infrastructure*: India's low-cost, high-quality information technology infrastructure can provide the necessary infrastructure to create electronic data capture systems, electronic audit and feedback reporting, just-in-time training and decision support that are part of learning health care systems. These systems and the resulting locally-derived data can inform contextualised, culture sensitive, equity promoting, cost-effective guidelines.

Future directions in cardiovascular health care quality improvement programmes

1. *Expansion beyond ischaemic heart disease and cerebro-vascular disease*: While Indian investigators have largely and appropriately, emphasised improving care of leading acute cardiovascular diseases, principally acute coronary syndrome and stroke, there are opportunities for improving outpatient care, surgical or procedure-based care (i.e. interventional cardiology and electrophysiology) and care in other disease states such as heart failure or atrial fibrillation.
2. *Increased regulation*: Hospital accreditation by quality and safety organisations, such as the National Accreditation Board of Hospitals and others, seems likely to increase and thereby increase regulation, initially within private and charity hospitals. This regulation will be driven by increasing private insurance coverage whereby payers will direct patients to accredited hospitals as a means of improving quality while managing costs paid on behalf of beneficiaries. Accreditation alone will not improve quality, but the goal will be to leverage the focus on processes of care to improve patient outcomes and experiences.
3. *Patients' voices will be louder*: Patient advocacy groups can and will disseminate their messages more widely and more easily through social media outlets. Physicians and hospitals will be evaluated and rated, fairly or not, on online platforms and many will challenge patients' abilities to perform such evaluations. This may influence the power dynamics between some patients and physicians toward a more shared decision-making model. On the other hand, supply-demand dynamics may limit the influence of these platforms given the relative dearth of health care professionals and even fewer specialists in some parts of the country.

CONCLUSION

Cardiovascular health care quality improvement programmes are emerging, yet crucially important areas to reduce the burden of cardiovascular diseases in India. Improving quality and safety requires broad engagement with patients, families, government, private insurance and non-physician health care workers to effect change on a large scale. Fundamental concepts related to quality improvement and safety appear universal, yet require contextu-alisation to the Indian setting to be most effective. Initial studies in India are promising yet complex, and scalability to state and national levels will be important next steps to capitalise on the opportunities that lay ahead.

ACKNOWLEDGEMENT

The author acknowledges the contribution of Dr Mark D. Huffman, MD, MPH, Associate Professor of Preventive Medicine (Epidemiology) and Medicine (Cardiology) of

Northwestern University Feinberg School of Medicine, Chicago, Illinois, in preparing this manuscript.

REFERENCES

1. Srinath Reddy K, Shah B, Varghese C, Ramadoss A. Responding to the threat of chronic diseases in India. *Lancet*. 2005;366:1744–1749.

2. Roth GA, Huffman MD, Moran AE et al. Global and regional Pat- terns in cardiovascular mortality from 1990 to 2013. *Circulation*. 2015; 132(17):1667–78.

3. Huffman MD, Prabhakaran D, Abraham AK et al. Optimal in-hospital and discharge medical therapy in acute coronary syndromes in Kerala: Results from the Kerala acute coronary syndrome registry. *Circ Cardiovasc Qual Outcomes*. Jul 2013;6(4):436–43.

4. Mohanan PP, Mathew R, Harikrishnan S et al. Presentation, management, and outcomes of 25 748 acute coronary syndrome admissions in Kerala, India: Results from the Kerala ACS Registry. *Eur Heart J*. Jan 2013;34(2):121–9.

5. Smith M, Saunders R, Stuckhardt L, McGinnis JM. *Best Care at Lower Cost: The Path to Continuously Learning Health Care in America*. 2013. The National Academies Press.

6. Hannan EL, Kilburn H, O'Donnell JF, Lukacik G, Shields EP. Adult open heart surgery in New York State. An analysis of risk factors and hospital mortality rates. *JAMA*. 5 Dec 1990;264(21):2768–74.

7. Hannan EL, Cozzens K, King SB, Walford G, Shah NR. The New York State cardiac registries: History, contributions, limitations, and lessons for future efforts to assess and publicly report healthcare outcomes. *J Am CollCardiol*. 19 Jun 2012;59(25):2309–16.

8. Brubakk K, Vist GE, Bukholm G, Barach P, Tjomsland O. A systematic review of hospital accreditation: The challenges of measuring complex intervention effects. *BMC Health Serv Res*. 2015;15(1):280.

9. Institute of Medicine (US) Committee on Quality of Health Care in America. *Crossing the Quality Chasm: A New Health System for the 21st Century*. Washington (DC): National Academies Press (US). 2001.

10. Emanuel L, Berwick D, Conway J, Combes J. What exactly is patient safety? In: Henrikson K, Battles JB, Keyes MA, Editors. *Advances in Patient Safety New Directions and Alternative Approaches*. Rockville, MD. 2008.

11. Berwanger O, Guimarães HP, Laranjeira LN et al. Effect of a multifaceted intervention on use of evidence-based therapies in patients with acute coronary syndromes in Brazil: The BRIDGE-ACS randomized trial. *JAMA*. 2012;307(19):2041–9.

12. Du X, Gao R, Turnbull F et al. Hospital quality improvement initiative for patients with acute coronary syndromes in China: A cluster randomized, controlled trial. *Circ Cardiovasc Qual Outcomes*. Mar 2014;7(2):217–26.

13. Wood DA, Kotseva K, Connolly S et al. Nurse-coordinated multidisciplinary, family-based cardiovascular disease prevention programme (EUROACTION) for patients with coronary heart disease and asymptomatic individuals at high risk of cardiovascular disease: A paired, cluster-randomised controlled trial. *Lancet*. 14 Jun 2008;371(9629):1999–2012.

14. Peterson ED, Roe MT, Mulgund J et al. Association between hospital process performance and outcomes among patients with acute coronary syndromes. *JAMA*. 26 Apr 2006;295(16):1912–20.

15. Balachandran R, Kappanayil M, Sen AC et al. Impact of the International Quality Improvement Collaborative on outcomes after congenital heart surgery: A single center experience in a developing economy. *Ann Card Anaesth*. Jan 2015;18(1):52–7.

16. CARRS Trial Writing Group, Shah S, Singh K, Ali MK et al. Improving diabetes care: Multi-component cardiovascular disease risk reduction strategies for people with diabetes in South Asia--the CARRS multi-center translation trial. *Diabetes Res ClinPract*. Nov 2012;98(2):285–94.

17. Ali MK, Singh K, Kondal D et al. Effectiveness of a multicomponent quality improvement strategy to improve achievement of diabetes care goals. *Ann Intern Med*. 12 Jul 2016;165(6):399–408.

18. Alexander T, Victor SM, Mullasari AS et al. Protocol for a prospective, controlled study of assertive and timely reperfusion for patients with ST-segment elevation myocardial infarction in Tamil Nadu: The TN-STEMI programme. *BMJ*. 2013;3(12):e003850–0.

19. Alexander T, Mullasari AS, Joseph G et al. A system of care for patients with st-segment elevation myocardial infarction in India. *JAMA Cardiol*. 2017;2(5):498–505.

20. Kamath DY, Xavier D, Gupta R et al. Rationale and design of a randomized controlled trial evaluating community health worker-based interventions for the secondary prevention of acute coronary syndromes in India (SPREAD). *Am Heart J*. Nov 2014;168(5):690–7.

21. Prabhakaran D, Jeemon P, Mohanan PP, Govindan U, Geevar Z, Chaturvedi V, Reddy KS. Management of acute coronary syndrome in secondary care settings in Kerala: Impact of a quality improvement programme. *Natl Med J India*. 2008;21(3):107–111.

22. Huffman MD, Mohanan PP, Devarajan R et al. Acute Coronary Syndrome Quality Improvement in Kerala (ACS QUIK): Rationale and design for a cluster randomized stepped wedge trial. *Am Heart J*. Mar 2017;185:154–160.

23. Mehndiratta MM, Singhal AB, Chaturvedi S, Sivakumar MR, Moonis M. Meeting the challenges of stroke in India. *Neurology*. 11 Jun 2013;80(24):2246–7.

26

Primary angioplasty
Basic principles

SRINIVASAN NARAYANAN AND AJIT S MULLASARI

INTRODUCTION

Sudden fibrous cap disruption of an atherosclerotic plaque or surface erosion in the absence of fibrous cap disruption can result in the formation of an occlusive thrombus in the coronary artery resulting in acute ST-elevation myocardial infarction (STEMI) [1]. Reperfusion of the infarcted coronary artery with either primary percutaneous coronary intervention (PPCI) or fibrinolytic therapy improves myocardial salvage and reduces mortality compared to no reperfusion if performed in a timely manner. This is especially important in the first few hours after onset of symptoms, when the amount of myocardium salvageable by reperfusion is greatest. As the benefits of reperfusion decline rapidly with time, reperfusion should be implemented as soon as possible.

Primary PCI when performed in a timely fashion is the reperfusion strategy of choice in patients who are having an acute STEMI or an MI with a new or presumed new onset of left bundle branch block (LBBB) or true posterior wall myocardial infarction.

VARIOUS TREATMENT STRATEGIES FOR ACUTE STEMI

Various treatment strategies [2] that have been used to achieve reperfusion in acute STEMI include:

1. Pharmacological reperfusion – Fibrinolysis
2. Mechanical reperfusion – Primary percutaneous coronary intervention (PPCI) with balloon angioplasty thrombosuction and stenting
3. Rescue PCI or salvage PCI for apparent failure of fibrinolysis
4. Facilitated PCI – Administration of pharmacological measures in order to achieve an open infarct-related artery before arrival at the catheterisation lab for angiography and PCI
5. Pharmaco-invasive strategy – Immediate transfer and or routine angiography with adjunctive PCI within 3–24 hours of successful pharmacological reperfusion
6. Ischaemia/symptom-guided PCI

The definitive goal in STEMI management is early, complete and sustained reperfusion, which in turn results in better short-term and long-term outcomes [3].

LIMITATIONS OF FIBRINOLYSIS

Since the primary role of thrombus is paramount in the patho-physiology of STEMI, the introduction of fibrinolytic therapy was a major advance in the treatment of acute STEMI. The net effect in major fibrinolytic trials was an approximate 30% reduction in the 7% to 10% short-term mortality in STEMI with fibrinolytic therapy.

The following limitations of fibrinolytic therapy provided the impetus for the role of PPCI in STEMI:

1. Since the resistance of cross-linked fibrin to fibrinolysis is time-dependent the benefit of fibrinolysis is greatest when therapy is given in the first 4 hours, especially in the first 70 minutes [3].
2. Attainment of TIMI 3 flow is much more common in PPCI 93%–96% as per the PAMI AND CADILLAC trials versus only 50%–60% with thrombolysis [4–6].
3. Major haemorrhagic complications with fibrinolysis are around 2% to 3%, with 1% of it being intracerebral haemorrhages [7].
4. Older adults presenting with acute STEMI are not candidates for fibrinolytics because of contraindications such as active internal bleeding, recent stroke or hypertension and constitute around 20% to 30% of acute MI [8].
5. Efficacy of fibrinolytics has not been demonstrated in patients with cardiogenic shock.

PRIMARY PCI: GOALS, TIME LOGISTICS, WHY AND IN WHICH SITUATIONS?

The goal of PPCI in STEMI is to achieve initial reperfusion with good coronary flows as early as feasible in a safe and effective manner so that ischaemic damage to the myocardium is minimised and to prevent coronary re-occlusion with stenting. A similar goal exists for patients who are first given fibrinolytics but who do not show signs of reperfusion as evidenced by clinical and ECG findings. Primary PCI should be the universally preferred strategy for prompt early reperfusion if there are no resource or logistical constraints. The American College of Cardiology/American Heart Association (ACC/AHA) and the European Society of Cardiology (ESC) STEMI guidelines recommend PCI as the initial approach to management of STEMI, at centres with a skilled PCI laboratory with rapid initiation [9,10].

The recommendation to prefer primary PCI is based on the results of multiple randomised trials comparing it to fibrinolytic therapy. In a meta-analysis of 23 such trials, the risk of short-term death was lower with primary PCI (7% vs. 9%; p = 0.0002), as was the risk of stroke or non-fatal MI [11].

BASIC TERMINOLOGIES RELATED TO PRIMARY PCI TIMING

Door-to-needle time refers to the time from presentation to the hospital/ambulance to administration of fibrinolytics [9,12].

Door-to-balloon time refers to the time from presentation to a PCI-capable centre to the first balloon inflation irrespective of stenting. PCI-related delay is the difference between the door-to-balloon time and the door-to-needle time. DIDO (Door In Door Out) is defined as the duration of time from arrival to discharge at the first STEMI referral hospital and has become a performance measure of spoke hospitals providing referral to PCI-capable hub hospitals. The 2008 ACC/AHA performance measures recommend a DIDO time of <30 minutes [11].

If high quality primary PCI can be delivered in <120 minutes of first medical contact (FMC) to a non-PCI-capable hospital after STEMI, then PPCI should be preferred over thrombolysis as per the ACC 2013 STEMI guidelines. If the patient presents to a PCI-capable centre then ideally PPCI should be performed within 90 minutes of FMC. STEMI guidelines indicate that thrombolysis is generally preferred over primary PCI when the door-to-balloon time minus door-to-needle time exceeds 1 hour.

The current ACC/AHA guidelines strongly recommend that all PCI hospital systems achieve a median door-to-balloon time for primary PCI of 90 minutes. PPCI may be preferred for some patients even when it cannot be performed in a timely manner. Examples of such indications include those in whom the diagnosis is in doubt, those with high bleeding risk and those in high risk of death such as those in cardiogenic shock. In the absence of ST-segment elevation, a primary PCI (PPCI) strategy is indicated in patients with suspected ongoing ischaemic symptoms suggestive of myocardial infarction and with at least one of the following criteria as per the 2017 ESC STEMI guidelines [10]:

1. Haemodynamic instability or cardiogenic shock
2. Recurrent angina or angina refractory to medications
3. Life-threatening arrythmias or cardiac arrest
4. Mechanical complications of MI
5. Acute heart failure
6. Dynamic ST-T segment changes especially intermittent ST-elevation

PROCEDURAL ASPECTS OF INTERVENTIONS DURING PPCI

In most of the patients undergoing primary PCI for STEMI, routine stent implantation with or without thrombosuction with or without prior balloon dilatation is performed according to current guidelines [9,10].

However, 12% to 37% of patients undergoing PPCI may not achieve tissue-level perfusion even after successful recanalisation of the epicardial coronary artery. Inadequate myocardial perfusion of a given coronary segment without angiographic evidence of epicardial vessel obstruction, flow-limiting dissection, conduit vessel spasm, or apparent in situ thrombosis is known as no-reflow or micro-vascular obstruction (MVO) [13].

The no-reflow phenomenon is caused by various mechanisms, and various predictors of no-reflow are shown in Table 26.1. No-reflow results in increased morbidity and mortality in patients of acute MI undergoing PPCI and hence needs to be recognised and effectively prevented [14,15].

Table 26.1 Predictors of no-reflow phenomenon

Demographics
- Male sex
- Elderly patient
- Diabetes mellitus
- Renal insufficiency

Clinical and investigations
- Absence of pre-infarct angina
- Killips classification >2
- Longer time to achieve reperfusion
- Elevated blood glucose anc cholesterol levels on admission
- Larger infarct size with higher cardiac biomarkers
- Higher initial neutrophil count and CRP levels
- Lower baseline ejection fraction on echo

Angiographic indicators (Yip et al.)
- Abrupt cut-off pattern of infarct artery with reference diameter >4 mm
- Floating thrombus
- >5 mm accumulated thrombus proximal to lesion
- Persistent dye stasis distal to lesion

PREVENTION OF DISTAL EMBOLISATION IN PPCI

Yip et al. [15] have shown that patients who present with angiographic high thrombus load have a higher risk of no-reflow and epicardial artery distal embolization, which clearly translates into a higher cardiac mortality rate at 30 days. There are several strategies for preventing distal embolisation of distal thrombus [16]:

- Use of adjunctive mechanical devices (thrombosuction/ embolic protection)

- Pharmacological approaches to dissolve thrombus role of glycoprotein IIb/IIIa inhibitors (GPI)
- Dedicated stents for thrombus entrapment, e.g. Mguard stent

THROMBUS ASPIRATION IN PPCI

Thrombus aspiration can be either mechanical aspiration with Angiojet, X-Sizer, etc., or the more commonly used manual thrombus aspiration using thrombosuction catheters. Figure 26.1 shows the commonly used thrombosuction catheters in PPCI.

The TAPAS [17] trial resulted in the wide adoption of manual thrombus aspiration in almost all PPCI patients. Figure 26.2 shows the effect of PPCI with thrombosuction followed by stenting in establishing TIMI flow in totally occluded RCA.

Based on the results of the TAPAS and EXPIRA trials and the metanalysis by Bavry et al., the 2013 ACC/AHA and the 2012 ESC STEMI guidelines give a class IIa indication for manual thrombus aspiration with level of evidence B. However, the last two trials (TASTE and TOTAL) did not demonstrate benefit with routine thrombosuction, the Thrombus Aspiration during ST-Segment Elevation (TASTE) myocardial infarction trial, which included more than 7000 participants was unable to document a mortality benefit from aspiration thrombectomy [18]. Also, the results from the randomised trial of routine aspiration ThrOmbecTomy with PCI versus PCI Alone (TOTAL) [19] in patients with STEMI undergoing primary PCI did not show any reduction in primary outcomes of cardiovascular death or recurrent myocardial infarction. The 2014 ESC ESC/EATS guidelines on myocardial revascularisation give a class IIb indication for thrombosuction in selected cases after considering the TASTE trial results [20]. Based on the results of the TASTE and TOTAL trials, the 2017 ESC guidelines for STEMI have

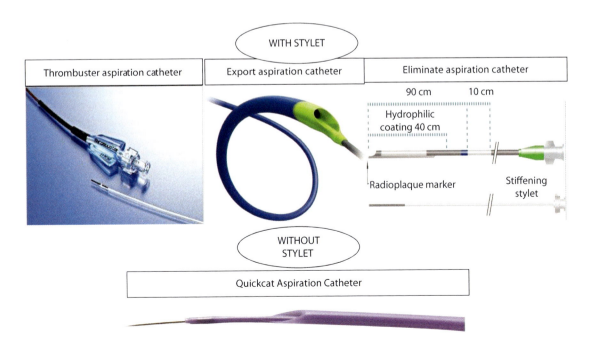

Figure 26.1 Commonly used thrombosuction catheters.

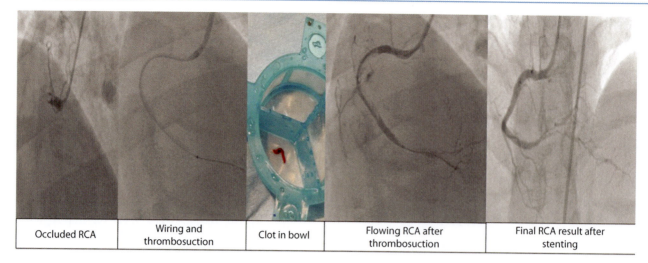

| Occluded RCA | Wiring and thrombosuction | Clot in bowl | Flowing RCA after thrombosuction | Final RCA result after stenting |

Figure 26.2 Thrombosuction followed by stenting of an occluded RCA resulting in TIMI three flow.

downgraded routine thrombosuction in STEMI to a class III indication [10].

ROLE OF COVERED STENTS AND DISTAL EMBOLISATION DEVICES IN PPCI

The Mguard™ stent, which consists of bare metal stent (BMS) platform covered with a polyethylene terephthalate mesh that aims to trap thrombus and hence prevent distal embolization, showed a trend towards reduced 1-year mortality in patients of STEMI undergoing primary PCI in the MASTER trial [21]. Embolic distal protection devices in the EMERALD and PROMISE trials did not show benefit in terms of ST resolution, final infarct size or the incidence of MACE at 6 months [21].

ROLE OF GLYCOPROTEIN IIB/IIIA INHIBITORS (GPIs) IN PPCI

Abciximab (large molecule), eptifibatide and tirofiban (small molecule) are the available GPI agents, and they are potent and effective intravenous platelet aggregation inhibitors and have been studied in the setting of ACS and in PCI with highly thrombotic lesions. In various randomised trials in patients with acute MI, the IIb/IIIa inhibitors abciximab, eptifibatide and tirofiban improved infarct size, ST resolution, TIMI flow grade, MBG, no-reflow by cardiac MRI, MCE perfusion score at 1 month, ejection fraction at 1 month and left ventricular remodelling at 6 months. However, in the post hoc analysis from the CADILLAC trial of patients undergoing PPCI with or without stenting and with or without abciximab there was a similar incidence of a normal post-procedure myocardial blush grade (17.3% with and 17.6% without abciximab) [22]. It is unclear whether GPI when infused peripherally reduce the incidence of no-reflow since data addressing this issue are limited and have inconsistent results. The 2017 ESC guidelines for STEMI recommend that GPI can be considered as a bailout for no-reflow or thrombotic complication with class IIa level C indication.

INTRACORONARY PHARMACOTHERAPY IN PPCI

Patients with high risk of no-reflow on the basis of the presence of predictors of reperfusion-related injury can be treated with drugs like nicorandil (2–5 mg boluses up to 15 mg), nitroprusside (50–200 mcg boluses as per blood pressure), adenosine and verapamil.

INTRACORONARY FIBRINOLYTICS

Intracoronary fibrinolytics in STEMI interventions are postulated to improve tissue level perfusion by dissolving thrombi at the micro-vascular level [23]. A pilot study by Sezer et al. [23] randomised 41 STEMI patients undergoing PCI to receive either 250 kU of IC streptokinase or no additional therapy and found that the measured various indices of micro-vascular function were better in the streptokinase arm at the end of 2 days after PCI. However, the initial enthusiasm with intracoronary thrombolysis with or without PCI was met with minimal success and high bleeding complication rates. Larger randomised controlled trials are needed to define the role of intracoronary fibrinolytics to document their benefit versus risk of their usage. There are currently no guideline recommendations for their use in PPCI.

TECHNICAL ISSUES IN PRIMARY PCI

RADIAL VERSUS FEMORAL APPROACH IN PPCI

Radial approach compared to the common femoral approach for PPCI has the potential to reduce the risk of major access site bleeding as the radial artery is smaller and readily compressible. The best evidence supporting better outcomes with radial catheterisation comes from a 2016 meta-analysis [24] of 24 trials (n = 22,843), including the four large, contemporary trials of acute coronary syndrome patients: RIVAL, MATRIX, RIFLE-STEACS, and STEMI RADIAL. Comparing radial with femoral access, the risk of major bleeding, all-cause mortality and major adverse cardiovascular events were all reduced with the radial approach [24].

STENTING IN PRIMARY PCI

Stenting is recommended over plain balloon angioplasty as class Ia indication as per the latest 2014 ESC/EATS guidelines on myocardial revascularisation. Direct stenting with low pressure dilatation reduces distal embolisation by avoiding balloon-induced thrombus fragmentation and by entrapping the athero-thrombus under the stent struts. Direct stenting has been shown to be superior to balloon pre-dilatation followed by stenting irrespective of aspiration in previous studies [25].

SELECTION OF STENT TYPE IN PPCI

The ACC 2013 and the ESC 2017 guidelines on the management of patients with STEMI recommend the use of DES as class IIa indication in all patients without contraindications to prolonged use of dual anti-platelet therapy. The 2014 ESC/EATS myocardial revascularisation give a class Ia indication for newer generation DES over BMS in primary PCI.

Newer second-generation DES with biodegradable polymers or polymer-free platforms are preferable over first-generation DES or BMS as evidenced from the EXAMINATION study [26] and COMFORTABLE AMI trial [27].

DEFERRED STENTING IN PPCI

Despite evidence of benefit in few early studies, deferred stenting is not recommended for patients of STEMI undergoing PPCI. Routine use of deferred stenting is a class III indication as per the 2017 ESC STEMI guidelines.

ROLE OF INTRA-AORTIC BALLOON PUMP (IABP) IN PPCI

Routine use of IABP is not recommended in PPCI unless complicated with cardiogenic shock or associated mechanical complications like acute mitral regurgitation or ventricular septal rupture.

ROLE OF INTRACORONARY IMAGING IN PPCI

The role of adjunctive intra-vascular imaging techniques, such as intravascular ultrasound (IVUS) and optical coherence tomography (OCT), has not been established in patients undergoing primary PCI. Several registries have found varying results. In the ADAPT–DES study of 813 STEMI patients, IVUS use was associated with improved outcomes in STEMI patients [28]. In the CREDO-Kyoto AMI Registry, 3028 patients with STEMI underwent PCI with or without IVUS. Following risk adjustment, there was no difference in target vessel failure between the groups (adjusted hazard ratio = 1.14; 0.86–1.51) [29]. However, the risk of stent thrombosis was lower with IVUS guidance. Likewise, a randomised, multicentre trial of angiographic compared with OCT-guided drug-eluting stent placement found that OCT guidance did not reduce the incidence of major adverse cardiac events. OCT guidance led to post-PCI stent optimisation in 29% of patients [30]. The use of OCT to identify plaque erosion versus plaque rupture as the cause of MI especially in young patients followed by strategy of treating erosions with thrombosuction alone without stenting has been studied in a small series of patients and is controversial [31,32].

PRIMARY PCI IN SPECIAL SITUATIONS

NON-CULPRIT LESION PCI IN STEMI

There are four principal strategies to manage non-culprit lesions:

1. Refer for CABG after the patient has recovered from acute STEMI
2. No further revascularisation unless standard indications for revascularisation in patients with stable coronary disease are met
3. PCI of non-culprit lesions at the time of primary PCI
4. PCI of non-culprit lesions prior to hospital discharge

There are nine published randomised trials of patients with multi-vessel disease that have compared culprit only with complete revascularization, with DANAMI3 PRIMULTI, PRAMI, CvLPRIT and COMPARE ACUTE being the four largest trials. In the DANAMI 3 PRIMULTI trial, 313 patients with one or more clinically significant coronary stenosis in addition to the culprit lesion were randomised to either no further invasive treatment or complete FFR guided revascularisation prior to discharge usually 2 days after PPCI.

The primary composite end point (all-cause mortality, non-fatal infarction and ischaemia-driven revascularisation of lesions in non-infarct-related arteries) occurred less often in the group with complete revascularisation (13% vs. 22%; hazard ratio [HR] 0.56%, 95% CI 0.38–0.83). The benefit was almost entirely attributable to a lower rate of subsequent revascularisation of non-infarct related arteries (HR 0.31%, 95% CI 0.18–0.53).

Approximately one-third of patients who were assigned to the complete revascularisation strategy did not undergo non-culprit PCI, as FFR values were above the discrimination value of 0.80, despite the fact that initial angiography suggested high-grade stenoses.

A 2017 meta-analysis of 10 randomised trials with 2285 patients compared four revascularisation strategies in STEMI patients with multi-vessel disease at the time of primary PCI: complete revascularisation at the index procedure; complete revascularisation as a staged procedure, with the non-culprit vessel(s) being treated prior to discharge; complete revascularisation as a staged procedure in which the non-culprit vessel(s) was treated within a few weeks after discharge (not symptom driven); and culprit-only PCI showed that complete revascularisation, either at the index procedure or as a staged procedure, compared with culprit-only PCI, was associated with a lower risk of major adverse cardiac events [33].

PPCI IN CARDIOGENIC SHOCK

STEMI with cardiogenic shock has 25%–50% mortality despite the best efforts to revascularise the patient. PPCI with mechanical support, e.g. IABP/Impella/ECMO offers the best chance of survival for these patients and hence patients with cardiogenic shock should be offered early revascularisation. Current ACC/AHA guidelines carry a class I indication for primary PCI in cardiogenic shock for patients <75 yrs old and class IIa for patients >75 yrs old. Immediate transfer for cardiogenic shock or severe acute HF is a class I indication for transfer for CAG irrespective of time delay from MI onset as per the 2013 ACC/AHA STEMI guidelines.

CONCLUSION

Timely PPCI can markedly help improve the prognosis and outcomes in patients with STEMI. Creating patient awareness and improving triage with early transport to a PPCI capable hospital will go a long way in improving outcomes.

REFERENCES

1. Falk E, Shah AC, Fuster V. Coronary plaque disruption. *Circulation* 1995;92:657–671.
2. Pakshirajan B, Vijaykumar S, Ajit S. Mullasari pharmaco invasive management in STEMI. *Intervent Cardiol Clin.* 2012;1:409–419.
3. Ndrepepa G, Mehilli J, Schulz S et al. Prognostic significance of epicardial blood flow before and after percutaneous coronary intervention in patients with acute coronary syndromes. *J Am Coll Cardiol.* 2008;52:512–517.
4. Boersma E, Maas AC, Deckers JW, Simoons ML. Early thrombolytic treatment in acute myocardial infarction: Reappraisal of the golden hour. *Lancet* 1996;348(9030):771–775.
5. The GUSTO Investigators. The effects of tissue plasminogen activator, streptokinase, or both on coronary-artery patency, ventricular function, and survival after acute myocardial function. *N Engl J Med.* 1993;329:1615–1622.
6. Mehta RH, Harjai KJ, Cox D et al. Clinical and angiographic correlates and outcomes of suboptimal coronary flow in patients with acute myocardial infarction undergoing primary percutaneous coronary intervention. *J Am Coll Cardiol.* 2003;42:1739.
7. Stone GW, Grines CL, Cox DA et al. Comparison of angioplasty with stenting, with or without abciximab, in acute myocardial infarction. *N Engl J Med.* 2002;346:957.
8. Gurwitz JH, Gore JM, Goldberg RJ et al. Risk for intracranial hemorrhage after tissue plasminogen activator treatment for acute myocardial infarction. Participants in the National Registry of Myocardial Infarction 2. *Ann Intern Med.* 1998;129:597.
9. O'Gara PT, Kushner FG, Ascheim DD et al. 2013 ACCF/AHA guideline for the management of ST-elevation myocardial infarction: A report of the American College of Cardiology Foundation/American Heart Association Task Force on Practice Guidelines. *Circulation* 2013;127:1–88.
10. 2017 ESC Guidelines for the management of acute myocardial infarction in patients presenting with ST-segment elevation The Task Force for the management of acute myocardial infarction in patients presenting with ST-segment elevation of the European Society of Cardiology (ESC). *Eur Heart J.* 2018;39:119–177.
11. Keeley EC, Boura JA, Grines CL. Primary angioplasty versus thrombolytic therapy for acute myocardial infarction: A quantitative review of 23 randomized trials. *Lancet* 2003;361:13–20.
12. Krumholz HM, Anderson JL, Bachelder BL et al. ACC/AHA 2008 performance measures for adults with ST-elevation and non-ST-elevation myocardial infarction: a report of the American College of Cardiology/American Heart Association Task Force on Performance Measures (Writing Committee to Develop Performance Measures for ST-Elevation and Non-ST-Elevation Myocardial Infarction) Developed in Collaboration with the American Academy of Family Physicians and American College of Emergency Physicians Endorsed by the American Association of Cardiovascular and Pulmonary Rehabilitation, Society for Cardiovascular Angiography and Interventions, and Society of Hospital Medicine. *J Am Coll Cardiol.* 2008;52:2046.
13. Jaffe R, Charron T, Puley G, Dick A, Strauss BH. Microvascular obstruction and the no reflow phenomenon after percutaneous coronary intervention. *Circulation* 2008;117:3152–3156.
14. Reffelmann T, Kloner RA. The 'no-reflow' phenomenon: basic science and clinical correlates. *Heart* 2002;87:162–168.
15. Yip HK, Chen MC, Chang HW et al. Angiographic morphologic features of infarct-related arteries and timely reperfusion in acute myocardial infarction: Predictors of slow-flow and no-reflow phenomenon. *Chest* 2002;122:1322–1332.
16. Dharma S, Kedev S, Jukema JW. Thrombus management in the catheterization laboratory in the setting of primary percutaneous coronary intervention: What is the current evidence. *Heart* 2013;99:279–284.
17. Svilaas T, Vlaar PJ, van der Horst IC et al. Thrombus aspiration during primary percutaneous coronary intervention. *N Engl J Med.* 2008;358:557–567.
18. Frobert O, Lagerqvist B, Olivecrona GK et al. Thrombus aspiration during ST segment elevation myocardial infarction. *N Engl J Med.* 2013;369:1587–1597.
19. Jolly SS, Cairns JA, Yusuf S et al. Randomized trial of primary PCI with or without routine manual thrombectomy. *N Engl J Med.* 2015;372:1389–1398.
20. Stephan W, Philippe K, Fernando A et al. 2014 ESC/EATS guidelines of myocardial revascularization. *Eur Heart J.* 2014;35(37):2541–2619.
21. Stone GW, Webb J, Cox DA et al. Distal microcirculatory protection during percutaneous coronary intervention in acute ST segment elevation myocardial infarction: A randomized controlled trial. *JAMA* 2005;293:1063–1072.

22. Costantini CO, Stone GW, Mehran R et al. Frequency, correlates, and clinical implications of myocardial perfusion after primary angioplasty and stenting, with and without glycoprotein IIb/IIIa inhibition, in acute myocardial infarction. *J Am Coll Cardiol.* 2004;44:305.

23. Sezer M, Olfaz H, Goren T et al. Intracoronary streptokinase after primary PCI. *N Engl Med.* 2007:356:1823–1834.

24. Ferrante G, Rao SV, Jüni P et al. Radial versus femoral access for coronary interventions across the entire spectrum of patients with coronary artery disease: A meta-analysis of randomized trials. *JACC Cardiovasc Interv.* 2016;9:1419.

25. Loubeyre C, Morice MC, Lefevre T, Piéchaud JF, Louvard Y, Dumas P. A randomized comparison of direct stenting with conventional stent implantation in selected patients with acute myocardial infarction. *J Am Coll Cardiol.* 2002;39:15–21.

26. Sabaté M, Brugaletta S, Cequier A et al. Clinical outcomes in patients with ST-segment elevation myocardial infarction treated with everolimus-eluting stents versus bare-metal stents (EXAMINATION): 5-year results of a randomised trial. *Lancet* 2016;387:357.

27. Räber L, Kelbæk H, Ostojic M et al. Effect of biolimus-eluting stents with biodegradable polymer vs. bare-metal stents on cardiovascular events among patients with acute myocardial infarction: The COMFORTABLE AMI randomized trial. *JAMA* 2012;308:777.

28. Witzenbichler B, Maehara A, Weisz G et al. Relationship between intravascular ultrasound guidance and clinical outcomes after drug-eluting stents: The assessment of dual antiplatelet therapy with drug-eluting stents (ADAPT-DES) study. *Circulation* 2014;129:463.

29. Nakatsuma K, Shiomi H, Morimoto T et al. Intravascular ultrasound guidance vs. angiographic guidance in primary percutaneous coronary intervention for ST-segment elevation myocardial infarction – long-term clinical outcomes from the CREDO-Kyoto AMI Registry. *Circ J* 2016;80:477.

30. Kala P, Cervinka P, Jakl M et al. OCT guidance during stent implantation in primary PCI: A randomized multicenter study with nine months of optical coherence tomography follow-up. *Int J Cardiol.* 2018;250:98.

31. Prati F, Uemura S, Souteyrand G et al. OCT-based diagnosis and management of STEMI associated with intact fibrous cap. *J Am Coll Cardiol Imag.* 2013;6:283–1287.

32. Holmes DR Jr, Lerman A, Moreno PR, King SB III, Sharma SK. Diagnosis and management of STEMI arising from plaque erosion. *JACC CV Imag.* 2013;6(3):283–287.

33. Elgendy IY, Mahmoud AN, Kumbhani DJ et al. Complete or culprit-only revascularization for patients with multivessel coronary artery disease undergoing percutaneous coronary intervention: A pairwise and network meta-analysis of randomized trials. *JACC Cardiovasc Interv.* 2017;10:315.

27

Management of acute coronary syndromes in acute phase in India
Relevance of Western guidelines

NITEEN VIJAY DESHPANDE

INTRODUCTION

Coronary artery disease (CAD) remains a leading cause of morbidity and mortality in India. Due to lack of indigenous data and guidelines, physicians in India rely heavily for management strategies on the Western guidelines. The European Society of Cardiology (ESC) and the American College of Cardiology (ACC)/American Heart Association (AHA) regularly update the practice guidelines for cardiac diseases taking into account the published data and advances made in the diagnostic and therapeutic area. The ACC/AHA guidelines [4] for management of non-ST-elevation acute coronary syndromes (NSTE-ACS) were published in 2014. The most recent guidelines for management of acute coronary syndromes (ACS) were published by ESC [5] in 2015.

However, these guidelines are designed for a Western population with all attendant corollaries with respect to availability of transport, communication, primary and secondary health care. The applicability of these guidelines to a third world nation with the health care delivery system peculiarities in India have not been reviewed or validated. Limited data on diagnosis and management of acute coronary syndromes exist from India. The Kerala ACS Registry [1] published in 2013 represents such large data on ACS limited to presentation, initial management and in-hospital outcomes. Other relevant data comes from the CREATE registry [2] and OASIS registry [3] and smaller studies. This chapter will attempt to discuss the Western guidelines, especially the European ones, and their applicability to the Indian population.

CLINICAL SPECTRUM

The clinical spectrum of non-ST-elevation acute coronary syndromes ranges from unstable angina (UA) to non-ST-elevation myocardial infarction (NSTEMI). Unstable angina is defined as myocardial ischaemia at rest or minimal exertion in the absence of cardiomyocyte necrosis as evidenced by lack of elevation of cardiac troponins, while NSTEMI is myocardial ischaemia associated with troponin elevation indicating myocyte necrosis. These definitions are standard and have applicability across populations and can easily be used in India.

DIAGNOSIS AND INITIAL ASSESSMENT

Anginal pain and atypical presentations are as described in the guidelines and these definitions are standard [6]. Atypical presentations include epigastric pain and indigestion-like symptoms and are reported more frequently by the elderly, women, patients with diabetes, chronic renal disease and dementia [7]. Physical examination is generally unremarkable but suggestive of heart failure and haemodynamic or electrical instability should be carefully observed. Detection of new murmurs indicates mechanical complications help in risk stratification. Physical examination also can help in identifying other causes of chest pain like musculoskeletal disorders.

Resting 12-lead ECG is the first diagnostic tool and the ESC guidelines recommend that ECG should be recorded and interpreted within 10 minutes of first medical contact. In India, many small medical establishments have no access to ECG and even if they do, the ability to interpret these within even the first 30 minutes is often not available. Additionally, it is important to remember that ECG may be normal in about one third of the patients. The guidelines also suggest recording of extended ECG leads V7 to V9 and V3R if signs and symptoms are suggestive of ACS and the standard ECG is non-diagnostic to rule out true posterior wall MI or right ventricular MI [8]. This is only possible in hospital-based practices and will thus be restricted to large metropolitan cities. Additionally, in patients with bundle branch blocks and paced rhythm, ECG is of no help in diagnosis of NSTE-ACS.

Biomarkers, especially the new generation high sensitivity troponins, must be estimated in patients with suspected NSTE-ACS and form the basis of the diagnostic algorithm in ACS. However, quantitative and qualitative troponins are not always available even in medium-sized establishments. The concept of emergency departments often does not exist, and serial troponins are expensive, and the described algorithms are financially challenging to implement.

When available, the point-of-care assays which are used commonly in emergency departments offer a quick result and rapid turn-around time. This comes at cost of lower sensitivity, lower diagnostic accuracy and lower negative predictive value as compared to automated assays. The 0/3 hours algorithm (Figure 27.1 ESC) is now suggested to rule-out/rule-in NSTE-ACS and 0/1 hour algorithm can be used if high sensitivity assay with validated algorithm is available. A comparison of the relative merits of the 0 h/1 h and 0 h/3 h algorithms is shown in Table 27.1.

Trans-thoracic echocardiography offers quick evaluation of left ventricular function with assessment of regional wall motion abnormalities. It also helps to identify the presence of mechanical complications, if any should exist. Additionally, echocardiography can help in proving alternative diagnoses like pulmonary embolism and dissection of aorta, pericardial effusion, hypertrophic cardiomyopathy and aortic stenosis. Availability in emergency departments is often a major limitation.

In patients at low risk of adverse events, further functional testing is advised. Stress imaging is preferred over stress ECG due to its better diagnostic yield [9]. Stress ECG, however, remains the most commonly done stress evaluation method in an Indian scenario due to limited availability of stress echocardiography and the high cost of myocardial perfusion imaging. Multi-detector CT angiography can be used to exclude obstructive coronary artery disease in patients at low risk presenting with chest pain syndromes. Severe calcification of coronary arteries and prior stent implantation are the two areas where MDCT angiography may have limited value.

RISK STRATIFICATION

Risk assessment is the cornerstone of management of ACS and needs to be done for both ischaemic risk and bleeding risk.

ISCHAEMIC RISK

The GRACE risk score [10] is recommended by the ESC guidelines and is based on age, systolic blood pressure, pulse rate, serum creatinine, Killip Class on presentation, cardiac arrest at admission, elevated cardiac biomarkers and ST-segment deviation. The online GRACE 2.0 calculator offers mortality while in hospital, at 6 months, 1 year and 3 years. It also indicates risk of death or

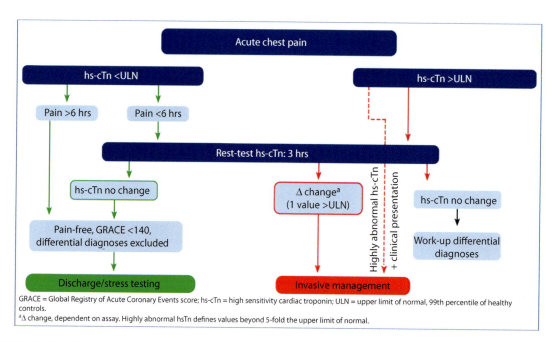

Figure 27.1 0 h/3 h Algorithm for ruling out acute coronary syndrome [5].

Table 27.1 Characteristics of 0 h/3 h and 0 h/1 h Algorithm [5]

	0 h/3 h Algorithm	0 h/1 h Algorithm
Negative predictive value for acute MI	98%–100%	98%–100%
Positive predictive value for acute MI	Unknown, depending on delta change and assay	75%–80%
Effectiveness	++	+++
Feasibility	++ requires GRACE score	+++
Challenges	Pain onset cannot be reliably quantified in many patients	Cut-off levels are assay-specific and different from the 99th percentile
Validation in large multicentre studies	+	+++
Additional advantages	Already used clinically	Shorter time to decision

myocardial infarction at 1 year. Alternatively, the TIMI risk score [11] can be used, which is a simple score but the discriminative accuracy is inferior to the GRACE score [12].

BLEEDING RISK

Major bleeding events increase risk of mortality in NSTE-ACS and hence bleeding risk needs to be assessed. The risk scores recommended by the ESC include the CRUSADE bleeding risk score [13] and ACUITY bleeding risk score [14]. The statistics for the ACUITY score appear better than that for the CRUSADE bleeding risk score. These scores are easily available online and need to be used to optimise outcomes in high-risk patients. Predictive value of these scores is not established in medically managed patients and patients receiving oral anti-coagulation.

Figure 27.2 shows ESC recommendations for diagnosis, risk stratification, imaging, rhythm monitoring in patients with suspected NSTE-ACS.

MANAGEMENT STRATEGIES FOR NSTE-ACS

Management strategies are guided by risk assessment, however, they are heavily influenced by available facilities and financial constraints. Data from Indian registries highlight these points very well. Patients often present late in India and tend to be older with more comorbidities. The use of evidence-based therapies is less. Accessibility of health care and literacy have significant impact in India, especially in rural areas while financial constraints play an important role in urban areas where accessibility to health care is not a great issue anymore.

GUIDELINE-MANDATED MANAGEMENT STRATEGIES

On diagnosis of NSTE-ACS patients should receive non-enteric coated aspirin (150–300 mg) along with a loading dose of clopidogrel (300 mg) and a high dose of atorvastatin (40–80 mg). Fibrinolytic therapy has no role in NSTE-ACS and upstream use of GP IIb/IIIa blockers is not recommended any longer.

PHARMACOLOGIC TREATMENT OF ISCHAEMIA

The main aim of anti-ischaemic therapy is to reduce myocardial oxygen demand or to increase myocardial oxygen supply. If the initial therapy fails to alleviate symptoms and signs of ischaemia, the patient should be immediately considered for invasive assessment. Oxygen should be administered when oxygen saturation is <90% and opiates help if symptoms persist (Figure 27.3).

Recommendations with respect to nitrates and beta-blockers are standard and can be implemented as recommended. Caution needs to be exercised in patients receiving phosphodiesterase 5 inhibitors, where nitrates can precipitate severe hypotension [15]. Early treatment with BB is associated with significant reduction in risk of in-hospital mortality [16] without increasing cardiogenic shock [17]. Early use of BB should be avoided in patients at risk of developing cardiogenic shock or when left ventricular function is unknown.

PLATELET INHIBITION

Aspirin has shown to reduce the risk of MI and death in trials conducted in the pre-PTCA era [18–20]. A lower maintenance dose of aspirin (75–100 mg) in patients undergoing invasive strategy is as effective as a higher dose (300–325 mg) as observed in the CURRENT-OASIS 7 study [21].

P2Y12 INHIBITORS

The current concept of dual anti-platelet therapy mandates the use of P2Y12 inhibitor in addition to aspirin for 1 year following NSTE-ACS. Clopidogrel (loading dose of 300 to 600 mg followed by maintenance dose of 75 mg) has been shown to reduce recurrent events as compared to aspirin alone [22,23]. Variability in clopidogrel response, however, is a major issue leading to suboptimal platelet inhibition and explaining residual risk even on DAPT with clopidogrel [24]. Prasugrel (60 mg loading dose followed by 10 mg daily maintenance dose) has a faster onset and more pronounced platelet inhibitory effect as compared to clopidogrel. Based on the current evidence from the TRITON-TIMI-38 study [25], this drug is recommended for patients with known coronary anatomy who are scheduled for PCI. Severe bleeding complications remain a major consideration with prasugrel. Prasugrel is contraindicated

Recommendations	Class	Level
Diagnosis and risk stratification		
It is recommended to base diagnosis and initial short-term ischaemic and bleeding risk stratification on a combination of clinical history, symptoms, vital signs, other physical findings, ECG and laboratory results.	I	A
It is recommended to obtain a 12-lead ECG within 10 min after first medical contact and to have it immediately interpreted by an experienced physician. It is recommended to obtain an additional 12-lead ECG in case of recurrent symptoms or diagnostic uncertainty.	I	B
Additional ECG leads (V_{3R}, V_{4R}, V_7–V_9) are recommended if ongoing ischaemia is suspected when standard leads are inconclusive.	I	C
It is recommended to measure cardiac troponins with sensitive or high-sensitivity assays and obtain the results within 60 min.	I	A
A rapid rule-out protocol at 0 h and 3 h is recommended if high-sensitivity cardiac troponin tests are available.	I	B
A rapid rule-out and rule-in protocol at 0 h and 1 h is recommended if a high-sensitivity cardiac troponin test with a validated 0 h/1 h algorithm is available. Additional testing after 3–6 h is indicated if the first two troponin measurements are not conclusive and the clinical condition is still suggestive of ACS.	I	B
It is recommended to use established risk scores for prognosis estimation.	I	B
The use of the CRUSADE score may be considered in patients undergoing coronary angiography to quantify bleeding risk.	IIb	B
Imaging		
In patients with no recurrence of chest pain, normal ECG findings and normal levels of cardiac troponin (preferably high-sensitivity), but suspected ACS, a non-invasive stress test (preferably with imaging) for inducible ischaemia is recommended before deciding on an invasive strategy.	I	A
Echocardiography is recommended to evaluate regional and global LV function and to rule in or rule out differential diagnoses.	I	C
MDCT coronary angiography should be considered as an alternative to invasive angiography to exclude ACS when there is a low to intermediate likelihood of CAD and when cardiac troponin and/or ECG are inconclusive.	IIa	A

Figure 27.2 ESC recommendation for diagnosis and risk stratification of NSTE-ACS [5].

in patients with prior TIA or stroke. In patients above 75 years of age and with low body weight (<60 kg), prasugrel may not offer benefits over clopidogrel and should not be used. Ticagrelor is the third P2Y12 inhibitor which has a reversible action with shorter plasma half-life of 6 to 12 hours mandating twice-a-day dosing.

Recommendations	Class	Level
Early initiation of beta-blocker treatment is recommended in patients with ongoing ischaemic symptoms and without contraindications.	I	B
It is recommended to continue chronic beta-blocker therapy, unless the patient is in Killip Class III or higher.	I	B
Sublingual or i.v. nitrates are recommended to relieve angina; i.v. treatment is recommended in patients with recurrent angina, uncontrolled hypertension or signs of heart failure.	I	C
In patients with suspected/confirmed vasospastic angina, calcium channel blockers and nitrates should be considered and beta-blockers avoided.	IIa	B

Figure 27.3 Recommendations for use of anti-ischaemic drugs in the acute phase of NSTE-ACS [5].

Like prasugrel, ticagrelor offers more consistent and faster platelet inhibition. Based on trial data from the PLATO study [26] this agent is recommended for patients undergoing invasive strategy as well as conservative management. Figure 27.4 shows ESC recommendations on use of platelet inhibitors in NSTE-ACS.

INITIATION, DURATION AND DISCONTINUATION OF P2Y12 INHIBITORS

Initiation of DAPT soon after diagnosis of ACS is recommended implying pre-treatment with DAPT prior to coronary angiography. Based on results of the ACCOAST trial [27], pre-treatment with prasugrel is not recommended. While both clopidogrel and ticagrelor can be used prior to coronary angiography, no data exists on optimal timing of ticagrelor prior to invasive strategy. Clopidogrel thus appears to be the safest agent to be administered immediately on diagnosis and may be switched to more potent agents like prasugrel or ticagrelor after coronary angiography depending on the modality of revascularisation. Currently recommended dual anti-platelet therapy duration following ACS is at least 1 year. Extended DAPT should be considered on an individual patient basis balancing the ischaemic benefit versus the bleeding risk [28]. No long-term trial data about duration of DAPT exists for medically managed patients following ACS. These patients form a large proportion in clinical practice in India and continuation of DAPT consisting of aspirin and clopidogrel beyond 1 year of the initial event extending up to 3 years may be a reasonable option if the bleeding risk is not excessive.

GLYCOPROTEIN IIB/IIIA INHIBITORS

GP IIb/IIIa inhibitors block the final common pathway of platelet aggregation. Addition of GP IIb/IIIa inhibitors to heparin in medically managed patients with ACS reduces risk of death or non-fatal MI by 9% [29]. However, the greatest benefit of IIb/IIIa inhibitors is seen in patients undergoing PCI [30,31]. Upstream use is also associated with increased risk of bleeding without significant increase in intra-cranial bleeding. With availability of more potent and reliable

Recommendations	Class	Level
Oral anti-platelet therapy		
Aspirin is recommended for all patients without contraindications at an initial oral loading dose of 150–300 mg (in aspirin-naive patients) and a maintenance dose of 75–100 mg/day long-term regardless of treatment strategy.	I	A
A P2Y12 inhibitor is recommended, in addition to aspirin, for 12 months unless there are contraindications such as excessive risk of bleeds.	I	A
• Ticagrelor (180 mg loading dose, 90 mg twice daily) is recommended, in the absence of contraindications, for all patients at moderate-to-high risk of ischaemic events (e.g. elevated cardiac troponins), regardless of initial treatment strategy and including those pretreated with clopidogrel (which should be discontinued when ticagrelor is started).	I	B
• Prasugrel (60 mg loading dose, 10 mg daily dose) is recommended in patients who are proceeding to PCI if no contraindication.	I	B
• Clopidogrel (300–600 mg loading dose, 75 mg daily dose) is recommended for patients who cannot receive ticagrelor or prasugrel or who require oral anticoagulation.	I	B
$P2Y_{12}$ inhibitor administration for a shorter duration of 3–6 months after DES implantation may be considered in patients deemed at high bleeding risk.	IIb	A
It is not recommended to administer prasugrel in patients in whom coronary anatomy is not known.	III	B
Intravenous antiplatelet therapy		
GPIIb/IIIa inhibitors during PCI should be considered for bailout situations or thrombotic complications.	IIa	C
Cangrelor may be considered in $P2Y_{12}$ inhibitor-naive patients undergoing PCI.	IIb	A
It is not recommended to administer GPIIb/IIIa inhibitors in patients in whom coronary anatomy is not known.	III	A
Long-term $P2Y_{12}$ inhibition		
$P2Y_{12}$ inhibitor administration in addition to aspirin beyond 1 year may be considered after careful assessment of the ischaemic and bleeding risks of the patient.	IIb	A

Figure 27.4 Recommendation for platelet inhibition in NSTE-ACS [5].

P2Y12 inhibitors like prasugrel and ticagrelor, IIb/IIIa inhibitors are recommended only for bailout during PCI or for thrombotic complications. Routine upstream usage is not recommended.

ANTI-COAGULATION

Anti-coagulants inhibit thrombin generation and activity, thereby decreasing the ischaemic events. Combination of anti-coagulants with anti-platelet agents is more effective than either therapy alone and should be used in patients with NSTE-ACS [32]. Unfractionated heparin (UFH), low molecular weight heparins (LMWH), fondaparinux (anti-Xa inhibitor) and bivalirudin (direct thrombin inhibitor) are the choices, and the agent used depends on the availability of the agent, whether the patient undergoes PCI or medical management. Crossing over to other anti-coagulants during PCI is strongly discouraged [33]. Benefit of LWMH over UFH is documented in a large number of trials and meta-analysis [34]. Fondaparinux is a selective Xa inhibitor and binds reversibly to anti-thrombin preventing thrombin generation. This agent is completely bioavailable and has long elimination half-life of 17 hours allowing once a day dosing. Unlike heparins, fondaparinux does not cause HIT. The OASIS-5 trial showed that fondaparinux was non-inferior to enoxaparin in treatment of NSTE-ACS [35]. Bivalirudin binds directly to thrombin inhibiting fibrin generation. This agent is recommended as an alternative to UFH/LMWH in patients undergoing urgent or elective PCI and has been shown to reduce bleeding complications. ESC recommendations for use of anticoagulants is shown in Figure 27.5.

Recommendations	Class	Level
Parenteral anticoagulation is recommended at the time of diagnosis according to both ischaemic and bleeding risks.	I	B
Fondaparinux (2.5 mg s.c. daily) is recommended as having the most favourable efficacy–safety profile regardless of the management strategy.	I	B
Bivalirudin (0.75 mg/kg i.v. bolus, followed by 1.75 mg/kg/h for up to 4 h after the procedure) is recommended as an alternative to UFH plus GPIIb/IIIa inhibitors during PCI.	I	A
UFH 70–100 IU/kg i.v. (50–70 IU/kg if concomitant with GPIIb/IIIa inhibitors) is recommended in patients undergoing PCI who did not receive any anticoagulant.	I	B
In patients on fondaparinux (2.5 mg s.c. daily) undergoing PCI, a single i.v. bolus of UFH (70–85 IU/kg, or 50–60 IU/kg in the case of concomitant use of GPIIb/IIIa inhibitors) is recommended during the procedure.	I	B
Enoxaparin (1 mg/kg s.c. twice daily) or UFH are recommended when fondaparinux is not available.	I	B
Enoxaparin should be considered as an anticoagulant for PCI in patients pretreated with s.c. enoxaparin.	IIa	B
Additional ACT-guided i.v. boluses of UFH during PCI may be considered following initial UFH treatment.	IIb	B
Discontinuation of anticoagulation should be considered after PCI, unless otherwise indicated.	IIa	C
Crossover between UFH and LMWH is not recommended.	III	B
In NSTEMI patients with no prior stroke/TIA and at high ischaemic risk as well as low bleeding risk receiving aspirin and clopidogrel, low-dose rivaroxaban (2.5 mg twice daily for approximately 1 year) may be considered after discontinuation of parenteral anticoagulation.	IIb	B

Figure 27.5 Recommendation for anti-coagulation in NSTE-ACS [5].

INVASIVE CORONARY ANGIOGRAPHY AND REVASCULARISATION

Invasive coronary angiography followed by revascularisation is performed in the majority of patients admitted with NSTE-ACS in well-developed health care systems. However, cost constraints and non-availability of the invasive procedures limit their use in the majority of India. With limited resources it is very important to risk stratify the patient quickly on admission (Table 27.2) and consider invasive treatment for at least the high-risk patients.

The indications for invasive approach and timing of revascularisation depend on multiple factors like clinical presentation, comorbidities, risk level, presence of high-risk features specific for revascularisation modality, frailty, estimated life expectancy and pattern of coronary artery disease. Additional factors like cost implications play a very important role in resource-limited settings like ours where the expenditure is mostly out-of-pocket for the patient. Routine invasive strategy as compared to selective invasive strategy has been shown to offer significantly better outcomes in patients with NSTE-ACS [36–38]. The timing for invasive strategy could be immediate (<2 hours of admission), early (<24 hours of admission) or delayed invasive (<72 hours of admission). The immediate invasive strategy must be considered for very high-risk patients with haemodynamic or electrical instability and has been shown to improve outcomes significantly in high-risk patients with a high GRACE score [39].

Table 27.2 Risk criteria mandating invasive strategy in NSTE-ACS [5]

Very high-risk criteria
- Haemodynamic instability or cardiogenic shock
- Recurrent or ongoing chest pain refractory to medical treatment
- Life-threatening arrhythmias or cardiac arrest
- Mechanical complications of MI
- Acute heart failure
- Recurrent dynamic ST-T wave changes, particularly with intermittent ST-elevation

High-risk criteria
- Rise or fall in cardiac troponin compatible with MI
- Dynamic ST or T wave changes (symptomatic or silent)
- GRACE score >140

Intermediate-risk criteria
- Diabetes mellitus
- Renal insufficiency (eGFR <60 mL/min/1.73 m^2)
- LVEF <40% or congestive heart failure
- Early post-infarction angina
- Prior PCI
- Prior CABG
- GRACE risk score >109 and <140

Low-risk criteria
- Any characteristics not mentioned previously

REVASCULARISATION STRATEGIES

Complete revascularisation should be the aim in most of the patients presenting with NSTE-ACS since it has been shown to be a very strong determinant of long-term outcomes [40]. This may mandate a staged procedure, especially in patients with complex coronary anatomy and comorbidities increasing the cost burden of treatment. Approximately 10% of patients presenting with NSTE-ACS may require coronary artery bypass graft surgery (CABG) during index hospitalisation [41]. Cost implications for complete revascularisation may tilt this balance more towards CABG in the Indian scenario. However, timing of the procedure remains the key as the bleeding risk versus ischaemic risk needs to be balanced carefully for CABG. While PCI can offer a faster revascularisation of the culprit lesion with lower risk of stroke, CABG may offer more complete revascularisation. In absence of data comparing CABG with PCI in patients with multi-vessel disease in NSTE-ACS, this decision is left to the discretion of the treating physician. This decision about revascularisation is also heavily influenced by the available local expertise for the required modality. It is suggested by the ESC guidelines that a heart team should discuss the possibilities of revascularisation in patients with multi-vessel CAD considering patient preferences before arriving to a specific modality. The SYNTAX score offers a useful guide to choose between PCI or CABG in patients with NSTE-ACS and should be used in light of the clinical situation [42]. A culprit vessel PCI followed either by staged PCI for other vessels of CABG may help to stabilise a high-risk NSTE-ACS patient and can be considered in high-risk unstable patients.

RELEVANCE OF THE GUIDELINES FOR CLINICAL PRACTICE IN INDIA

Limited data on management and outcomes of NSTE-ACS is published from India. The Kerala ACS Registry is the most contemporary data available on the subject, which includes 7857 patients admitted with diagnosis of ACS. Only 18.6% of patients underwent coronary angiography during hospitalisation and 11.7% patients were treated with PCI, while CABG was performed in 1.2%. Interestingly, 26.6% patients received thrombolysis. This data shows the low percentage of patients undergoing an invasive approach in ACS. This also means that most of the patients were managed medically, and thus it is imperative that we update our practices towards a more guideline-oriented approach. Catheterisation laboratory facilities have expanded rapidly over the last decade in India, and physicians have to change their orientation towards using these facilities for quicker diagnosis and treatment planning. Until these numbers increase to comparable numbers in the Western population, it is imperative for us to offer other guideline-mandated strategies including early risk stratification using validated scores like the GRACE and TIMI scores and offering appropriate initial medical management. The use of aspirin and clopidogrel was 92.5% and 94.9% in the Kerala ACS Registry with close to 70% patients receiving any of the heparins. Availability of more potent P2Y12 inhibitors, especially ticagrelor, can offer better outcomes, and practice needs to change in favour of these drugs. Prasugrel, although not recommended without knowledge of coronary anatomy, can be a cheaper alternative. Usage of other agents like beta-blockers, statins and ACE inhibitors was also significantly high in the Kerala ACS Registry, but may not be the case for many other states which have lower literacy rates and lower socio-economic status.

Extended use of DAPT with either clopidogrel or ticagrelor as documented by studies can prevent recurrent events in medically managed ACS patients if the bleeding risk is low and they tolerate DAPT during first year without bleeding complications. Use of appropriate dose LMWH/fondaparinux can ease the burden of continuous intravenous administration of UHF and also offer a consistent anti-coagulant effect. High intensity statins to lower LDL cholesterol >50% from baseline are also an important aspect of medical management both in patients managed with invasive as well as conservative strategy [43]. Ezetimibe offers additional LDL lowering to high-intensity statin therapy as documented by the IMPROVE-IT trial [44] and should be kept in mind if patients fail to achieve the LDL target with statin therapy alone.

CONCLUSION

NSTE-ACS is a leading cause of mortality and morbidity. ESC guidelines outline therapies and indicate pathways to improve outcomes in these high-risk patients. Clinical practice in India, however, is quite different than the guidelines mandated therapies and needs to catch up, especially with the invasive management. It is imperative for us to at least offer optimal medical management with frequent follow-up and medical supervision to optimise outcomes in our resource limited setting.

REFERENCES

1. Mohanan PP, Mathew R, Harikrishnan S et al. Presentation, management, and outcomes of 25 748 acute coronary syndrome admissions in Kerala, India: Results from the Kerala ACS Registry. *Eur Heart J.* 2013;34(2):121–129.
2. Xavier D, Pais P, Devereaux PJ et al. CREATE registry investigators: Treatment and outcomes of acute coronary syndromes in India (CREATE): A prospective analysis of registry data. *Lancet* 2008;371(9622):1435–1442.
3. Prabhakaran D, Yusuf S, Mehta S et al. Two-year outcomes in patients admitted with non-ST elevation acute coronary syndrome: Results of the OASIS registry 1 and 2. *Indian Heart J.* 2005;57:217–225.
4. Amsterdam EA, Wenger NK, Brindis RG et al. American College of Cardiology; American Heart Association Task Force on Practice Guidelines; Society for Cardiovascular Angiography and Interventions; Society of Thoracic Surgeons; American Association for Clinical Chemistry. 2014 AHA/ACC Guideline for the Management of Patients with Non-ST-Elevation Acute Coronary Syndromes: A report of the American College of Cardiology/American Heart Association Task Force on Practice Guidelines. *J Am Coll Cardiol.* 2014;64:e139–e228.
5. Roffi M, Patrono C, Collet JP et al. Management of Acute Coronary Syndromes in Patients Presenting without Persistent ST-Segment Elevation of the European Society of Cardiology. 2015 ESC Guidelines for the management of acute coronary syndromes in patients presenting without persistent ST-segment elevation: Task Force for the Management of Acute Coronary Syndromes in Patients Presenting without Persistent ST-Segment Elevation of the European Society of Cardiology (ESC). *Eur Heart J.* 2016;37:267–315.
6. Campeau L. Letter: Grading of angina pectoris. *Circulation* 1976;54:522–523.
7. Canto JG, Fincher C, Kiefe CI et al. Atypical presentations among Medicare beneficiaries with unstable angina pectoris. *Am J Cardiol.* 2002;90:248–253.
8. Thygesen K, Alpert JS, Jaffe AS et al. Third universal definition of myocardial infarction. *Eur Heart J.* 2012;33:2551–2567.
9. Montalescot G, Sechtem U, Achenbach S et al. 2013 ESC guidelines on the management of stable coronary artery disease: The Task Force on the Management of Stable Coronary Artery Disease of the European Society of Cardiology. *Eur Heart J.* 2013;34:2949–3003.
10. Fox KA, Fitzgerald G, Puymirat E et al. Should patients with acute coronary disease be stratified for management according to their risk? Derivation, external validation and outcomes using the updated GRACE risk score. *BMJ Open* 2014;4:e004425.
11. Antman EM, Cohen M, Bernink PJ et al. The TIMI risk score for unstable angina/non-ST elevation MI: A method for prognostication and therapeutic decision making. *JAMA* 2000;284:835–842.
12. Aragam KG, Tamhane UU, Kline-Rogers E et al. Does simplicity compromise accuracy in ACS risk prediction? A retrospective analysis of the TIMI and GRACE risk scores. *PLoS One* 2009;4:e7947.
13. Subherwal S, Bach RG, Chen AY et al. Baseline risk of major bleeding in non-ST-segment-elevation myocardial infarction: The CRUSADE (Can Rapid risk stratification of Unstable angina patients Suppress ADverse outcomes with Early implementation of the ACC/AHA guidelines) bleeding score. *Circulation* 2009;119:1873–1882.
14. Mehran R, Pocock SJ, Nikolsky E et al. A risk score to predict bleeding in patients with acute coronary syndromes. *J Am Coll Cardiol.* 2010;55:2556–2566.
15. Schwartz BG, Kloner RA. Drug interactions with phosphodiesterase-5 inhibitors used for the treatment of erectile dysfunction or pulmonary hypertension. *Circulation* 2010;122:88–95.
16. Yusuf S, Wittes J, Friedman L. Overview of results of randomized clinical trials in heart disease. I. Treatments following myocardial infarction. *JAMA* 1988;260:2088–2093.
17. Chatterjee S, Chaudhuri D, Vedanthan R et al. Early intravenous beta-blockers in patients with acute coronary syndrome—a meta-analysis of randomized trials. *Int J Cardiol.* 2013;168:915–921.
18. The RISC group. Risk of myocardial infarction and death during treatment with low dose aspirin and intravenous heparin in men with unstable coronary artery disease. *Lancet* 1990;336:827–830.

19. Lewis HD Jr, Davis JW, Archibald DG et al. Protective effects of aspirin against acute myocardial infarction and death in men with unstable angina. Results of a Veterans Administration cooperative study. *N Engl J Med.* 1983;309:396–403.

20. Theroux P, Ouimet H, McCans J et al. Aspirin, heparin, or both to treat acute unstable angina. *N Engl J Med.* 1988;319:1105–1111.

21. Mehta SR, Bassand JP, Chrolavicius S et al. Dose comparisons of clopidogrel and aspirin in acute coronary syndromes. *N Engl J Med.* 2010;363:930–942.

22. Yusuf S, Zhao F, Mehta SR et al. Effects of clopidogrel in addition to aspirin in patients with acute coronary syndromes without ST-segment elevation. *N Engl J Med.* 2001;345:494–502.

23. Mehta SR, Yusuf S, Peters RJ et al. Effects of pretreatment with clopidogrel and aspirin followed by long-term therapy in patients undergoing percutaneous coronary intervention: The PCI-CURE study. *Lancet* 2001;358:527–533.

24. Aradi D, Storey RF, Komocsi A et al. Expert position paper on the role of platelet function testing in patients undergoing percutaneous coronary intervention. *Eur Heart J.* 2014;35:209–215.

25. Wiviott SD, Braunwald E, McCabe CH et al. Prasugrel versus clopidogrel in patients with acute coronary syndromes. *N Engl J Med.* 2007;357:2001–2015.

26. Wallentin L, Becker RC, Budaj A et al. Ticagrelor versus clopidogrel in patients with acute coronary syndromes. *N Engl J Med.* 2009;361:1045–1057.

27. Montalescot G, Bolognese L, Dudek D et al. Pretreatment with prasugrel in non-ST-segment elevation acute coronary syndromes. *N Engl J Med.* 2013;369:999–1010.

28. Mauri L, Kereiakes DJ, Yeh RW et al. Twelve or 30 months of dual antiplatelet therapy after drug-eluting stents. *N Engl J Med.* 2014;371:2155–2166.

29. Roffi M, Chew DP, Mukherjee D et al. Platelet glycoprotein IIb/IIIa inhibition in acute coronary syndromes. Gradient of benefit related to the revascularization strategy. *Eur Heart J.* 2002;23:1441–1448.

30. Stone GW, Bertrand ME, Moses JW et al. Routine upstream initiation vs deferred selective use of glycoprotein IIb/IIIa inhibitors in acute coronary syndromes: The ACUITY timing trial. *JAMA* 2007;297:591–602.

31. Giugliano RP, White JA, Bode C et al. Early versus delayed, provisional eptifibatide in acute coronary syndromes. *N Engl J Med.* 2009;360:2176–2190.

32. Eikelboom JW, Anand SS, Malmberg K et al. Un-fractionated heparin and low-molecular-weight heparin in acute coronary syndrome without ST elevation: A meta-analysis. *Lancet* 2000;355:1936–1942.

33. Ferguson JJ, Califf RM, Antman EM et al. Enoxaparin vs unfractionated heparin in high-risk patients with non-ST-segment elevation acute coronary syndromes managed with an intended early invasive strategy: Primary results of the SYNERGY randomized trial. *JAMA* 2004;292:45–54.

34. Murphy SA, Gibson CM, Morrow DA et al. Efficacy and safety of the low-molecular weight heparin enoxaparin compared with unfractionated heparin across the acute coronary syndrome spectrum: A meta-analysis. *Eur Heart J.* 2007;28:2077–2086.

35. Yusuf S, Mehta SR, Chrolavicius S et al. Comparison of fondaparinux and enoxaparin in acute coronary syndromes. *N Engl J Med.* 2006;354:1464–1476.

36. Bavry AA, Kumbhani DJ, Rassi AN et al. Benefit of early invasive therapy in acute coronary syndromes: A meta-analysis of contemporary randomized clinical trials. *J Am Coll Cardiol.* 2006;48:1319–1325.

37. O'Donoghue M, Boden WE, Braunwald E et al. Early invasive vs conservative treatment strategies in women and men with unstable angina and non-ST-segment elevation myocardial infarction: A meta-analysis. *JAMA* 2008;300:71–80.

38. Katritsis DG, Siontis GC, Kastrati A et al. Optimal timing of coronary angiography and potential intervention in non-ST-elevation acute coronary syndromes. *Eur Heart J.* 2011;32:32–40.

39. Mehta SR, Granger CB, Boden WE et al. Early versus delayed invasive intervention in acute coronary syndromes. *N Engl J Med.* 2009;360:2165–2175.

40. Farooq V, Serruys PW, Bourantas CV et al. Quantification of incomplete revascularization and its association with five-year mortality in the SYNergy between percutaneous coronary intervention with TAXus and cardiac surgery (SYNTAX) trial validation of the residual SYNTAX score. *Circulation* 2013;128:141–151.

41. Ranasinghe I, Alprandi-Costa B, Chow V et al. Risk stratification in the setting of non-ST elevation acute coronary syndromes 1999–2007. *Am J Cardiol.* 2011;108:617–624.

42. Palmerini T, Genereux P, Caixeta A et al. Prognostic value of the SYNTAX score in patients with acute coronary syndromes undergoing percutaneous coronary intervention: Analysis from the ACUITY (Acute Catheterization and Urgent Intervention Triage strategY) trial. *J Am Coll Cardiol.* 2011;57:2389–2397.

43. Grundy SM, Stone NJ, Bailey AL et al. 2018 AHA/ACC/AACVPR/AAPA/ABC/ACPM/ADA/AGS/APhA/ASPC/NLA/PCNA guideline on the management of blood cholesterol: A report of the American College of Cardiology/American Heart Association Task Force on Clinical Practice Guidelines. *J Am Coll Cardiol.* 2018 Nov 8. doi: 10.1016/j.jacc.2018.11.003. [Epub ahead of print].

44. Cannon CP, Blazing MA, Giugliano RP et al., for the IMPROVE-IT Investigators. Ezetimibe Added to Statin Therapy after Acute Coronary Syndromes. *N Eng J Med.* 2015;372:2387–e002397.

Index

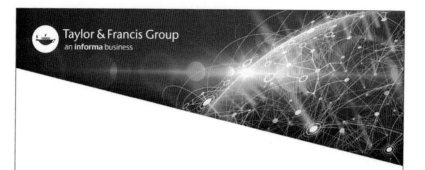